AJPH

A PUBLICATION OF THE
AMERICAN PUBLIC HEALTH ASSOCIATION

AMERICAN JOURNAL of PUBLIC HEALTH
JANUARY 2026
Issue 1

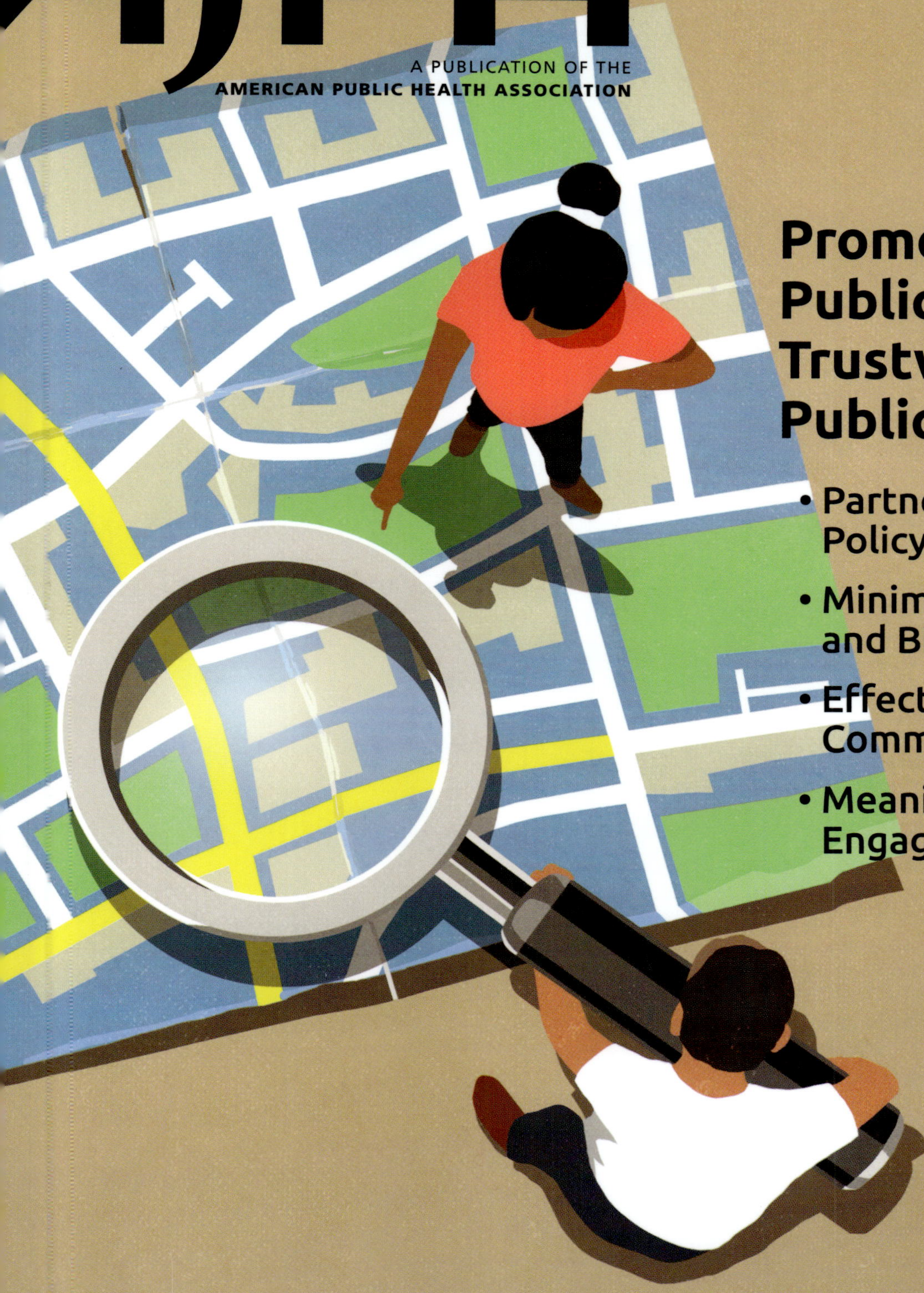

Promoting Public Trust and Trustworthiness in Public Health

- Partnerships With Policymakers
- Minimal Undue Influences and Biases
- Effective and Consistent Communication
- Meaningful Community Engagement

AMERICAN PUBLIC HEALTH ASSOCIATION
For science. For action. For health.

AJPH®, published monthly, is the official Journal of the American Public Health Association®, 800 I St NW, Washington, DC 20001-3710; (202) 777- APHA; TDD (202) 777-2500. APHA is a nongovernmental professional society founded in 1872, representing all disciplines and specialties in public health.

The *American Journal of Public Health*® (*AJPH*) (print ISSN: 0090-0036; electronic ISSN: 1541- 0048), first published in 1911, is the official journal of the American Public Health Association® (APHA). The oldest and largest organization of public health professionals in the world, APHA represents approximately 30 000 members from more than 50 occupations of public health.

Submissions: Visit www.editorialmanager.com/ajph for online manuscript preparation and submission guidelines. Contributions of original unpublished research, social science analyses, scholarly essays, critical commentaries, departments, and letters to the editor are welcome. Questions? Write ajph.submissions@apha.org or call APHA at (202) 777-2469.

Print plus online subscriptions: Institutional price (print copy with online access) for a single institution and all authorized users, regardless of geographic location varies by size of organization; multiple campuses not permitted without special arrangement. To order, write apha.subscriptions@apha.org.

Online-only subscriptions: Institutional price for one US federal institution and its authorized users is $1,015–$1,510. To order, write apha.subscriptions@apha.org. For academic, non-US federal consortia, or multisite subscriptions, contact apha.subscriptions@apha.org or visit http://research.ebsco.com for pricing information.

Print-only subscriptions: Institutional price is US $970, $1,065 international.

Back print issues: A limited number of print issues are for sale. Single copies are US $80, $90 international (air delivery). Shipping and handling fees will apply; prepay only. To order, write apha.subscriptions@apha.org.

Reprints: For prices and ordering information on 50 or more reprints, check the Reprints section at www.ajph.org. To order smaller quantities of reprints (rush delivery), use the "Purchase Article" link on the article site itself.

Electronic access: Online articles more than 10 years old are available free for personal use at www.ajph.org. Recent articles are available through pay-per-view: single PDF article for $24, single issue access for 24 hours for $33, or entire site access for 24 hours for $38.

Postal information: Periodicals postage paid at Washington, DC, and additional mailing offices. Postmaster: Send address changes to American Journal of Public Health, 800 I St NW, Washington, DC 20001-3710.

Address changes: Send to AJPH, Membership Department (members) or AJPH Subscriptions (subscribers), APHA, 800 I St NW, Washington, DC 20001-3710. Or write to membership.mail@apha.org (members) or apha.subscriptions@apha.org (subscribers).

Advertising: For pricing and other information, see www.ajph.org. Please write to brian.selzer@apha.org or call (202) 777-2464 for other advertising opportunities. Ask about special exhibit packages and sponsorships. Acceptance of advertising by the *Journal* does not imply endorsement of products.

Indexes: Publications that index or abstract articles from *AJPH* include the following: Ageline, Assia (Applied Social Science Index and Abstracts), Biological Abstracts, Chemical Abstracts, CINAHL, Criminal Justice Abstracts, EMBASE, EMCare, Environmental Abstracts, e-psyche, ERIC, ETOH (Alcohol and Alcohol Problems Science Database), Excerpta Medica, Food Science and Technology, General Science Index, Grateful Med, Hospital Literature Index, Human Resources Abstracts, International Pharmaceutical Abstracts (IPA), Medline, Physical Education Index, Pollution Abstracts, Psychological Abstracts, PsychINFO, Safety Science Abstracts, Sage Family Studies Abstracts, Sage Human Resources Abstracts, Science Citation Index, SCOPUS, SIIC Data Bases, Social Work Research and Abstracts, and Statistical Reference Index (SRI)/LexisNexis.

AJPH

A PUBLICATION OF THE
AMERICAN PUBLIC HEALTH ASSOCIATION

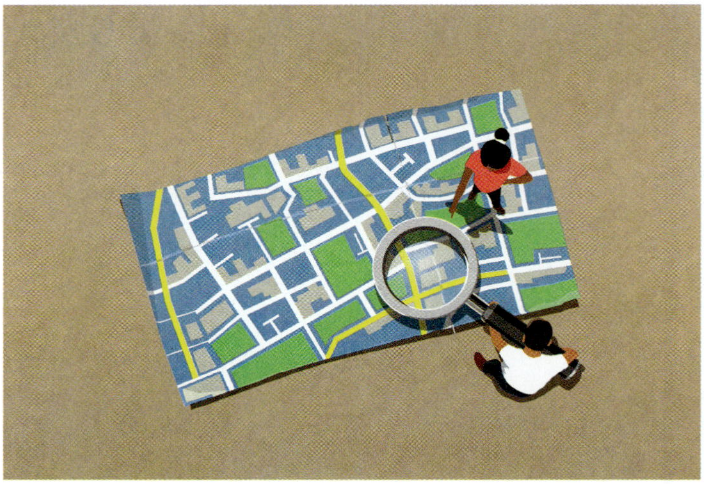

COVER: It is a critical time to rebuild trust and trustworthiness in public health through strategies informed by both science and community voices. Working in partnerships with policymakers and community members across geopolitical divides, we can build a new map for the future.

Cover design and selection by Aleisha Kropf. Cover image by Malte Mueller/Getty Images. Printed with permission.

APHA
AMERICAN PUBLIC HEALTH ASSOCIATION
For science. For action. For health.

Promoting public health research, policy, practice, and education is the *AJPH* mission. As we widen our scope to embrace global issues, we also sharpen our focus to support the needs of public health practitioners. We invite contributions of original unpublished research, opinion and commentary, and letters to the editor.

The *Journal* is printed on acid-free recycled paper.

OPEN ACCESS ONLINE ONLY PODCAST DATA SUPPLEMENT AVAILABLE

EDITOR'S CHOICE

4 Scientific Independence and Public Health Trustworthiness
D. T. Lau and J. D. Schoendorf

OPINIONS, IDEAS, & PRACTICE

PERSPECTIVES

6 Misrepresentation in Data Collection as a Form of Institutional Discrimination
D. Claudio, D. L. Comey, E. Aghbashian, and S. Moyce

12 The Need to Invest in Infrastructure and Partnerships to Achieve Complete Public Health Data
T. D. McCaffrey, C. Bland, L. Merchant, L. Richidt, M. Wamsley, and L. Williamson

14 Funding and Defunding of NIH Research Should Be Based on Real Science and Not Politics or Amorphous Constructs
K. Resnicow, K. E. Gamarel, J. S. Ahluwalia, D. R. Williams, S. Naar, and D. M. Griffith

18 Fixing Up Places Is Easier Than Fixing People
J. MacDonald

21 A Renewed Effort to Control and Eliminate Congenital Syphilis in the United States
C. Stafylis and J. D. Klausner

24 The Patients Are Ready, but the System Is Not: Closing the Gap Between Opioid Overdose Prevention and Recovery
S. G. Henry and A. Moulin

26 Extreme Polarization Is a Threat to US Health
J. B. Nuzzo

29 Homeownership as a Determinant of Health: A Broader Consideration of Housing and Homelessness Amid Current Challenges
D. K. Padgett

TRUST IN PUBLIC HEALTH

31 Restoring and Expanding Public Trust in Public Health
D. T. Lau

35 The Role of Uncertainty in Rebuilding Trust in Science
K. McCain

38 Public Health, Science, and the Public's Trust
K. Rochel de Camargo

42 Lessons Learned From the COVID-19 Pandemic: "Those Who Cannot Remember the Past Are Condemned to Repeat It"
R. J. Kim-Farley

47 Relationships Matter: Rebuilding Policymaker Trust in Public Health Leadership
S. A. Hearne and K. M. Pollack Porter

51 Public Health Policymaking Outside of the Federal Government: Reflections on Authority and Trust-Building Challenges
L. A. Taylor and A. L. Caplan

57 Public Trust, Private Data: Four Considerations for the Future of Health
N. Dasgupta, J. D. Schoendorf, D. T. Lau, and L. Thorpe

62 Restoring Trust in Public Health by Preventing Financial Conflicts of Interest in the Scientific Literature and Government Decision-Making
N. Chartres, T. J. Woodruff, and L. A. Bero

67 Building Trust in Public Health Information Through Transparency, Inclusivity, and Community Engagement
S. Landers and S. C. Fiala

70 Freedom, Fairness, and Trust: Speaking the Language of Public Health Across the Political Divide
B. C. Castrucci, J. M. Rivera, and A. Kwong

74 "What We've Got Here Is Failure to Communicate": The Need for Crisis Communication Skills Training in Public Health Graduate Programs
P. J. A. Kelly and S. B. Bass

79 The Challenge of Trust in Public Health Institutions Among Communities of Color: Where Do We Go From Here?
T. J. Padamsee and J. C. Allen

82 Stop Asking Communities to Trust You: Make Public Health Trustworthy
C. Nnaji and L. Bowleg

86 To Demonstrate Trustworthiness, Public Health Must Listen, Reflect, Act, and Revisit
P. M. Alberti, J. K. Bretsch, D. Oto-Kent, and K. M. King

90 Fostering Collaboration and Trust to Address COVID-19–Related Disparities and Misinformation in South Central Texas
T. Ravi, J. Rodriguez, R. L. Ferrer, A. Estacio, A. Gomez, P. Winkler, and E. L. Thompson

RESEARCH & ANALYSIS

OPEN-THEMED RESEARCH

95 The Association Between Vacant Lot Redevelopment and Violent/Firearm Violent Crime: A Difference-in-Difference Analysis From 2007 to 2023
N. Asa, H. Y. Zewdie, A. Rowhani-Rahbar, B. H. Wagenaar, and S. J. Mooney

103 Congenital Syphilis: From Near-Elimination to Crisis
C. J. Abresch, I. A. Stafford, R. M. Johnson, K. Olabanji, A. M. Sutphen, H. E. Cejtin, and A. Hoover

113 Opioid Overdose Mortality Among Patients Receiving a Peer-Delivered, Emergency Department–Based Nonfatal Opioid Overdose Intervention in New York City, 2017–2022
K. L. Kepler, A. E. Welch, E. Tuazon, D. Chambless, J. Kennedy, and A. Jeffers

124 Political Polarization During Disease Outbreaks: A Meta-Analysis of Archival Survey Data From Polio to COVID-19
C. L. McMurtry and R. Cheu

137 Housing Status and Health in the United States: A National Study of Homeownership, Health Outcomes, and Access to Care
S. Rahman

Scientific Independence and Public Health Trustworthiness

See also Trust in Public Health, pp. 31–94.

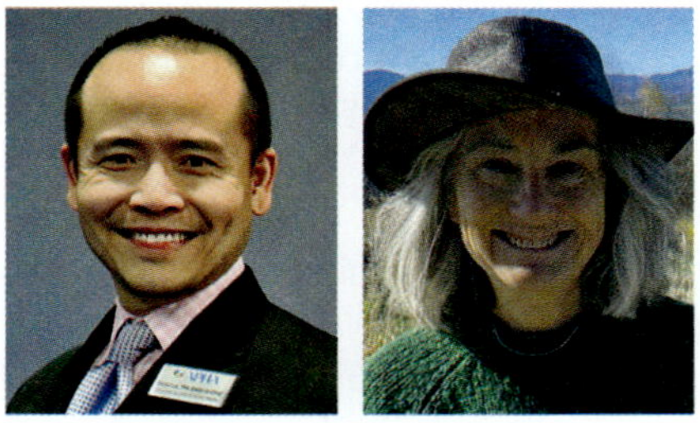

Denys T. Lau, PhD
AJPH Editor-in-Chief
Jennifer D. Schoendorf, PhD
AJPH Senior Deputy Editor

AJPH January 2026, Vol. 116, No. 1

Freedom from undue influence, or independence, has been a priority since the early days of our nation to ensure government trustworthiness and public trust. Having endured tyranny under the British monarchy, the founders framed the Constitution of the United States on the principles of independence and a system of checks and balances among the three branches of government. This design allows each branch to function without undue influence while providing the authority to monitor and restrain the others. This independence and inherent oversight compel government branches and public institutions to make decisions with limited influence of partisan politics or special interests, thereby strengthening public confidence in the fairness and integrity of the system. Similarly, scientific independence—shielding public health institutions from political, ideological, or commercial interference—is critical for ensuring evidence-based decisions to remain objective and rigorous, and maintaining public trust and cooperation with public health measures.

Scientific independence is necessary when federal public health institutions, such as those within the US Department of Health and Human Services, are working to protect and improve the public's health by monitoring health status, investigating health problems, and developing policies to promote health. However, tension can arise between scientific independence of public health institutions and political priorities of the executive branch. As part of the executive branch, public health agencies must balance their reliance on independent, scientific expertise with their duty to serve the policy priorities of the federal administration. While the executive branch has the authority and responsibility to set broad policy goals, political overreach and discourse that undermine scientific integrity and objective data can be detrimental to public health. When public health science and institutions are politicized, political divide widens and public trust in public institutions further erodes. This is happening under the current federal administration, which is reducing the federal scientific workforce and replacing them with political loyalists (go.nature.com/4nulX8a and nyti.ms/4oDXDBz), eliminating entire public health work units, suppressing or undermining health data, and altering scientific findings (bit.ly/4qDSCuW).

Furthermore, public health officials seek input from independent expert advisory panels to help appraise evidence and make recommendations. Such practice is a key mechanism to mitigate political interference and check internal biases. However, the credibility of these expert panels is severely undermined when members are appointed based on political or ideological reasons or for having a known predetermined scientific stance.

Independence alone is but one component of public trust. The effectiveness of federal health agencies is contingent upon their ability to maintain transparent decision-making processes and foster meaningful engagement with the public and political leaders. Political leaders and public health officials would need to transcend the political divide to repair and strengthen public confidence by working together toward the goal of improving population health and creating inclusive processes to develop policy solutions with bipartisan support (bit.ly/49s8REZ). Furthermore, strict scrutiny of financial conflicts of interest is also necessary to avoid commercial bias. The public needs to know that their interests are not compromised by corporation influence or political ideologies.

As *AJPH* editors, we have the responsibility to ensure that the *Journal* is a trusted source of public health information. Our editorial decisions have always been and will remain independent of political, commercial, professional, and other external influences. We employ different methods to further the *Journal*'s trustworthiness. For example, all research submissions undergo a rigorous peer-review process that involves external scientific experts and community leaders, as appropriate. We publish diverse topics and perspectives relevant to different audiences. To ensure transparency, we will continue developing and adhering to our *Journal*'s policies and engage meaningfully with policymakers at all levels to build stakeholder confidence in the *AJPH*. AJPH

DOI: https://doi.org/10.2105/AJPH.2025.308332

Misrepresentation in Data Collection as a Form of Institutional Discrimination

David Claudio, PE, PhD, Danika Lee Comey, MPH, Elizabeth Aghbashian, MPH, and Sally Moyce, RN, PhD

ABOUT THE AUTHORS

David Claudio is an associate professor in the Department of Mechanical & Industrial Engineering, University of Massachusetts Lowell, Lowell, MA. Danika Lee Comey is the research lead for Proyecto SALUD (Scientists And Latinos United against Disparities), Mark and Robyn Jones College of Nursing, Montana State University, Bozeman. Elizabeth Aghbashian is a retired public health professional living in Bozeman, MT. Sally Moyce is an associate professor in the Mark and Robyn Jones College of Nursing, Montana State University, Bozeman.

See also McCaffrey et al., p. 12.

AJPH January 2026, Vol. 116, No. 1

Let's travel to an ideal future: The year is 2045, and the public health system has transformed into a model of equity, inclusion, and accessibility. For the past two decades, public health programs across the United States collected comprehensive data to capture the full spectrum of participation in federal cancer-screening programs. Data sets differentiate among qualifying individuals who completed the screening, are currently undergoing the screening process, started but did not complete it, and are eligible but have not initiated screenings.

Each data set includes critical information, such as age, ethnicity, race, socioeconomic status, language preferences, geographic location, education level, employment status, household income, health insurance coverage, access to transportation, and caregiving responsibilities. These rich data enable policymakers, researchers, and health care providers to identify disparities and design interventions that address the root causes of health inequities.

In this future state, people report overwhelmingly positive experiences with cancer-screening programs. The process is free, simple, and streamlined, with minimal wait times between stages. Every participant is treated with dignity, ensuring that everyone feels valued and respected throughout the process. Instructions and reminders are available in multiple languages, supported by culturally congruent materials and on-site interpreters.

Patient navigators play a critical role, guiding patients through the process, addressing concerns, and advocating patient needs. Free transportation services eliminate logistical barriers, ensuring that no one is left out because they lack resources or accessibility.

Because of these efforts, communities report a strong sense of belonging and trust in a system that truly cares about their health and well-being. Cancer-screening programs are no longer seen as daunting bureaucratic processes but as empowering community-centered initiatives.

This vision reflects health care systems that have eradicated institutional discrimination. Programs prioritize cultural humility, equity, and respect for all individuals. They foster trust by engaging directly with communities, addressing historical injustices, and ensuring that every voice is heard and respected. This is how our health care systems should function.

This vision will remain aspirational as long as institutional discrimination persists in public health systems. The current reality is far from this ideal.

WHEN LOCAL REALITIES AND STATE DATA DIVERGE

Data serve as the foundation for public health research, policy development, program implementation, and funding decisions. However, when data are misrepresented or when crucial data are not properly collected, they can unintentionally perpetuate institutional discrimination by omitting the realities of marginalized populations, thus contributing to inequities in care.

In our recent analysis of breast and cervical cancer-screening data for Hispanic and non-Hispanic women in Montana, we identified significant gaps between state-reported outcomes and county-level records. The Centers for Disease Control and Prevention (CDC) National Breast and Cervical Cancer Early Detection Program funds states to offer free breast and cervical cancer screenings to low-income, uninsured, and underinsured women.[1] In Montana, program administrators at county health departments report data on enrollment and screening completion rates to the Montana Department of Health and Human Services, which supplies the information to the CDC.

Our analysis of state-level data over a seven-year period (2016–2022) revealed no statistically significant differences in cancer-screening completion rates between non-Hispanic and Hispanic women. For breast cancer screening, reported completion rates were 96.97% for non-Hispanic women and 96.54% for Hispanic women. Similarly, for cervical cancer screening, rates were 98.73% and 98.11%, respectively. It is important to note that we excluded open (i.e., ongoing) cases from all analyses.

These figures contrast sharply with data obtained from a single county. County-level records for the same period showed that 95.52% of non-Hispanic women completed the screening program compared with only 84.54% of Hispanic women. Notably, during the 2021 to 2022 period, only 74.20% (23 of 31) of Hispanic women in the county who initiated the screening process completed it.

Our review of patient records from the same county health department revealed that 28 Hispanic women failed to complete either breast or cervical cancer screening after beginning the process between 2016 and 2022. By contrast, the state database reported only 26 such noncompletions for Hispanic women across all 56 counties during that same period. In several cases, we were unable to locate patients in the state-provided data set who were documented in the county records, particularly those who started and dropped the screening process.

These inconsistencies raise important methodological questions. How can a single county, where program oversight and data tracking were closely managed, report more noncompletions than the entire statewide system?

A qualitative study based on interviews with data analysts and county health department officials revealed inconsistencies in data collection practices, reporting accuracy, and oversight mechanisms. Broader concerns about data quality in Montana further contextualize these findings,[2] highlighting longstanding challenges in statewide health data infrastructure.

Although program administrators typically collect the minimum data required by federal agencies as outlined by the CDC, our study found that they are often not required to capture data on program attrition. Some administrators report only the number of vouchers issued and screenings completed, without accounting for individuals who began but did not finish the screening process. As a result, data sets are frequently incomplete and unreliable. Moreover, women are not receiving their cancer screenings.

These limitations place a burden on data analysts, who must create complex workarounds to approximate outcomes that should be directly reported. To compensate, analysts often define program noncompletion indirectly, for example, by identifying women who enrolled but failed to use their voucher within one year of enrollment. However, this approach redefines noncompletion based on timing rather than actual disengagement from the screening pathway and does not accurately reflect attrition. As a result, it remains unclear how many women could benefit from the program but are unable to access or finish it. This limited reporting scope may unintentionally understate the true need and, in turn, affect resource allocation.

This practice conceals critical dropout points in the continuum of care and ultimately limits the ability of public health systems to identify where and why patients are falling through the cracks. The issue is further compounded by a broader lack of awareness about the importance of collecting and reporting comprehensive data beyond minimal federal requirements. Without these insights, public health systems struggle to identify institutional barriers to equitable care or to design programs that support those who face challenges in accessing and completing essential screening services.

We aimed to highlight how common data limitations, such as underreporting and inconsistent definitions of program completion, can reinforce inequities in care delivery. While the importance of disaggregated data and the impact of selective reporting have been identified in the broader literature on health equity,[3,4] we believe our research offers a novel contribution by applying these concerns to a concrete, underexamined context: cancer-screening data in a rural state with a small but growing Hispanic population.

Our integration of real program data with quantitative and qualitative evidence and community-engaged insights highlights how well-intentioned data systems can inadvertently perpetuate racial inequities. We believe this framing, and our focus on how these issues manifest in rural, low-diversity contexts, is a meaningful and timely addition to the discourse.

HOW FAULTY DATA REFLECT INSTITUTIONAL DISCRIMINATION

For this research, we defined institutional discrimination not as overt prejudice but as the cumulative effect of institutional practices and data policies that unintentionally exclude or misrepresent marginalized populations. While this form of discrimination contributes to many structural inequities in health care access, we distinguished between barriers related to care delivery and those rooted in data governance, collection, and reporting.

Our findings suggest that institutional discrimination in care access and methodological flaws in data collection contribute to the disparities observed in cancer-screening outcomes. Although it can be challenging to isolate their individual effects, together they reinforce persistent health inequities.

Figure 1 illustrates a recurring cycle of institutional discrimination, as identified through our quantitative and qualitative analyses. The boxes outlined in red represent two distinct types of institutional discrimination: we identified the first, related to care delivery, in our previous research; the second, related to data systems, is the focus of the present study. The yellow boxes highlight the consequences of these discriminatory practices within the cycle.

Hispanic women face well-documented barriers to health care access, including language obstacles, limited transportation, distrust in the health care system, cultural insensitivities, and fear of deportation.[1,5,6] According to our data, they are approximately 3.5 times more likely than are non-Hispanic women to drop out of the screening process once it is initiated. These drop-offs are often not reflected in state-level data sets, which prioritize completed cases and do not systematically track attrition by reporting cases in which women enroll but do not complete screenings.

Additionally, the state's definition of program completion is based on whether a screening occurs within one year of enrollment, rather than on clinical engagement or follow-through. This narrow definition risks misclassifying delayed or disrupted care as nonparticipation, further distorting the data. As a result, the high reported completion rates may overstate program effectiveness and underrepresent those facing the most significant barriers. Inflated metrics mask disparities and undermine efforts to advocate targeted interventions.[7,8] When these barriers are not accounted for, public health data sets misrepresent the true scale of disparities.[9,10] This misrepresentation can contribute to fewer resources being directed to Hispanic women, reinforcing the very obstacles that impede access to care.

This pattern of exclusion is part of what scholars term "data inequity,"[3] which refers to the systematic exclusion of certain groups from data sets, contributing to invisibility in the public health domain. Incomplete data limit the ability of health systems to recognize the needs of underserved groups and design targeted interventions. This is especially concerning in rural and underresourced areas, where

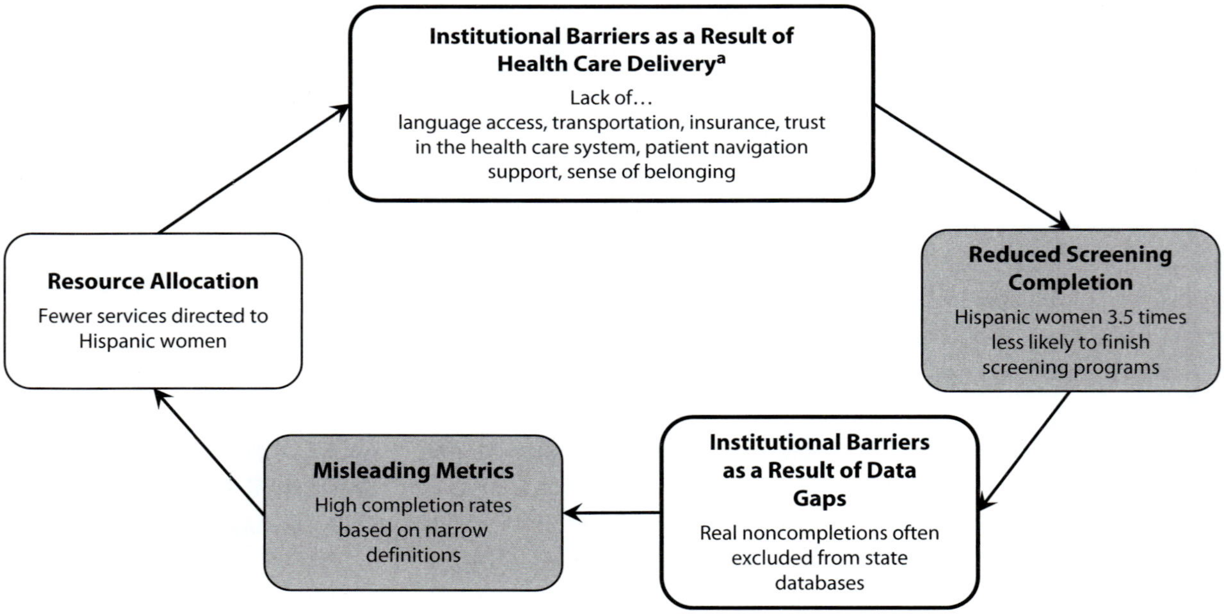

FIGURE 1— Cycle of Institutional Discrimination Affecting Hispanic Women's Participation in Breast and Cervical Cancer Screening Programs: Montana, 2016–2022

[a]See Moyce et al.[1]

institutional barriers disproportionately affect marginalized populations.[11]

Although Hispanic individuals currently make up less than 5% of Montana's population, they are a rapidly growing demographic. Investing in improved data collection practices now can help build a more inclusive and accurate foundation for serving this population and others more effectively in the future.

HOW MISREPRESENTATION PERPETUATES INEQUITIES

We recognize that many of the institutional barriers stemming from data collection gaps are likely unintentional and may result from poor planning, the desire to present favorable outcomes, or limited communication among those who collect, analyze, and report data. Throughout our investigations, we worked with data stakeholders and analysts at multiple levels, including county and state administrators. Many were responsive and willing to share data and explore inconsistencies.

Despite this collaborative spirit, we encountered persistent systemic barriers that limited our ability to fully understand and address discrepancies across the state. These included challenges such as rigid data structures, limited standardization of data definitions and collection (i.e., the right people collecting the right data, in the right format, at the right time, through the right processes[12]), and a general reluctance to make changes, often attributed to a lack of resources, lack of ownership, or the perception that "this would be too difficult to implement." Some stakeholders expressed that the current system was "good enough" or implied that improving data collection was someone else's responsibility.

While the previous statement may come across as critical, we believe it is important to share our lived experiences to contribute meaningfully to change. Omitting these observations would risk reinforcing the very forms of institutional discrimination that our work seeks to dismantle. Ultimately, the way data systems are designed and maintained can either perpetuate inequities or serve as a foundation for accountability and reform.

Failing to acknowledge or address institutional barriers because of data gaps perpetuates and reinforces systemic inequities in four ways:

1. *Justifying inaction.* When data inaccurately suggest that screening rates are equitable, the perceived urgency to address systemic barriers is diminished. Policymakers and public health officials may be less inclined to pursue targeted interventions, as it appears no problem exists. This illusion of equity fosters complacency.[13] Furthermore, the absence of nuanced, disaggregated data leads to funding decisions that fail to reflect the structural challenges Hispanic women face, ultimately reinforcing existing disparities.
2. *Skewing policy and funding decisions.* Data drive public health policies and funding. Misrepresented data divert resources away from marginalized communities, perpetuating disparities. Hispanic women in Montana, for example, are less likely to benefit from targeted outreach or culturally competent care if the data suggest they do not face unique challenges.[8,14]
3. *Undermining trust.* Lived experiences of marginalized populations contradicting official data erode trust in public health institutions. Communities are less likely to engage in future data collection efforts or health programs, further exacerbating disparities.[10]
4. *Limiting research opportunities.* Inaccurate data undermine the credibility of research and hinder the ability to conduct robust analyses. Researchers (as we experienced firsthand) are left without the tools to document disparities or advocate systemic change effectively.[9,15]

TOWARD INCLUSIVE AND ACCURATE DATA

Addressing institutional discrimination in data collection requires intentional and sustained efforts grounded in community insight and structural change. Drawing on recent studies that highlight effective strategies for uncovering and reducing disparities, we propose the following actionable recommendations:

- *Community-informed data practices.* Engage directly with Hispanic communities and other underrepresented populations to codesign data collection tools that reflect their realities. This will encourage accurate data on completion and noncompletion rates. We advocate participatory approaches, focus groups, and partnerships with trusted community organizations.[8,14,16,17]
- *Culturally competent data collection.* Ensure that survey instruments are culturally and linguistically appropriate, including translating materials into Spanish and Indigenous languages,[1] hiring bilingual and bicultural data collectors, and conducting surveys in safe and

familiar community settings.[10] Ensure that survey instruments are legible and understandable to the populations completing the surveys.

- *Disaggregated data.* Avoid lumping diverse populations into single categories. Collect and report data disaggregated by ethnicity, language proficiency, and socioeconomic indicators to uncover hidden disparities.[6,7,13] If the data are too detailed to support reliable decision-making, data can be aggregated to increase sample sizes. It is far easier to aggregate disaggregated data than to attempt to disaggregate data that were never collected in detail.
- *Auditing and validation.* Regularly audit data sets to ensure accuracy. Validate quantitative findings through triangulation with qualitative research and community feedback.[9] This was the approach we used in our research, as we attempted to validate state-reported data through quantitative and qualitative analyses conducted at the county level. This process revealed significant inconsistencies in data collection and data-mining practices.
- *Oversampling underrepresented groups.* To address underreporting and sampling bias, oversample underrepresented groups in surveys and programs. This can help ensure that the data reflect the experiences of those most affected by systemic barriers.[8,15]
- *Accountability in reporting.* Public health agencies must be transparent about data limitations and avoid overstating success metrics. This includes acknowledging gaps in representation and highlighting areas for improvement.[7]

CONCLUSIONS

Misrepresentation in data collection may be unintentional or stem from resource limitations; it nonetheless functions as a form of institutional discrimination and perpetuates health inequities by overlooking the experiences of marginalized communities. Accurate, inclusive, and transparent data are essential for advancing equity in public health research and practice. To ensure that public health efforts reflect the realities of those most in need, researchers must critically examine data systems, challenge flawed practices, and amplify the voices of underrepresented populations through systemic change. AJPH

CORRESPONDENCE

Correspondence should be sent to Danika Lee Comey, PO Box 173560, Bozeman, MT 59717 (e-mail: danika.comey@montana.edu). Reprints can be ordered at https://www.ajph.org by clicking the "Reprints" link.

PUBLICATION INFORMATION

Full Citation: Claudio D, Comey DL, Aghbashian E, Moyce S. Misrepresentation in data collection as a form of institutional discrimination. *Am J Public Health.* 2026;116(1):6–11.

Acceptance Date: July 14, 2025.

DOI: https://doi.org/10.2105/AJPH.2025.308249

ORCID iDs:
Danika Lee Comey https://orcid.org/0000-0001-7000-4777

Sally Moyce https://orcid.org/0000-0003-0995-6239

CONTRIBUTORS

D. Claudio led the conceptualization and design of the study, guided the analytical framework, and led the writing and revision of the article. D. L. Comey participated in the analyses and contributed to drafting the article. E. Aghbashian collected data and conducted preliminary analyses, completed the literature review, supported data interpretation, and contributed to editing and formatting the article. S. Moyce coordinated the research activities, provided oversight, and critically reviewed and revised the final version of the article. All authors read and approved the final version of the article and agree to be accountable for all aspects of the work.

ACKNOWLEDGMENTS

This research was funded by the Robert Wood Johnson Foundation under the Interdisciplinary Research Leaders Program (grant A-79693).

CONFLICTS OF INTEREST

The authors have no financial, personal, or professional affiliations that could be perceived as influencing the content of this work and no conflicts of interest regarding the publication of this article.

HUMAN PARTICIPANT PROTECTION

The Montana State University institutional review board reviewed and approved this study. The study was conducted in accordance with the ethical principles outlined in the Declaration of Helsinki and complied with all relevant regulations concerning the protection of human research participants.

REFERENCES

1. Moyce S, Claudio D, Aghbashian E, Keenan K, Comey DL, Chavez-Reyes G. Barriers and facilitators to breast and cervical cancer screenings for Hispanic women in a rural state. *J Racial Ethn Health Disparities.* 2024;12(4):2145–2153. https://doi.org/10.1007/s40615-024-02037-6
2. Sakariassen A. Montana only state missing from national childhood immunization reports. *Bozeman Daily Chronicle.* December 6, 2024. Available at: https://www.bozemandailychronicle.com/news/montana-only-state-missing-from-national-childhood-immunization-reports/article_09a51d22-b421-11ef-9802-5bbfc1dbdca7.html. Accessed January 6, 2025.
3. Kauh TJ, Read JG, Scheitler AJ. The critical role of racial/ethnic data disaggregation for health equity. *Popul Res Policy Rev.* 2021;40(1):1–7. https://doi.org/10.1007/s11113-020-09631-6
4. Zambrana RE, Amaro G, Butler C, DuPont-Reyes M, Parra-Medina D. Analysis of Latina/o sociodemographic and health data sets in the United States from 1960 to 2019: findings suggest improvements to future data collection efforts. *Health Educ Behav.* 2021;48(3):320–331. https://doi.org/10.1177/10901981211011047
5. Metcalf M, Comey D, Hines D, Chavez-Reyes G, Moyce S. "Because we are afraid": voices of the undocumented in a new immigrant destination in the United States. *J Public Health Policy.* 2024;45(2):367–377. https://doi.org/10.1057/s41271-024-00475-4
6. Hacker K, Anies M, Folb BL, Zallman L. Barriers to health care for undocumented immigrants: a literature review. *Risk Manag Healthc Policy.* 2015;8:175–183. https://doi.org/10.2147/RMHP.S70173
7. Marmot M, Bell R. Fair society, healthy lives. *Public Health.* 2012;126(suppl 1):S4–S10. https://doi.org/10.1016/j.puhe.2012.05.014
8. Weinstein JN, Geller A, Negussie Y, Baciu A, eds. *Communities in Action: Pathways to Health Equity.* Washington, DC: National Academies Press; 2017. https://doi.org/10.17226/24624

9. Krieger N. Measures of racism, sexism, heterosexism, and gender binarism for health equity research: from structural injustice to embodied harm—an ecosocial analysis. *Annu Rev Public Health.* 2020;41:37–62. https://doi.org/10.1146/annurev-publhealth-040119-094017
10. Braveman PA, Kumanyika S, Fielding J, et al. Health disparities and health equity: the issue is justice. *Am J Public Health.* 2011;101(suppl 1): S149–S155. https://doi.org/10.2105/AJPH.2010.300062
11. Claudio D. Residuals (or on the use of statistical analysis to perpetuate systemic racism). *Health Promotion Practice.* 2025;26(3):419–420. https://doi.org/10.1177/15248399251320984
12. Bell S. *Lean Enterprise Systems: Using IT for Continuous Improvement.* Hoboken, NJ: Wiley-Interscience; 2005.
13. Bailey ZD, Krieger N, Agénor M, Graves J, Linos N, Bassett MT. Structural racism and health inequities in the USA: evidence and interventions. *Lancet.* 2017;389(10077):1453–1463. https://doi.org/10.1016/S0140-6736(17)30569-X
14. Williams DR, Mohammed SA. Discrimination and racial disparities in health: evidence and needed research. *J Behav Med.* 2009;32(1):20–47. https://doi.org/10.1007/s10865-008-9185-0
15. López N, Gadsden VL. Health inequities, social determinants, and intersectionality. In: *Perspectives on Health Equity and Social Determinants of Health.* Washington, DC: National Academies Press; 2017. Available at: https://www.ncbi.nlm.nih.gov/books/NBK595256. Accessed January 9, 2025.
16. Moyce S, Claudio D, Velazquez M. Using the PDCA cycle to uncover sources of mental health disparities for Hispanics. *Int J Ment Health Nurs.* 2023;32(2):556–566. https://doi.org/10.1111/inm.13100
17. Moyce S, Comey D, Claudio D, Velazquez M, Reyes GC, Aghbashian E. A community-engaged approach to reducing barriers to breast and cervical cancer screening: the use of mapping tools. *J Particip Res Methods.* 2024;5(2). https://doi.org/10.35844/001c.118575

The Need to Invest in Infrastructure and Partnerships to Achieve Complete Public Health Data

Ty D. McCaffrey, MSc, Colby Bland, MS, Leah Merchant, Lisa Richidt, MPH, Mark Wamsley, MBA, and Laura Williamson, MPH

ABOUT THE AUTHORS

All authors are with the Chronic Disease Prevention and Health Promotion Bureau, Public Health and Safety Division, Montana Department of Public Health and Human Services, Helena, MT.

See also Claudio et al., p. 6.

AJPH January 2026, Vol. 116, No. 1

In this month's issue of *AJPH*, the article "Misrepresentation in Data Collection as a Form of Institutional Discrimination" by Claudio et al. (p. 6) reports that misrepresentation in data collection may perpetuate systemic racism and notes a specific example from a single breast and cervical cancer screening program in a rural state to illustrate this point. As public health practitioners at the Montana Department of Public Health and Human Services (DPHHS), we share the authors' vision for a society that achieves health for all, and we agree that investment in high-quality data plays a pivotal role in guiding public health initiatives. Furthermore, we know, firsthand, that systematic biases in the collection and reporting of public health data can obscure health disparities across underrepresented populations. These systematic biases may further contribute to the disparities experienced by racial or ethnic groups both in the United States and in Montana.[1,2] However, we believe the authors' analysis of the problem is misdirected and overlooks the practical realities of public health data collection and use.

DATA PURPOSE AND STRUCTURE

The Montana Breast and Cervical Cancer Early Detection Program (hereafter the "cancer screening program") collects specific programmatic data to monitor and assess its performance, as established by the Centers for Disease Control and Prevention's National Breast and Cervical Cancer Early Detection Program's Minimum Data Elements.[3] The cancer screening regularly reports demographic characteristics and clinical outcomes of enrolled women following its established definitions. The quality and completeness of Montana's cancer screening data are evaluated by the Centers for Disease Control and Prevention semiannually to ensure that data standards are met, as described in the program's Minimum Data Elements.[4]

As highlighted by Claudio et al., the data collected by the cancer screening program do not suggest any substantial differences in breast and cervical cancer screening completion among non-Hispanic White and Hispanic women in Montana. The DPHHS calculates screening completion as the number of women enrolled in the cancer screening program who were screened for breast or cervical cancer divided by the total number of women who are enrolled in the program. Screening tests with this definition include clinical breast exams, screening mammography, and Papanicolaou tests. We estimated that from 2016 through 2021, 96% (5483/5696) of non-Hispanic women completed breast and cervical cancer screening through the cancer screening program compared with 94% (586/624) of Hispanic women. Although the authors' finding that a single county showed a higher number of noncompletions is a concern, they did not provide sufficient methodological detail for DPHHS to validate this claim or determine the reason for the reported incongruity.

DATA INFRASTRUCTURE AND PUBLIC HEALTH PARTNERSHIPS

It is crucial to recognize that administrative data sets, such as the Montana cancer screening program data, have historically been rigid, collecting only federally required information. This is largely because state and local public health departments often lack the funding or technology to gather additional state-specific data. Consequently, these administrative data sets can be limited in their ability to answer key questions. To address these limitations and ensure equitable health outcomes, we need sustained investment to modernize the public health data infrastructure.[5] This will enable public health researchers to collect, analyze, and report critical information in a timely manner to take effective public health action.

The Montana Cancer Control Program values the responsible use of our data by academic and nongovernmental partners. We see these collaborations as vital for describing and addressing health challenges for all Montanans. An effective way to address pressing public health issues is through direct collaboration between public health agencies and academic institutions.[6] Given our history of close collaboration with academic and nongovernmental partners, we would have welcomed the opportunity to speak directly with Claudio et al. on data complexity with an eye to developing data-driven improvements to our data collection systems. We believe that direct and transparent dialogue with data stewards can be an effective approach to addressing public health data concerns. We see this as an opportunity to reevaluate our lines of communication with those who use the Montana cancer screening program data to ensure that these data are not only accessible but also put into context for those who are accessing it.

Continuous evaluation of public health data systems is required to identify critical data gaps. The authors' efforts to highlight activities that can help identify institutional racism and improve data systems are necessary for contemporary public health discourse. However, singling out individual health programs in this manner is not. Through close collaboration between academic institutions and governmental public health agencies, we can continue to identify areas for improvement, actualize them through investment, and address systemic health disparities. AJPH

CORRESPONDENCE

Correspondence should be sent to Ty McCaffrey, 1400 Broadway, Room 314, Helena, MT 59620-2951 (e-mail: Ty.McCaffrey@mt.gov). Reprints can be ordered at https://www.ajph.org by clicking the "Reprints" link.

PUBLICATION INFORMATION

Full Citation: McCaffrey TD, Bland C, Merchant L, Richidt L, Wamsley M, Williamson L. The need to invest in infrastructure and partnerships to achieve complete public health data. *Am J Public Health*. 2026;116(1):12–13.

Acceptance Date: October 1, 2025.

DOI: https://doi.org/10.2105/AJPH.2025.308308

ORCID iDs:

Ty D. McCaffrey https://orcid.org/0009-0000-2145-9003

Laura Williamson https://orcid.org/0000-0002-9022-0642

CONTRIBUTORS

The authors contributed equally to drafting this response.

ACKNOWLEDGMENTS

This project is funded by the Centers for Disease Control and Prevention of the US Department of Health and Human Services (HHS) and the Montana Department of Public Health and Human Services (DPHHS; cooperative agreement 6NU58DP007106).

Note. The contents herein do not necessarily reflect the official views and policies of the HHS or the DPHHS.

CONFLICTS OF INTEREST

The authors have no conflicts of interest to declare.

REFERENCES

1. Krieger N. Structural racism, health inequities, and the two-edged sword of data: structural problems require structural solutions. *Front Public Health*. 2021;9:655447. https://doi.org/10.3389/fpubh.2021.655447
2. Centers for Disease Control and Prevention. COVID-19 incidence and mortality among American Indian/Alaska Native and White persons—Montana, March 13–November 30, 2020. *MMWR Morb Mortal Wkly Rep*. 2021;70(14):510–513. https://doi.org/10.15585/mmwr.mm7014a2
3. Centers for Disease Control and Prevention. *National Breast and Cervical Cancer Early Detection Program (NBCCEDP) Data User's Manual: MDE Version 7.0*. August 2019. Available at: https://www.chfs.ky.gov/agencies/dph/dwh/Documents/CDCMDEManual.pdf. Accessed October 22, 2025.
4. Centers for Disease Control and Prevention. *National Breast and Cervical Early Detection Program DP22-2202 Data User's Manual*. 2022. Available at: https://www.cdc.gov/breast-cervical-cancer-screening/index.html. Accessed October 22, 2025.
5. Singletary V, Richards CL Jr, Ross DA, O'Carroll P, Baker EL. Modernizing our nation's public health information system: toward an integrated approach. *J Public Health Manag Pract*. 2021;27(5):521–525. https://doi.org/10.1097/PHH.0000000000001400
6. Erwin PC, Grubaugh JH, Mazzucca-Ragan S, Brownson RC. The value and impacts of academic public health departments. *Annu Rev Public Health*. 2023;44:343–362. https://doi.org/10.1146/annurev-publhealth-071421-031614

Funding and Defunding of NIH Research Should Be Based on Real Science and Not Politics or Amorphous Constructs

Ken Resnicow, PhD, Kristi E. Gamarel, PhD, Jasjit S. Ahluwalia, MD, MPH, David R. Williams, PhD, Sylvie Naar, PhD, LP, and Derek M. Griffith, PhD

ABOUT THE AUTHORS

Ken Resnicow is with the University of Minnesota School of Public Health, Minneapolis. Kristi E. Gamarel is with the University of Michigan School of Public Health, Ann Arbor. Jasjit S. Ahluwalia is with the School of Public Health and the Alpert Medical School, Brown University, Providence, RI. David R. Williams is with the Harvard T. H. Chan School of Public Health, Harvard University, Boston, MA. Sylvie Naar is with the Florida State University College of Medicine, Tallahassee. Derek M. Griffith is with the School of Nursing and Perelman School of Medicine, University of Pennsylvania, Philadelphia.

AJPH January 2026, Vol. 116, No. 1

The current presidential administration and leadership of the Department of Health and Human Services (HHS) have dramatically redefined what is considered allowable and valuable federally sponsored research. Since January 2025, thousands of grants from the National Institutes of Health (NIH) and the National Science Foundation have been terminated, rejected before review, or delayed. The reasons for these actions are often opaque. Following, for example, is the verbatim language that appeared in a "termination letter" sent to two of the authors as well as many of our colleagues:

> Effective with this Notice of Award, this project is terminated It is the policy of NIH not to prioritize research programs related to DEI. Research programs based primarily on artificial and non-scientific categories, including amorphous equity objectives, are antithetical to the scientific inquiry, do nothing to expand our knowledge of living systems, provide low returns on investment, and ultimately do not enhance health, lengthen life, or reduce illness. Worse, so-called diversity, equity, and inclusion ("DEI") studies are often used to support unlawful discrimination on the basis of race and other protected characteristics, which harms the health of Americans. Therefore, it is the policy of NIH not to prioritize such research programs. Therefore, no additional funding will be awarded for this project, and all future years have been removed (F. L. Cross, PhD, email to K. Resnicow, PhD, May 12, 2025; S. Naar, PhD, e-mail to K. Resnicow, PhD, March 21, 2025; K. E. Gamarel, PhD, email to K. Resnicow, PhD, March 24, 2025).

Defunding letters note "amorphous" objectives that are "antithetical to the scientific inquiry" that "do nothing to expand our knowledge of living systems." Ironically, these criteria seem themselves a bit amorphous and lacking rigor. Letters inform grantees that their research "no longer effectuates the program goals or agency priorities" (F. L. Cross, email to K. Resnicow, PhD, May 12, 2025; S. Naar, PhD, e-mail to K. Resnicow, PhD, March 21, 2025; K. E. Gamarel, PhD, email to K. Resnicow, PhD, March 24, 2025).

The provided quote is from one of the DEI form letters. Variations of these defunding letters have similarly been used to terminate grants related to lesbian, gay, bisexual, transgender, and queer (LGBTQ+) health disparities having little to do with DEI. Reasons cited include unscientific views of "gender identity," lack of an "identifiable return on investment," and "ignoring rather than seriously examining, biological realities" (letter from NIH to K. E. Gamarel, PhD, March 20, 2025). To retain NIH funding, investigators have been asked to exclude transgender participants or eliminate gender identity measures. Beyond DEI and LGBTQ+ (as well as HIV) research termination letters, one of the authors (K. R.) had an NIH-funded vaccine study defunded because it "attempts to influence the public's opinion" (letter from NIH to E. Marsh and K. Resnicow, May 9, 2025). Could not every behavioral intervention arguably be tarred with the same brush?

DEFUNDING DISPARITY RESEARCH

Of note, many grants have been defunded despite having little to do with DEI. This includes projects focusing on health disparities. Disparity research, a major focus of public health research, seems to have been swept up into the dismantling of DEI.

The rationale for defunding disparity science is further articulated by NIH director Jay Bhattacharya, in a May interview in *Politico Magazine* (http://bit.ly/48jTIVI):

> The second principle is that we want to focus on real scientific ideas that actually improve health. So, I want to distinguish that from ideological constructs like DEI that in many ways are not even in principle falsifiable. If you believe structural racism is the primary reason why minorities are in lower health, how would you disprove that? What experiment could you do to disprove that? If you can't think of an experiment to disprove something, then that's not a scientific idea.

There are a few flaws in this argument. First, it seems to conflate DEI programs with those studying health disparity and health equity, particularly studies on structural racism. And second, this position seems to ignore the large body of rigorous correlational and intervention research in this space—"real science" that has narrowed racial and ethnic gaps in life expectancy and other health outcomes.[1,2]

Let us return to the first issue. DEI and health disparity and health equity research are distinct domains. DEI refers to organizational practices that promote full and fair access to jobs and education, equitable treatment, and a sense of belonging for all people—not only in hiring, promotion, retention, and termination but also across institutional culture, policies, and systems. In contrast, health disparities is a scientific discipline within social and medical science, which according to the National Institute on Minority Health and Health Disparities (NIMHD; http://bit.ly/4nVfzrl) entails

> largely preventable health differences that adversely affect populations who experience greater challenges to optimal health and are closely linked with intergenerational social, economic, and/or environmental disadvantages—primarily based on identification as an individual from a racial and/or ethnic minority group and/or by low socioeconomic status (SES) in society.
>
> Health disparities may be observed in the risks, prevalence, or problems resulting from specific behaviors, as well as the incidence, prevalence, and mortality from conditions, diseases, and/or disorders. Health disparities also can be observed in health care access, quality, and utilization, and within the delivery of clinical care.

BENEFITS OF DISPARITY RESEARCH

For more than 20 years, the NIH has prioritized disparity research through various mechanisms including targeted funding opportunities announcements, minority supplements, and training grants. These activities were largely bipartisan. Investigators were required to recruit diverse samples. Disparity research is not only about race and ethnicity but also includes underserved rural residents (from all racial and ethnic groups), sexual and gender minority people, and, more recently, individuals with disabilities. Moreover, disparity is generally studied through an intersectional lens that considers the interaction of social determinants and identity(ies) and examines how interlocking systems of power create and sustain health inequities.[3]

Race and racism, both interpersonal and structural, remain key drivers of health inequities.[3,4] While we have made considerable progress, racial and ethnic health disparities continue to harm families, harm the economy, and harm America. From 1999 through 2020, an estimated 997 623 excess deaths occurred among US Black males and 628 464 excess deaths among US Black females relative to their White counterparts—accounting for around 1.63 million excess deaths. This equates to more than 74 000 Black people dying unnecessarily each year.[5] These excess deaths equal 47 million and 35 million excess years of potential life lost among Black males and Black females, respectively.[5] Large and persistent inequities in health are evident for American Indians and Alaska Natives as well as Hispanic Americans, albeit in patterns somewhat different than those for Black Americans.[6–9]

The economic burden of racial and ethnic health disparities in the United States is immense, more than $400 billion annually.[9] Closing the racial equity gap in the United States would save $135 billion annually from reduced health care costs ($93 billion) and improved productivity ($24 billion). A healthier workforce spends more, pays more taxes, and uses fewer safety net services and resources.[10] Reducing the racial gap in health, education, incarceration, and employment would generate an additional $191 billion spent on food, $500 billion on housing, $52 billion on apparel, $259 billion on transportation, and $77 billion on entertainment each year. Federal tax revenues would increase by $450 billion, and state and local tax revenues would increase by $100 billion annually.[10] Equity will improve conditions for everyone, including many poor and working-class White Americans.

Disparities are also costly in terms of social impacts.[11] For example, Black children are three times as likely to lose a mother by age 10 years and twice as likely to lose a child by age 30 years and a spouse by age 60 years. Immigrants and their children have high levels of stress that impacts their health.[12]

Another cornerstone of the defunding rationale is that topics such as structural racism (and presumably other disparity and equity research) are not worthy of NIH funding because they are not falsifiable by any single "experiment." This is a red herring. It is the sum of disparity and equity research that provides proof of concept, not any single study. The effects of structural and interpersonal racism have been rigorously examined.[2,13–16] Moreover, culturally tailored interventions have been studied through randomized trials.[17–20] This includes studies that experimentally isolated the impact of cultural tailoring and racial message framing.[17,18,21,22] Furthermore, mediation analyses or causal modeling can be used to understand the psychological and behavioral mechanisms through which disparity and equity interventions work.

Consider the observation that access to health care is a major determinant of health outcomes. Yet, no single study can prove or disprove this. So, too, self-efficacy is a major determinant of behavioral outcomes, but again, no single study can prove or disprove it. Does that mean these topics are not worthy of federal research?

Robust cohort studies such as the Jackson Heart Study, the Black Women's Health Study, the Multi-Ethnic Study of Atherosclerosis, the Multiethnic Cohort Study, Chicago Health and Life Experiences of Women, and RADAR Cohort Study, as well as individual studies, have produced an impressive array of publications documenting the impact of racism, discrimination, segregation, identity, and social determinants on health outcomes.[2,9,15,23,24] We have learned that race is an independent predictor of health outcomes, not just a marker for lower socioeconomic status.[25] This is an important scientific matter, not a political or DEI issue.

There are legitimate criticisms of disparity research, including an overemphasis on describing the problem (correlational research) and not enough research to fix the problem (intervention research). And, similar to other research domains, not all disparity research is adequately rigorous, reproducible, and beneficial. We should take this opportunity to raise our standards and focus more on solutions than problems. We welcome an opportunity to work with our federal partners to improve the quality and impact of the disparity research they fund. However, throwing out this entire domain of research because of its putative connection to DEI seems to be tossing the baby with the bathwater.

Interestingly, cultural tailoring, a foundation of equity interventions,[19] is standard practice in corporate America. It is essentially a form of audience segmentation and target marketing. Virtually every industry, from automobiles and food to insurance and alcohol, uses targeting and audience segmentation strategies to determine where they advertise and how they frame their appeals. Subaru has famously targeted sexual minority women with tongue-in-cheek ads focusing on getting "out" and about while McDonald's employed the Williams sisters for the "365" campaign targeting Black Americans. Tailoring appeals to cultural values, beliefs, and practices is "usual care" in corporate America. It would be sad if it were prohibited at HHS.

NEXT STEPS

Documenting the adverse effects of racism and discrimination and designing studies to ameliorate their insidious effects should be prioritized at NIH, not canceled.

We ask our new leaders at HHS and NIH to collaborate with the disparity research and practice communities to advance high-quality, high-impact research. Despite decades of bipartisan support for health disparity research, there are few, if any, binding statutory protections to prevent politically motivated grant terminations and funding reallocations. Regulations to prevent any future dismantling of public health research are needed. Strengthening federal science governance—including codifying protections for priority research areas, establishing independent review bodies, and formalizing fair and transparent appeals processes—is essential. The NIMHD should be protected and adequately funded. Without systemic reform, long-standing public health priorities will remain vulnerable to the shifting ideologies of those in power. The fact that several of the authors' previously terminated grants have been recently reinstated is encouraging. Nonetheless, the terminations, even if reversed, have significant adverse consequences.

We welcome our new leaders' emphasis on using a data-driven approach and their desire to improve health outcomes. We believe the public health community can help in this regard. Replicable, rigorous research on race, racism, discrimination, and disparity will save lives, boost our economy, and improve life for all Americans. Let us finish the work we have started. AJPH

CORRESPONDENCE

Correspondence should be sent to Ken Resnicow, PhD, University of Minnesota, School of Public Health, EpiCH, West Bank Office Building, 1300 S Second St, Suite 300, Minneapolis, MN 55454-1015 (e-mail: kresnic@umich.edu). Reprints can be ordered at https://doi.org by clicking the "Reprints" link.

PUBLICATION INFORMATION

Full Citation: Resnicow K, Gamarel KE, Ahluwalia JS, Williams DR, Naar S, Griffith DM. Funding and defunding of NIH research should be based on real science and not politics or amorphous constructs. *Am J Public Health*. 2026;116(1):14–17.

Acceptance Date: August 5, 2025.

DOI: https://doi.org/10.2105/AJPH.2025.308268

ORCID iDs:

Ken Resnicow https://orcid.org/0000-0003-1416-9627

Kristi E. Gamarel https://orcid.org/0000-0001-9405-7515

Jasjit S. Ahluwalia https://orcid.org/0000-0003-1756-3646

David R. Williams https://orcid.org/0000-0002-8654-6228

Derek M. Griffith https://orcid.org/0000-0003-0018-9176

CONTRIBUTORS

All authors contributed to the conceptual development of this opinion piece, and all read and approved the final version.

CONFLICTS OF INTEREST

The authors declare no conflicts of interest.

REFERENCES

1. Griffith D, Twinamatsiko A. 'Divisive concepts' prohibitions: implications for health and health equity. *Health Affairs Health Policy Brief.* January 16, 2025. https://doi.org/10.1377/hpb20241230.689698
2. Bailey ZD, Krieger N, Agenor M, Graves J, Linos N, Bassett MT. Structural racism and health inequities in the USA: evidence and interventions. *Lancet.* 2017;389(10077):1453–1463. https://doi.org/10.1016/S0140-6736(17)30569-X
3. Abubakar I, Gram L, Lasoye S, et al. Confronting the consequences of racism, xenophobia, and discrimination on health and health-care systems. *Lancet.* 2022;400(10368):2137–2146. https://doi.org/10.1016/S0140-6736(22)01989-4
4. Selvarajah S, Corona Maioli S, Deivanayagam TA, et al. Racism, xenophobia, and discrimination: mapping pathways to health outcomes. *Lancet.* 2022;400(10368):2109–2124. https://doi.org/10.1016/S0140-6736(22)02484-9
5. Caraballo C, Massey DS, Ndumele CD, et al. Excess mortality and years of potential life lost among the Black population in the US, 1999–2020. *JAMA.* 2023;329(19):1662–1670. https://doi.org/10.1001/jama.2023.7022
6. Cullen MR, Lemeshow AR, Russo LJ, Barnes DM, Ababio Y, Habtezion A. Disease-specific health disparities: a targeted review focusing on race and ethnicity. *Healthcare (Basel).* 2022;10(4):603. https://doi.org/10.3390/healthcare10040603
7. Zavala VA, Bracci PM, Carethers JM, et al. Cancer health disparities in racial/ethnic minorities in the United States. *Br J Cancer.* 2021;124(2):315–332. https://doi.org/10.1038/s41416-020-01038-6
8. Muller C, Ihionkhan E, Stoffel EM, Kupfer SS. Disparities in early-onset colorectal cancer. *Cells.* 2021;10(5):1018. https://doi.org/10.3390/cells10051018
9. LaVeist TA, Pérez-Stable EJ, Richard P, et al. The economic burden of racial, ethnic, and educational health inequities in the US. *JAMA.* 2023;329(19):1682–1692. https://doi.org/10.1001/jama.2023.5965
10. Turner A. *Business Case for Racial Equity: A Strategy for Growth.* Publication 590-A. Battle Creek, MI: W. K. Kellogg Foundation/Altarum Institute; 2018.
11. Umberson D. Black deaths matter: race, relationship loss, and effects on survivors. *J Health Soc Behav.* 2017;58(4):405–420. https://doi.org/10.1177/0022146517739317
12. Fleming PJ, Patel MR, Green M, et al. Fear of deportation and associations with mental health among Michigan residents of Middle Eastern & North African descent. *J Immigr Minor Health.* 2023;25(2):382–388. https://doi.org/10.1007/s10903-022-01394-w
13. Resnicow K, Patel M, Green M, et al. The association of unfairness with mental and physical health in a multiethnic sample of adults: cross-sectional study. *JMIR Public Health Surveill.* 2021;7(5):e26622. https://doi.org/10.2196/26622
14. Williams DR, Mohammed SA. Discrimination and racial disparities in health: evidence and needed research. *J Behav Med.* 2009;32(1):20–47. https://doi.org/10.1007/s10865-008-9185-0
15. Williams DR, Neighbors HW, Jackson JS. Racial/ethnic discrimination and health: findings from community studies. *Am J Public Health.* 2008;98(9 suppl):S29–37. https://doi.org/10.2105/ajph.98.supplement_1.s29
16. Borrell LN, Kiefe CI, Williams DR, Diez-Roux AV, Gordon-Larsen P. Self-reported health, perceived racial discrimination, and skin color in African Americans in the CARDIA study. *Soc Sci Med.* 2006;63(6):1415–1427. https://doi.org/10.1016/j.socscimed.2006.04.008
17. Webb Hooper M, Antoni MH, Okuyemi K, Dietz NA, Resnicow K. Randomized controlled trial of group-based culturally specific cognitive behavioral therapy among African American smokers. *Nicotine Tob Res.* 2017;19(3):333–341. https://doi.org/10.1093/ntr/ntw181
18. Webb Hooper M, Carpenter KM, Salmon EE, Resnicow K. Enhancing tobacco quitline outcomes for African American adults: an RCT of a culturally specific intervention. *Am J Prev Med.* 2023;65(6):964–972. https://doi.org/10.1016/j.amepre.2023.06.005
19. Griffith DM, Efird CR, Baskin ML, Webb Hooper M, Davis RE, Resnicow K. Cultural sensitivity and cultural tailoring: lessons learned and refinements after two decades of incorporating culture in health communication research. *Annu Rev Public Health.* 2024;45(1):195–212. https://doi.org/10.1146/annurev-publhealth-060722-031158.
20. Resnicow K, Campbell MK, Carr C, et al. Body and soul. A dietary intervention conducted through African-American churches. *Am J Prev Med.* 2004;27(2):97–105. https://doi.org/10.1016/j.amepre.2004.04.009
21. Langford AT, Larkin K, Resnicow K, Zikmund-Fisher BJ, Fagerlin A. Understanding the role of message frames on African-American willingness to participate in a hypothetical diabetes prevention study. *J Health Commun.* 2017;22(8):647–656. https://doi.org/10.1080/10810730.2017.1339146
22. Nollen N, Ahluwalia JS, Mayo MS, et al. A randomized trial of targeted educational materials for smoking cessation in African Americans using transdermal nicotine. *Health Educ Behav.* 2007;34(6):911–927. https://doi.org/10.1177/1090198106294652
23. Williams DR, Neighbors HW, Jackson JS. Racial/ethnic discrimination and health: findings from community studies. *Am J Public Health.* 2003;93(2):200–208. https://doi.org/10.2105/ajph.93.2.200
24. Krieger N, Rowley D, Herman A, Avery B, Phillips M. Racism, sexism, and social class, implications for studies of health, disease, and well-being. *Am J Prev Med.* 2022;62(6):816–863. https://doi.org/10.1016/S0749-3797(18)30666-4
25. Williams DR. Miles to go before we sleep: racial inequities in health. *J Health Soc Behav.* 2012;53(3):279–295. https://doi.org/10.1177/0022146512455804

Fixing Up Places Is Easier Than Fixing People

John MacDonald, PhD

ABOUT THE AUTHOR

The author is with the Department of Criminology, University of Pennsylvania, Philadelphia.

See also Asa et al. p. 95.

Serious violent crime and firearm violence represent a major public health challenge in the United States. Firearm homicide is a leading cause of death in the United States, with substantial racial disparities documented over time. Serious crime and violence in the United States are also spatially concentrated in the most socially and economically disadvantaged urban neighborhoods. Hebrew University criminologist David Weisburd has referred to this empirical reality as the "law of crime concentration."[1]

Several study authors have noted that place-based approaches offer an effective means of reducing the concentration of serious crime and gun violence in the most economically disadvantaged communities.[2] There is a growing body of high-quality controlled and randomized trials showing that remediation of blighted vacant land and abandoned housing helps mitigate serious crime and firearm violence.[3,4]

However, absent from this research has been a focus on what happens to blighted vacant land or abandoned housing once there is reinvestment with new properties. Although structural repairs to abandoned and occupied housing have been shown to help reduce serious crime and gun violence in controlled and randomized trials,[5–7] to date there are few causal studies that show whether investments in new housing and occupied structures help alleviate the concentration of serious crime and gun violence.

Asa et al. (p. 95) take up this issue in their study of the effect of the redevelopment of 254 vacant lots in Philadelphia, Pennsylvania, over a 16-year period (2007–2023) on serious violent crime and violent crimes committed with firearms. The exposure in this case was the specific repurposing of vacant lots into permanent structures, largely housing, as compared with lots that remained vacant and blighted. This study is ideal because the authors rely on a rigorous difference-in-difference design that attributes changes in violent crime and gun violence to the timing of when the vacant lot was repurposed for new housing or a building structure. Useful for public health policy, they found that among the subset of vacant lots repurposed into permanent housing or business structures, there was a statistically significant effect on aggravated assault (i.e., a reduction of 30%) and overall violence committed with firearms (a reduction of 14.7%). The gun violence reduction benefits of repurposing vacant lots, however, occurred only with permanent housing or business structures, not parking lots or fenced-off vacant lots that were maintained.

The mechanisms by which building new structures on blighted vacant lots reduces gun violence are not explained, because the study authors could not observe human activities changing around the places before and after they were repurposed. However, the study offers a view into what could be done in the future. Following the same methodology, it is possible to use cell phone data that are available to researchers to examine how, if at all, human activity around vacant lots changes after they are repurposed. Perhaps new foot traffic arrives, the level of guardianship at locations changes, or some combination of new residents and the dynamics of the places shifts after vacant lots are converted to housing and business structures.

The Asa et al. study shows no evidence that repurposed vacant lots lead to displacement of aggravated assaults and overall gun violence to nearby areas. These findings are consistent with a growing body of evidence showing minimal displacement from place-based crime prevention interventions.[8] Places that attract gun violence may not be easily transferred elsewhere. Situational dynamics of places attracting gun violence such as open air drug markets, for example, may not easily be relocated from a vacant lot on one block to another location.

Sprucing up vacant lots to keep them in a stable and maintained condition until they can be repurposed for housing or commercial use benefits both Philadelphians and the city's tax base. To that end, the Pennsylvania Horticultural Society's LandCare program cleans, greens, and maintains vacant lots. New structures mean that new property taxes can be collected and neighborhoods can attract reinvestment. Although gentrification is often a concern, the more housing that is developed, the lower on average the price per unit. In short, the only way to secure more affordable housing in

AJPH January 2026, Vol. 116, No. 1

cities such as Philadelphia is to build more housing.

The available evidence from the Asa et al. study and others suggests, contrary to conventional wisdom in many circles, that redevelopment that spurs some degree of gentrification lowers serious crime.[9] At the same time, it is important to recognize that gentrification can lead to displacement of existing residents if new housing and businesses lead to rising property values and higher local tax assessments. To mitigate this issue, policies such as homestead exemptions should be in place to reduce the assessed value of existing homes near new developments.

The Asa et al. study adds to the growing body of high-quality studies demonstrating that abating vacant land in an urban neighborhood can dramatically reduce serious crime and gun violence. The changes do not require large-scale structural investments from taxpayers. Rather, they require cities to provide access to vacant properties in a way that allows them to be repurposed into housing and business structures in a cost-effective way to spur redevelopment. Although this may, in some circumstances, change the social fabric of neighborhoods, it is an inevitable process of neighborhood change when new generations of residents move into a place. The alternative is stagnation and decline.

Public health policy can gain considerably from focusing on place-based changes such as those emphasized in the Asa et al. study. Redevelopment of properties may be seen as a real estate or urban planning issue; considering the degree to which gun violence and serious crime are concentrated in cities and how this issue affects population health, however, public health policies should view place-based approaches as part of the portfolio of interventions to study, test, and advocate.[2]

In fact, place-based public health interventions were central to the foundation of public health. Dr. John Snow shutting off the water pump at Southwark/Vauxhall after showing evidence that the cholera outbreak was worse around that location where residents obtained their water than around Lambeth is a foundational example of a place-focused public health intervention. Given that gun violence is a leading cause of morbidity and mortality in the United States, place-based interventions that focus on improving the built environment should be central to public health policy. Epidemiologists working in public health agencies should be partnering with their local housing, code enforcement, and redevelopment authorities; mapping serious crime and gun violence; and assessing the role that each of these agencies can have in helping address the concentration of such problems in cities through place-based interventions that are within their purview.

Given that serious crime and gun violence are highly concentrated in the same places, strategic planning can have large-scale population health benefits. Imagine a scenario in which a thousand blocks in a city are responsible for 75% of all serious crime and gun violence. A set of place-based interventions could be launched, including redeveloping vacant lots, cleaning streets, improving sidewalks, and condemning abandoned structures for repurposing into new housing or businesses. If addressing the blighted built environment in this way produced a 30% reduction in serious crime and gun violence in these thousand blocks, the entire city would experience a 22.5% reduction in serious crime and gun violence.

In the United States, public health policy undervalues place-based interventions such as vacant lot repurposing and housing remediation as methods for reducing gun violence and serious crime. Although social programs have demonstrated promise in reducing serious crime, they are resource intensive and often hinge on a charismatic leader or a specialized programmatic model that is difficult to scale. Place-based interventions also require planning, overcoming inertia, and leadership, but they are easily scaled and achievable. The reality is that serious crime and gun violence are hyperconcentrated, suggesting that changes to the built environment could be a particularly salient non–criminal justice approach to prevention. AJPH

CORRESPONDENCE

Correspondence should be sent to John MacDonald, Department of Criminology, 558 McNeil Building, 3718 Locust Walk, University of Pennsylvania, Philadelphia, PA 19104-6286 (e-mail: johnmm@upenn.edu). Reprints can be ordered at https://www.ajph.org by clicking the "Reprints" link.

PUBLICATION INFORMATION

Full Citation: MacDonald J. Fixing up places is easier than fixing people. *Am J Public Health*. 2026;116(1):18–20.

Acceptance Date: October 14, 2025.

DOI: https://doi.org/10.2105/AJPH.2025.308319

ORCID iD:
John MacDonald https://orcid.org/0000-0001-6714-8905

ACKNOWLEDGMENTS

The author receives funding from Arnold Ventures, a philanthropic foundation.

CONFLICTS OF INTEREST

The author has no conflicts of interest to disclose.

REFERENCES

1. Weisburd D. The law of crime concentration and the criminology of place. *Criminology*. 2015;53(2):133–157.
2. MacDonald J, Stokes R, Branas CC. *Changing Places: The Science and Art of New Urban Planning*. Princeton University Press; 2019.

3. Branas CC, South E, Kondo MC, et al. Citywide cluster randomized trial to restore blighted vacant land and its effects on violence, crime, and fear. *Proc Natl Acad Sci U S A.* 2018;115(12):2946–2951.
4. MacDonald J, Nguyen V, Jensen ST, Branas CC. Reducing crime by remediating vacant lots: the moderating effect of nearby land uses. *J Exp Criminol.* 2022;18(3):639–664.
5. South EC, MacDonald JM, Tam VW, Ridgeway G, Branas CC. Effect of abandoned housing interventions on gun violence, perceptions of safety, and substance use in Black neighborhoods: a citywide cluster randomized trial. *JAMA Intern Med.* 2023;183(1):31–39.
6. South EC, MacDonald J, Reina V. Association between structural housing repairs for low-income homeowners and neighborhood crime. *JAMA Netw Open.* 2021;4(7):e2117067.
7. Kondo MC, Keene D, Hohl BC, MacDonald JM, Branas CC. A difference-in-differences study of the effects of a new abandoned building remediation strategy on safety. *PLoS One.* 2015;10(7):e0129582.
8. Johnson SD, Guerette RT, Bowers K. Crime displacement: what we know, what we don't know, and what it means for crime reduction. *J Exp Criminol.* 2014;10(4):549–571.
9. MacDonald JM, Stokes RJ. Gentrification, land use, and crime. *Annu Rev Criminol.* 2020;3:121–138.

A Renewed Effort to Control and Eliminate Congenital Syphilis in the United States

Chrysovalantis Stafylis, MD, MPH, and Jeffrey D. Klausner, MD, MPH

ABOUT THE AUTHORS

Chrysovalantis Stafylis and Jeffrey D. Klausner are with the Department of Population & Public Health Sciences, Keck School of Medicine, University of Southern California, Los Angeles.

See also Abresch et al., p. 103.

Congenital syphilis in the United States has risen sharply over the past decade after near elimination, with reported cases increasing from 362 in 2013 to more than 3900 in 2024,[1] according to the Centers for Disease Control and Prevention's (CDC's) most recent Sexually Transmitted Infections Surveillance Report. Apart from a transient increase between 1990 and 1992 attributable to the crack cocaine epidemic, there has not been nearly 4000 cases in congenital syphilis in United States since the 1950s. The infection, caused by *Treponema pallidum* and transmitted from the mother to the fetus during pregnancy or delivery, is entirely preventable through timely screening and treatment.[2] However, important gaps in the prevention of congenital syphilis persist as 40% of mothers of affected infants receive no prenatal care, and 88% of cases were born to mothers without adequate testing or treatment.[3] Untreated maternal infection can result in stillbirth or neonatal death,[4] and surviving infants may have lifelong neurological and other complications.

LESSONS FROM THE PAST

In this issue of *AJPH*, Abresch et al. present the summary of recommendations from the Congenital Syphilis Summit in Atlanta, Georgia (2025), gathering past experiences and opinions of public health experts and stakeholders (p. 103). Drawing from the past syphilis elimination efforts, the authors identified five critical and interconnected system failures that have impeded our response:

1. cyclical boom-and-bust funding,
2. workforce deterioration,
3. fragmented surveillance,
4. disconnected health care systems, and
5. health inequities.

More importantly, the authors propose strategies to rebuild and maintain the prevention infrastructure. This conference summary adds to the increasing number of calls to action from major public health and medical organizations, such as the American Academy of Pediatrics, urging immediate action and resource allocation to address the rising rates of congenital syphilis. It is also a call to rethink our approach to congenital syphilis prevention and control. We wish to highlight a few key points.

MOVING FORWARD TO ELIMINATION

Congenital syphilis is a modern public health crisis. Addressing it will require a renewed multidisciplinary and multifaceted Congenital Syphilis Elimination Plan. Similar to previous elimination efforts, the Plan will set priorities and strategies coordinated at the highest level by national health agencies, like the National Syphilis and Congenital Syphilis Syndemic Federal Task Force. Partnerships are necessary to bring together public health organizations: the American Public Health Association, the Council of State and Territorial Epidemiologists, the National Association of City and County Health Officers; government entities, like the Substance Abuse and Mental Health Services Administration; expert associations, such as the American College of Obstetricians and Gynecologists and the American Academy of Pediatrics; policy organizations; and local, state, county, and city governments. It is important to highlight that this effort cannot succeed without community participation. Program and policy development must include the affected community across all stages of implementation. Advocates play an important role in the design and adaptation of the programs to the local context and needs of the communities they represent.

We agree on the importance of breaking the "deadly cycle of panic and neglect."[5] Providing short-term, emergency funding to address an outbreak to only scale back once contained is shortsighted; this approach is practical

AJPH January 2026, Vol. 116, No. 1

for acute infections with single event exposures but may not be adequate for syphilis—a chronic endemic infection that is often asymptomatic. Long-term funding with a focus on maintaining public health systems and workforce is needed, which will enable constant vigilance through effective surveillance, early identification, active case management, and treatment. Another approach is to integrate funding for maternal health programs with other related prevention services, as the authors recommend. Perinatal syphilis screening combined with HIV screening is a cost-effective approach[5] and could include programs on gonorrhea and chlamydia screening, hepatitis B, substance use, or mental health. Stakeholders will request cost-effective and budget-maximizing strategies for allocating resources efficiently within systems and communities. Research will be necessary to indicate optimal ways to allocate funds.

Testing and treating cases are the cornerstones of the public health response to control an infectious disease epidemic. Universal prenatal screening, along with expanded access to care in underserved areas and populations, should play a central role in our efforts. According to the CDC, all pregnant women should be screened serologically for syphilis at the first prenatal visit, and tested at a later stage during pregnancy depending on risk factors and previous serological test results.[7] However, the American College of Obstetricians and Gynecologists recommends universal first visit and third trimester screening for all women.[8] In fact, many states mandate syphilis screening during pregnancy, but there is variability in additional screening recommendations state by state.[9] We need consistent screening recommendations and a proactive system to monitor screening practices and hold providers and care systems accountable. Solutions such as simple automated medical record screening prompts could help. Considering that only 80% of pregnant women in care are tested for syphilis even once, testing must be expanded in traditional and nonclinical environments to reach underserved and disproportionately burdened communities. Pilot projects have demonstrated the feasibility of screening in emergency departments[10] and jails[11]; however, innovative approaches, such as testing in community sites, immigrant detention facilities, and homeless service programs or the provision of home self-test kits, should also be explored.

A "test and treat" approach, where treatment is administered at the time of a positive test result, could be highly effective in decreasing mother-to-child syphilis transmission. A single dose of penicillin is 98% effective in preventing congenital syphilis. Laboratory-based serological testing, which is the current cornerstone of current syphilis diagnosis and management, requires extensive infrastructure (i.e., collection sites, trained phlebotomists, specimen transportation, laboratory equipment, information systems, and certified staff), and the extended time to test result notification may result in delayed or no treatment. Recent advances in syphilis rapid point-of-care tests can increase the opportunities for wider screening with quick results.[12] Rapid tests require a single drop of blood, can be performed by staff without specialized training, and yield results within 10 minutes. In people with no history of syphilis or syphilis treatment, a positive test result is sufficient for immediate treatment.

Considering the uneven burden of syphilis among different communities, we must adapt our clinical work to alleviate the impact of societal factors that drive congenital syphilis. Homelessness, substance misuse and addiction, partner violence, and incarceration pose significant obstacles to receiving timely management[13] and may be both risk factors for acquiring syphilis and factors that keep women from accessing testing and treatment. We advocate "safe haven" clinics and policies of "hold harmless," where pregnant women are taken care of in safe environments, without stigma, fear of criminal persecution, or fear of losing custody of their child, regardless of substance use or immigration status. We will need a holistic approach to maternal–child health beyond syphilis treatment, including harm reduction and partner violence support services, along with appropriately educated expert health care personnel.

It is apparent that congenital syphilis will require a multisector approach. It is necessary to develop local teams of disease intervention specialists, community health care workers, and clinicians to increase opportunities for education and collaboration. At the clinical level, we need to ensure close interaction between infectious disease, maternal health, and child health professionals. We will need to further integrate public health with medical care with almost "live" data exchange and regularly disseminate surveillance data to monitor progress.

By reviewing past successes, Abresch et al. showed that there is enough evidence to implement interventions for congenital syphilis elimination and control; however, what may be lacking is sufficient political will. While research gaps exist, we have the current tools to control and eliminate congenital syphilis. Congenital syphilis has been successfully eliminated in 19 countries to date. What prevents us from doing so in the United States? We must work to protect the health of mothers and children, but we need to ensure that we do not repeat past mistakes once that goal is achieved. AJPH

CORRESPONDENCE

Correspondence should be sent to Chrysovalantis Stafylis, 1845 N Soto St, Los Angeles, CA 90033 (e-mail: chrysovalantis.stafylis@med.usc.edu). Reprints can be ordered at https://www.ajph.org by clicking the "Reprints" link.

PUBLICATION INFORMATION

Full Citation: Stafylis C, Klausner JD. A renewed effort to control and eliminate congenital syphilis in the United States. *Am J Public Health*. 2026; 116(1):21–23.

Acceptance Date: October 10, 2025.

DOI: https://doi.org/10.2105/AJPH.2025.308316

ORCID iD:
Chrysovalantis Stafylis https://orcid.org/0000-0002-1486-1130

CONTRIBUTORS

Both authors contributed to the development of the article.

ACKNOWLEDGMENTS

J. D. Klausner received funding from National Institutes of Health (NIH) R01AI139265 and NIH R01AI196655.

Note. The funding source had no input in the development of this article.

CONFLICTS OF INTEREST

The authors report no conflicts of interest.

REFERENCES

1. Centers for Disease Control and Prevention. Sexually Transmitted Infections Surveillance, 2024 (Provisional). September 24, 2025. Available at: https://www.cdc.gov/sti-statistics/annual/index.html. Accessed October 20, 2025.
2. Stafford IA, Workowski KA, Bachmann LH. Syphilis complicating pregnancy and congenital syphilis. *N Engl J Med.* 2024;390(3):242–253. https://doi.org/10.1056/NEJMra2202762
3. McDonald R, O'Callaghan K, Torrone E, et al. Vital signs: Missed opportunities for preventing congenital syphilis—United States, 2022. *MMWR Morb Mortal Wkly Rep.* 2023;72(46):1269–1274. https://doi.org/10.15585/mmwr.mm7246e1
4. Carlson JM, Sancken CL, Nguyen K, et al. Birth outcomes among women with syphilis during pregnancy in six US states, 2018–2021. *Obstet Gynecol.* May 2 2025;146(1):121–128. https://doi.org/10.1097/AOG.0000000000005913
5. Syphilis is resurging in the US, a sign of public health's funding crisis. NPR. November 1, 2021. Available at: https://www.npr.org/transcripts/1050568646. Accessed October 21, 2025.
6. Zhang M, Zhang H, Hui X, et al. The cost-effectiveness of syphilis screening in pregnant women: a systematic literature review. *Front Public Health.* 2024;12:1268653. https://doi.org/10.3389/fpubh.2024.1268653
7. Workowski KA, Bachmann LH, Chan PA, et al. Sexually Transmitted Infections Treatment Guidelines, 2021. *MMWR Recomm Rep.* 2021; 70(4):1–187. https://doi.org/10.15585/mmwr.rr7004a1
8. American College of Obstetricians and Gynecologists. Updated ACOG Recommendation. Screening for Syphilis in Pregnancy. 2025. Available at: https://www.acog.org/clinical/clinical-guidance/practice-advisory/articles/2024/04/screening-for-syphilis-in-pregnancy. Accessed September 12, 2025.
9. Emerson B, Tao G, Hufstetler K, Cramer R, Pearson WS. Syphilis screening during pregnancy in 18- to 49-year-old women in commercially insured claims data, 2022. *Sex Transm Dis.* 2025; 52(5):295–303. https://doi.org/10.1097/OLQ.0000000000002089
10. Stafford I, Bakunas C, Haydamous J, et al. Implementation of an opt-out and rapid point-of-care syphilis testing program for pregnant patients presenting to the emergency department. *Sex Transm Dis.* 2025;52(6):352–355. https://doi.org/10.1097/OLQ.0000000000002131
11. Harmon JL, Dhaliwal SK, Burghardt NO, et al. Routine screening in a California jail: effect of local policy on identification of syphilis in a high-incidence area, 2016–2017. *Public Health Rep.* 2020;135(1 suppl):57s–64s. https://doi.org/10.1177/0033354920928454
12. Kojima N, Klausner JD. Is it time to test and treat for syphilis? *J Gen Intern Med.* 2025;40(10): 2421–2422. https://doi.org/10.1007/s11606-025-09547-x
13. Smullin C, Wagman J, Mehta S, Klausner JD. A narrative review of the epidemiology of congenital syphilis in the United States from 1980 to 2019. *Sex Transm Dis.* 2021;48(2):71–78. https://doi.org/10.1097/OLQ.0000000000001277

The Patients Are Ready, but the System Is Not: Closing the Gap Between Opioid Overdose Prevention and Recovery

Stephen G. Henry, MD, and Aimee Moulin, MD

ABOUT THE AUTHORS

The authors are with the University of California, Davis School of Medicine, Sacramento, CA.

See also Kepler et al., p. 113.

AJPH January 2026, Vol. 116, No. 1

In 2024, nearly 80 000 people died of opioid-related overdose in the United States.[1] The most effective overdose prevention strategies implemented over the past two decades involve expanding access to medications to treat opioid use disorder (OUD). These medications (especially buprenorphine and methadone) are highly effective at reducing overdose risk but remain grossly underused; in 2023 fewer than one in five patients with OUD received medication treatment.[2] A major reason for this underuse is that outpatient treatment programs have traditionally erected substantial barriers to access (e.g., lengthy wait times, requiring 100% abstinence from drugs for continued treatment) that disproportionately affect patients with the greatest overdose risk: those who are poor, unhoused, or have difficulty reaching outpatient clinics owing to lack of transportation, telephone service, or social instability.

As a result, clinical and public health researchers have long advocated lowering barriers to OUD treatment. One major focus of these efforts has been initiating medication for OUD in hospital emergency departments (EDs). EDs are well suited for providing OUD treatment. They are open 24 hours a day, can be used by patients who lack health insurance or primary care, and can easily monitor and support patients during withdrawal and treatment initiation. As a result, initiating OUD treatment in EDs has become a recommended best practice in emergency medicine.[3]

In this issue of *AJPH*, Kepler et al. (p. 113) from the New York City Department of Health and Mental Hygiene report data from Relay, a city-funded opioid overdose prevention program that employs wellness advocates (i.e., drug and alcohol counselors with lived experience of substance use). Wellness advocates respond to patients with suspected opioid overdose at 1 of 14 hospital EDs. They offer support, overdose prevention education, naloxone, and—for patients who accept them—referral to treatment and up to 90 days of follow-up support after patients leave the ED. Peer support provided by patients with lived experience of substance use is an effective strategy for nonjudgmentally engaging patients with OUD in care, is as effective as interventions by more highly trained clinicians,[4] and is an important strength of the Relay program.

Kepler et al. analyzed data from patients served by the Relay program over more than five years (June 2017–December 2022). Their primary analyses involved identifying characteristics associated with (1) agreeing to and receiving post-ED follow-up from wellness advocates, and (2) subsequent fatal opioid overdose. Both analyses controlled for patient age, sex, and race/ethnicity. The authors linked data collected during patients' ED visits to death certificate and medical examiner records, allowing them to identify patients who died from opioid overdose during the 12 months after receiving Relay services.

A major finding from this study was that 93% of the 5702 eligible patients accepted Relay services during their ED visits, and 69% accepted follow-up support. These results underscore that patients with OUD are eager to get care when it is offered to them, which is consistent with findings from other states that highlight the value of hospital EDs as low-barrier locations to engage patients in OUD treatment.[5] These numbers are in stark contrast to the one in five patients who receive medication for OUD nationally. Clearly, there is a gap between the motivated postoverdose ED patients and their ability to access outpatient medication.

Importantly, this observational study cannot provide conclusions about whether receiving Relay program services is effective in reducing patients' subsequent opioid overdose risk. Results from a parallel randomized trial of the Relay program are needed to answer this question and should be published soon.[6] This study has other important limitations. It did not report how many patients received medication for OUD during their ED visit or how many patients were referred to outpatient OUD treatment after they left the ED.

The authors' analysis of patient characteristics associated with accepting post-ED follow-up and at least one successful follow-up contact by wellness advocates indicates that patients who are most likely to accept follow-up services are also the least likely to be successfully contacted after they leave the ED, highlighting an important gap in services. Patients who reported unstable or temporary housing conditions, previous overdose, and participation in New York City's needle exchange program were significantly more likely to request follow-up but significantly less likely to actually be contacted. These same characteristics were also associated with significantly greater risk of death from opioid overdose at 12 months.

As the authors note, the most likely explanation for these findings is that the patients who are at greatest risk for fatal overdose (and so would benefit most from follow-up services) tend to request services but are also the most difficult to reach and engage in treatment after they leave the ED. Our current systems of care are not designed to effectively engage these high-risk patients. This is an important area for future study. Unfortunately, the same factors that make it challenging to engage these high-risk patients for OUD treatment also make it difficult to engage them in research. Indeed, the landmark trial that established the effectiveness of ED-initiated OUD treatment also found that the benefits of treatment initiation disappeared once patients were not regularly engaged by research teams.[7]

The findings of Kepler et al. suggest that ED-based OUD treatment and overdose prevention services are unlikely to be effective unless they are coupled with strategies that keep patients engaged in outpatient treatment after they leave the ED.

Accomplishing this may require supporting outpatient treatment options that have some of the flexibility of EDs (e.g., clinics that allow walk-in or same day outpatient visits). Maintaining patients in treatment is already difficult because the US outpatient OUD treatment infrastructure is underfunded and uneven. Recent federal efforts to weaken Medicaid are likely to make it even more difficult for Medicaid beneficiaries to access outpatient treatment.

The results from the study by Kepler et al. of the Relay program highlight both the promise and the limitations of current overdose prevention strategies. Our current systems of care and research efforts have difficulty reaching people at the highest risk for overdose and other harms. To change the trajectory of poor OUD outcomes, public health leaders need to reimagine outpatient OUD treatment as a continuum that begins in the ED but does not end there. This means investing in research on high-risk populations who may visit the ED but are not otherwise engaged in care. It means investing in flexible, low-barrier outpatient clinics and supporting peer-based engagement. By reshaping our systems to meet patients where they are and support them as they transition across care settings, we can close the fatal gap between patients' motivations to receive life-saving treatment and their ability to access it. AJPH

CORRESPONDENCE

Correspondence should be sent to Stephen G. Henry, 4150 V St, Suite 2400, Sacramento, CA 95817 (e-mail: sghenry@health.ucdavis.edu). Reprints can be ordered at https://www.ajph.org by clicking the "Reprints" link.

PUBLICATION INFORMATION

Full Citation: Henry SG, Moulin A. The patients are ready, but the system is not: closing the gap between opioid overdose prevention and recovery. *Am J Public Health*. 2026;116(1):24–25.

Acceptance Date: October 10, 2025.

DOI: https://doi.org/10.2105/AJPH.2025.308314

ORCID iD:
Stephen G. Henry https://orcid.org/0000-0002-5643-0881

CONTRIBUTORS

The authors contributed equally to the work and approved the final published version.

CONFLICTS OF INTEREST

The authors have no conflicts of interest to disclose.

REFERENCES

1. National Center for Health Statistics. Provisional drug overdose death counts. Available at: https://www.cdc.gov/nchs/nvss/vsrr/drug-overdose-data.htm. Accessed August 1, 2025.
2. Center for Behavioral Health Statistics and Quality, Substance Abuse and Mental Health Services Administration. Key substance use and mental health indicators in the United States: results from the 2023 National Survey on Drug Use and Health (NSDUH). 2024. Available at: https://www.samhsa.gov/data/sites/default/files/reports/rpt47095/National%20Report/National%20Report/2023-nsduh-annual-national.pdf. Accessed October 18, 2025.
3. Hawk K, Hoppe J, Ketcham E, et al. Consensus recommendations on the treatment of opioid use disorder in the emergency department. *Ann Emerg Med*. 2021;78(3):434–442. https://doi.org/10.1016/j.annemergmed.2021.04.023
4. Chambers LC, Li Y, Hallowell BD, et al. Effect of a peer-led emergency department behavioral intervention on non-fatal opioid overdose: 18-month outcome in the Navigator randomized controlled trial. *Addiction*. 2024;119(12):2116–2128. https://doi.org/10.1111/add.16581
5. Kalmin MM, Goodman-Meza D, Anderson E, et al. Voting with their feet: social factors linked with treatment for opioid use disorder using same-day buprenorphine delivered in California hospitals. *Drug Alcohol Depend*. 2021;222:108673. https://doi.org/10.1016/j.drugalcdep.2021.108673
6. Doran KM, Welch AE, Jeffers A, et al. Study protocol for a multisite randomized controlled trial of a peer navigator intervention for emergency department patients with nonfatal opioid overdose. *Contemp Clin Trials*. 2023;126:107111. https://doi.org/10.1016/j.cct.2023.107111
7. D'Onofrio G, Chawarski MC, O'Connor PG, et al. Emergency department-initiated buprenorphine for opioid dependence with continuation in primary care: outcomes during and after intervention. *J Gen Intern Med*. 2017;32(6):660–666. https://doi.org/10.1007/s11606-017-3993-2

Extreme Polarization Is a Threat to US Health

Jennifer B. Nuzzo, DrPH, SM

ABOUT THE AUTHOR

Jennifer B. Nuzzo is inaugural director of the Pandemic Center, and professor of epidemiology at the Brown University School of Public Health, Providence, RI.

See also McMurtry and Cheu, p. 124.

The COVID-19 pandemic harmed the United States in multiple, profound ways. More than a million people died, resulting in historic declines in US life expectancy.[1] Many who survived their infection continue to suffer from long-term, in some cases disabling, symptoms. But one lingering impact of the pandemic—extreme political polarization—is poised to erode the health of people in the United States far beyond even these staggering tolls. We urgently need evidence-based solutions to repair our social rifts and to prevent such polarization in future public health emergencies.

UNPRECEDENTED COVID-19 POLARIZATION

In an article in this issue of *AJPH* (p. 124), McMurtry and Cheu analyzed political polarization during the COVID-19 pandemic and in previous infectious disease emergencies. Comparing polls conducted in the United States during 13 infectious disease emergencies that occurred over nearly 70 years, they looked for partisan differences in responses to questions about infection risk perception and vaccine hesitancy. While historic trends would predict some degree of partisan differences during the pandemic, polarization regarding public concern about infection and vaccine hesitancy during the pandemic were 5 and 12 times greater than seen in previous infectious disease emergencies.

Though we cannot infer from McMurtry and Cheu's analysis the cause of such extreme polarization during the pandemic, we should be concerned about its persistence. Differences in support for public health priorities and approaches can lead to legislative gridlock that hinders the government's ability to respond to outbreaks. Polarization can erode public trust in government and risk perception, both of which may affect protective behaviors.

Extreme polarization during the pandemic may help us to understand why the tolls of the COVID-19 in the United States exceeded those in peer countries. Though it was ranked by the Global Health Security Index as among the best prepared countries in the world, the United States experienced more than eight times higher pandemic-associated mortality than other highly prepared countries.[2] Polarization may not have been the only reason for the United States' exceptional losses, but partisan differences in how Americans perceived risk and chose to protect themselves using vaccines and nonpharmaceutical interventions like masks have been well documented.[3]

PREVIOUS BIPARTISAN EFFORTS TO STRENGTHEN US PUBLIC HEALTH

Political decisions involved in protecting public health during emergencies do not always produce extreme political polarization. After the United States lost nearly 3000 people on September 11, 2001, and the anthrax attacks that followed, Congress passed bipartisan legislation giving public health a massive infusion of funding to modernize public health agencies at the federal, state, and local level. The US Department of Health and Human Services established a new office focused on public health preparedness (presently known as the Administration for Strategic Preparedness and Response) and expanded federal grant programs for state and local public health agencies and hospitals.[4,5]

But five years after COVID-19's start, the United States has not responded with a serious bipartisan effort to assess what went wrong during the pandemic and to implement improvements, as happened after the tragic events of 2001. Instead, political leaders continue to dispute facts about COVID-19, its harms, and the vaccines that protect against them. Major programs established after previous public health emergencies to prepare for future ones are being shuttered.[6] For example, massive staff cuts to and proposed reorganization at the Administration for Strategic Preparedness and Response raise serious questions about the ability of the office to function.

The United States continues to struggle to respond to infectious disease emergencies after the pandemic. The country is currently in the throes of the largest and deadliest measles outbreak

AJPH January 2026, Vol. 116, No. 1

that it has experienced since elimination of the disease 25 years ago. In the last year, multiple states have battled record high levels of whooping cough. The scale and severity of these trends will only worsen if partisan political efforts currently underway to weaken vaccine access and evidence-based vaccine recommendations are successful.

We urgently need evidence-based approaches to mend social rifts that threaten to erode decades of progress in improving and extending Americans' health. In reviewing past outbreaks, McMurtry and Cheu conclude that "high levels of polarization do not appear endemic to disease outbreaks, suggesting such division may be preventable in the future" (p. 124). This provides a note of hope that we may break these self-destructive trends.

But in seeking solutions, we must use caution in how we interpret polarization resulting from the US COVID-19 experience. There are no recent public health emergencies that were as severe in terms of disruptions and harm or were as pervasive and protracted as the COVID-19 pandemic. The pandemic was extraordinary in a multitude of ways—from the tolls of the disease to the sacrifices that millions of people in the United States had to make forgoing school and work in usual settings. The COVID-19 vaccines, which saved hundreds of thousands of US lives,[7] were without precedent. The first Trump administration's Operation Warp Speed applied great political will and resources to enable the development of safe and effective vaccines that used a novel technological approach. Though more than two thirds of people in the United States got vaccinated with at least one dose by the end of 2021,[8] it is understandable that not everyone was as quick to embrace these new tools.

COVID-19 DISAGREEMENTS SHOULD NOT UNDO HEALTH PROTECTIONS

It would not be correct to infer from COVID-19 that Americans are now hopelessly divided about all public health matters. Rather, polling indicates that there is broad support across party lines for routine childhood immunizations. For example, recent data from the Kaiser Family Foundation and the *Washington Post* show that an overwhelming majority of people in the United States, regardless of political affiliation, support and value routine childhood immunizations, like measles, mumps, and rubella (MMR) and polio vaccines, and believe they are safe.[9] Other polling shows that across the United States, parents of all political parties overwhelmingly support laws that require children to have routine immunizations to attend school.[10] Even in Florida, where political leaders recently announced an intention to remove school-based vaccine requirements, an overwhelming majority of parents support vaccines and laws that require children to receive routine immunizations to attend school.[11]

Still, there are some significant points on which people in the United States do disagree when it comes to vaccines and the protection of public health. For example, views and support for influenza and COVID-19 vaccines are generally lower and more partisan than for routine immunizations. The share of children who received an exemption for one or more required vaccines increased to 3.6% in 2024 to 2025 from 2.5% in 2019 to 2020.[11] Though a small change, any increase in vaccine exemptions should prompt concern given many communities across the United States have an MMR vaccination coverage that is lower than the 95% target that is required to prevent outbreaks of measles.

Political leaders, not recognizing important distinctions in Americans' views, may feel COVID-19 frustrations give them political license to weaken other public health protections. For example, Secretary Robert F. Kennedy Jr recently cited poor uptake of COVID-19 boosters to justify firings at the Centers for Disease Control and Prevention (CDC) and to dismiss the entire membership of the Advisory Committee on Immunization Practices (ACIP), the independent committee of external experts that provides nonpartisan, evidence-based advice regarding vaccines.[12] The secretary also cited lack of trust in the CDC as the cause of the United States' anomalous levels of COVID-19 deaths, without acknowledging that partisan politics may worsen polarization and distrust. Several states have responded to the dismissal of qualified experts from ACIP and the subsequent appointment to a reconstituted ACIP of individuals without vaccine-relevant expertise, by forming multistate coalitions to make alternative vaccine policy recommendations for their regions.[13]

Any effort that is not aligned with majority public sentiment will only increase polarization. While there are some public health questions on which the US public does not agree, there are still many areas of commonality. To protect public health, we must build on this common ground and be guided by evidence, not partisan politics. Even if federal leadership were more committed to bolstering public health preparedness, this would still likely require a bottom-up approach. State and local health agencies should work to engage with the public via the organizations and leaders that represent them—community groups, businesses, faith-based organizations, etc.—to define both the needs and values that should shape responses to future infectious disease emergencies. In addition to ensuring that responses are aligned with communities' interests, such continued, positive engagement is a necessary step to building trusted relationships. AJPH

CORRESPONDENCE

Correspondence should be sent to Jennifer B. Nuzzo, 621 E Pratt St, Providence, RI 02903 (e-mail: jennifer_nuzzo@brown.edu). Reprints can be ordered at https://www.ajph.org by clicking the "Reprints" link.

PUBLICATION INFORMATION

Full Citation: Nuzzo JB. Extreme polarization is a threat to US health. *Am J Public Health*. 2026; 116(1):26–28.

Acceptance Date: October 9, 2025.

DOI: https://doi.org/10.2105/AJPH.2025.308311

ORCID iD:

Jennifer B. Nuzzo https://orcid.org/0000-0002-7137-6625

CONFLICTS OF INTEREST

J. B. Nuzzo previously participated in a two-day scientific advisory meeting for CSL Seqirus for which she received a one-time honorarium.

REFERENCES

1. Silva S, Goosby E, Reid MJA. Assessing the impact of one million COVID-19 deaths in America: economic and life expectancy losses. *Sci Rep*. 2023;13:3065. https://doi.org/10.1038/s41598-023-30077-1
2. Nuzzo JB, Ledesma JR. Why did the best prepared country in the world fare so poorly during COVID? *J Econ Perspect*. 2023;37(4):3–22. https://doi.org/10.1257/jep.37.4.3
3. Mehlhaff ID, Tarillo MC, Vanegas A, Hetherington MJ. Partisanship and the pandemic: how and why Americans followed party cues on COVID-19. *J Health Polit Policy Law*. 2024;49(3):351–374. https://doi.org/10.1215/03616878-11066336
4. Watson CR, Watson M, Sell TK. Public health preparedness funding: key programs and trends from 2001 to 2017. *Am J Public Health*. 2017; 107(suppl 2):S165–S167. https://doi.org/10.2105/AJPH.2017.303963
5. US Department of Health and Human Services. HHS historical highlights. June 19, 2006. Available at: https://www.hhs.gov/about/historical-highlights/index.html. Accessed September 15, 2025.
6. Mandavilli A. Kennedy cancels nearly $500 million in mRNA vaccine contracts. *New York Times*. August 5, 2025. Available at: https://www.nytimes.com/2025/08/05/health/rfk-jr-vaccine-funding.html. Accessed September 15, 2025.
7. Steele MK, Couture A, Reed C, et al. Estimated number of COVID-19 infections, hospitalizations, and deaths prevented among vaccinated persons in the US, December 2020 to September 2021. *JAMA Netw Open*. 2022;5(7):e2220385. https://doi.org/10.1001/jamanetworkopen.2022.20385
8. USA Facts. US Coronavirus vaccine tracker. Available at: https://usafacts.org/visualizations/covid-vaccine-tracker-states. Accessed October 24, 2025.
9. Kearney A, Montero A, Valdes I, Hamel L, and Kirzinger A. KFF/The Washington Post Survey of Parents. KFF. October 10, 2025. Available at: https://www.kff.org/public-opinion/kff-the-washington-post-survey-of-parents. Accessed October 24, 2025.
10. Kearney A. Most parents nationally and in Florida want schools to require vaccines. KFF. September 4, 2025. Available at: https://www.kff.org/quick-take/most-parents-nationally-and-in-florida-want-schools-to-require-vaccines. Accessed September 15, 2025.
11. Williams E, Kates J, Michaud J. Kindergarten routine vaccination rates continue to decline. KFF. August 5, 2025. Available at: https://www.kff.org/medicaid/kindergarten-routine-vaccination-rates-continue-to-decline. Accessed September 15, 2025.
12. Kennedy RF Jr. Robert F. Kennedy Jr.: We're restoring public trust in the CDC. *WSJ*. September 2, 2025. Available at: https://www.wsj.com/opinion/robert-f-kennedy-jr-were-restoring-public-trust-in-the-cdc-6f26c176. Accessed September 15, 2025.
13. Rutschman A, Penrod J. The new vaccine federalism in the US. *Health Aff Forefr*. October 7, 2025. https://doi.org/10.1377/forefront.20251001.617873

Homeownership as a Determinant of Health: A Broader Consideration of Housing and Homelessness Amid Current Challenges

Deborah K. Padgett, PhD

ABOUT THE AUTHOR

Deborah K. Padgett is with the Silver School of Social Work, New York University, New York.

Note. The views and opinions expressed in this editorial are those of the author and do not necessarily reflect the views of their institutions or affiliates.

See also Rahman, p. 137.

Extensive research on the physical health and mental health consequences of homelessness helped to establish stable housing's legitimacy as a social determinant of health.[1] In his article in this issue of *AJPH*, Rahman (p. 137) makes a credible argument that homeownership (vs renting) has a substantially greater positive impact on health. At the harshest end of a continuum of housing's benefits, homelessness brings life-threatening exposures to contaminated water and food, physical violence, and skin and tissue infections. Undertreated conditions such as diabetes, kidney infections, and periodontal disease take their toll. For those living with a mental health condition, hit-or-miss access to psychiatric treatment is destabilizing, to say the least. Finally, prolonged proximity to illicit drugs and alcohol on the streets threatens the fragile grasp of abstention for a considerable proportion of those who are unhoused.[1]

Rahman's findings emerge from extensive analyses of a nationally representative sample of 407 916 US residents of whom 72.3% were homeowners. Perhaps not surprisingly, renters were younger, were more racially diverse, and had lower incomes. Renters were found to have greater health risks and lower access to health care services, including preventive care. The finding that homeowners have consistently better health outcomes even when controlling for differences in income, race, and education reveals a potent structural determinant of health.

The material conditions of housing as health have been the focus of public health initiatives in recent years. In addition to the physical health benefits of having a secure and stable place to live, having a home extends into the psychosocial realm of ontological security.[2] The phrase "ontological security" has its origins in Anthony Giddens's notions of modernity and the rising need for a sense of place and constancy in a rapidly changing world.[3] Interestingly, early research on ontological security focused on the advantages of homeownership.[4] Such benefits have been substantiated as even greater when obtaining a home after being homeless.[2] Defined as giving (1) a sense of constancy and daily routine, (2) privacy and freedom from surveillance, and (3) a secure foundation for identity development and self-actualization, ontological security transcends the material environment even as it is rooted in it.[2] Such benefits are akin to those found emerging from the lowest level of Maslow's pyramid depicting a hierarchy of needs.

Homeownership has long been a manifestation of the US value placed on private property that intensified as the nation's territorial borders were pushed to the West Coast in the late 1800s. Meanwhile, Jim Crow laws that had subverted freed slaves' legitimate claims to land were expanded in scope by restrictive policies that rendered land and homeownership out of reach for most African Americans.[5] Racial segregation was not the result of happenstance; it was a carefully cultivated conspiracy of the "haves" to ensure White control over land. The American dream of owning a home was cemented in place for White citizens through single-family zoning laws and redlining by banks and realtors determined to enforce racial segregation. Even wealthy African Americans were disproportionately forced into renting rather than owning a home.[5]

The single most influential factor in growing a family's generational assets was and is homeownership; it is no accident that White families' financial assets are 10 times greater than the accumulated assets of

AJPH January 2026, Vol. 116, No. 1

African American families.[5] It is also no accident that African Americans are roughly 13% of the US population and 40% of unhoused Americans. The historic conditions that bestow greater economic security on one racial group and amplify the deprivations of another create a continuum of socioeconomic well-being with homeownership at the top, followed by renting, and ending with the ultimate destitution of homelessness. The article by Rahman offers a detailed depiction of health benefits that align with this top-down continuum.

The success of an approach to ending homelessness known as Housing First is predicated on a simple, demonstrably cost-effective course of action: provide unhoused persons with a stable place to live (i.e., a rental apartment) and surround them with support services designed to heal both physical and psychological wounds.[6] It is Maslow's pyramid in action—exiting the streets for a home breaks the costly cycle of hospital emergency rooms, jail cells, and shelter beds and positively affects physical and mental health.[6]

Recent trends in land ownership and homeownership do not bode well for a nation with more than 700 000 citizens unhoused and many more experiencing housing precarity. Over the past decade, private equity and hedge funds have been engaged in massive buyouts of large rental properties in major US cities.[7] Rather than focus on long-term investment, these companies—hidden from view as limited liability corporations—reap sizable profits in the short term by letting the properties deteriorate, raising rents, and imposing additional fees. In states where single-family dwellings are the common standard, private equity firms purchase mortgages, increase rates, and become landlords.[7]

As it stands now, homeownership offers protection and stability—until it does not. The housing collapse that instigated the recession of 2008 was a not-so-subtle reminder that the benefits of homeownership—a harmonic convergence of US values and promising health outcomes—are fragile wins.[8] Meanwhile, wealthy tech billionaires are funding think tank–like institutes dedicated to, inter alia, ending support for Housing First in government funding of homeless services. The White House executive order of July 24, 2025, follows the script to the letter. Describing Housing First as a reckless enablement of personal irresponsibility, the intent is to ensure unhoused persons clean up their act (so to speak). Serious mental illness, misuse of alcohol or drugs, and other forms of behavioral nonconformity must be forcibly treated after being moved to an internment camp located on government property away from cities (to remove "urban blight"). At this writing, local homeless service providers are awaiting funding allocations from the Department of Housing and Urban Development that are a fraction of 2024 funding and tied to a stipulation of no support for Housing First initiatives.

This politically fraught picture of serious mental illness and addiction obscures the much greater diversity of those in the United States who are unhoused as well as the structural factors that make housing an increasingly scarce commodity.[9] A large subgroup are young families—typically a young mother and one or two small children. And the most effective assistance for them? Government-subsidized rental vouchers. Rahman's study further establishes that there is truly no place like home. AJPH

CORRESPONDENCE

Correspondence should be sent to Deborah K. Padgett, PhD, Silver School of Social Work, New York University, 1 Washington Square North, New York, NY 10003 (e-mail: dkp1@nyu.edu). Reprints can be ordered at http://www.ajph.org by clicking the "Reprints" link.

PUBLICATION INFORMATION

Full Citation: Padgett DK. Homeownership as a determinant of health: a broader consideration of housing and homelessness amid current challenges. *Am J Public Health*. 2026;116(1):29–30.

Acceptance Date: October 10, 2025.

DOI: https://doi.org/10.2105/AJPH.2025.308315

ORCID iD:
Deborah K. Padgett https://orcid.org/0000-0003-1483-2513

CONFLICTS OF INTEREST

The author has no conflicts of interest pertaining to this article.

REFERENCES

1. Brown RT, Evans JL, Valle K, Guzman D, Chen YH, Kushel MB. Factors associated with mortality among homeless older adults in California: The HOPE HOME study. *JAMA Intern Med*. 2022;182(10):1052–1060. https://doi.org/10.1001/jamainternmed.2022.3697
2. Padgett DK. There's no place like (a) home: ontological security among persons with serious mental illness in the United States. *Soc Sci Med*. 2007;64(9):1925–1936. https://doi.org/10.1016/j.socscimed.2007.02.011
3. Giddens A. *Consequences of Modernity*. Cambridge, UK: Polity Press; 1990.
4. Dupuis A, Thorns DC. Home, home ownership, and the search for ontological security. *Sociol Rev*. 1998;46(1):24–47. https://doi.org/10.1111/1467-954X.00088
5. Rothstein R. *The Color of Law: A Forgotten History of How Our Government Segregated America*. New York, NY: Liveright; 2017.
6. Padgett DK, Henwood BF, Tsemberis S. *Housing First: Ending Homelessness, Transforming Systems and Changing Lives*. Oxford, UK: Oxford Press; 2016.
7. Ross A. *Sunbelt Blues: The Failure of American Housing*. New York, NY: Metropolitan Books; 2021.
8. Sowell T. *The Housing Boom and Bust*. New York, NY: Basic Books; 2009.
9. Colburn G, Aldern CP. *Homelessness Is a Housing Problem*. Oakland: University of California Press; 2024.

Restoring and Expanding Public Trust in Public Health

Denys T. Lau, PhD

ABOUT THE AUTHOR

Denys T. Lau is Editor-in-Chief of AJPH. *He also has adjunct faculty appointments at Johns Hopkins University, Baltimore, MD, George Washington University, Washington, DC, and University of Illinois at Chicago.*

See also Trust in Public Health, p. 35–94.

The success of public health and medical sciences relies on public trust. When health professionals are trusted, the public is more willing to participate in prevention and treatment efforts designed to control outbreaks, manage pandemics, and improve health outcomes. Public trust fosters a shared sense of responsibility to adopt healthy behaviors and promote prevention practices for the greater good of community well-being. When trust declines, however, skepticism grows, and communities may question the legitimacy of public health guidance and challenge recommended treatment plans. Erosion of trust, over time, can lead to widespread antiscience sentiments and false medical claims, threatening the ability of even the best-designed public health measures to address future emergencies.

Since the start of the COVID-19 pandemic, trust in public health has declined significantly. The proportion of US adults who reported "a lot" of trust in physicians and hospitals decreased significantly from 72% in April 2020 to 40% in January 2024.[1] Federal public health agencies witnessed a drop in public confidence. For example, a September 2025 poll on health information and trust,[2] conducted after the Trump administration claimed that Tylenol could cause autism in children despite no scientific evidence of a causal link, found that half of those sampled said they trusted the Centers for Disease Control and Prevention (CDC) to provide reliable information about vaccines, a drop from 63% in September 2023.

Historical injustices and systemic inequities have created deep-seated mistrust in public health and health care systems among marginalized communities. Trust tends to be lower among certain racial and ethnic groups, particularly Black and Hispanic adults.[3] Individuals with lower income, with less education, and living in rural areas tend to have mistrust in health institutions and medical sciences.[4]

Partisan divide in trust has widened since the COVID-19 pandemic. Trust in scientists and health information among Democrats remained relatively stable during the pandemic, while trust among Republicans decreased significantly.[2] With new federal health leadership changes under the Trump administration, Republicans report that their confidence in public health recommendations will increase, while Democrats report

HISTORY CORNER

10 YEARS AGO

Public Health, Science, and Policy Debate: Being Right Is Not Enough

[C]ontemporary life in most of the world depends on complex technologies that are scarcely, if at all, understood even in superficial terms by most people. These technologies, labeled by British sociologist Anthony Giddens as "expert systems," are nevertheless trusted, in Giddens' view, through a kind of pragmatic faith. How the general population comes to trust such technologies is partially a matter of their effectiveness, but it also involves the way in which the public discourse about them is constructed. [C]onsidering the diversity of scientific and technological domains that are involved in understanding how any given expert system functions, this means that public opinion at some point has to rely on the word of experts. This is particularly true for most public health issues. A majority of health risks, for instance, are not self-evident, and identifying these risks requires a somewhat sophisticated epidemiological machinery that is fully understood by relatively few, even among health professionals. This means that the issue of what to trust usually becomes an issue of whom to trust.

From *AJPH*, February 2015, p. 232

that their trust will drop.[5] In fact, the September 2025 KFF poll shows that 67% of Republican respondents trusted Health and Human Services Secretary Robert F Kennedy Jr, while only 39% trusted the CDC. Among Democrats, 64% trusted the CDC and 13% trusted Kennedy.[2]

Trust also differs by source of public health information. During the pandemic, state and local public health agencies saw more stable levels of public trust compared with their federal counterparts, such as the CDC and the National Institutes of Health, which were perceived as more politically influenced and inconsistent over time.[6] Although personal medical doctors remain the most trusted source of health information for most people, recent data suggest a decrease in trust of physicians, possibly reflecting a broader declining trend across health professionals.[2] Health information from private sources and social networks was relied on more by non-White and younger populations, while government sources were trusted more by White and older populations.[7]

The epidemiology of mistrust in public health science, professionals, and policies is complex, as it is shaped by historical and ongoing systemic inequalities, as well as factors like public health institutional practices, misinformation, and political polarization. In this special section, *AJPH* has curated papers that answer the question, "How can we promote public trust and confidence in public health science, policies, and actions?" The collection of articles compiled in this section suggests that building partnerships with policymakers, minimizing influences and biases, improving communication, and increasing community engagement are key to answering this question.

CONTEXT

The COVID-19 pandemic was an unprecedented public health crisis in modern times, revealing the strengths and weaknesses in public health preparedness and response in the United States and worldwide. Rochel de Camargo (p. 38) discusses how public trust in public health and science were actively undermined by political, economic, and social interests during the pandemic. Kim-Farley (p. 4) provides an overview of the lessons learned during the pandemic—in preparedness, response, communication, and equity—that can help us chart a path forward to a more resilient, equitable, and unified response to future public health emergencies.

PARTNERSHIPS WITH POLICYMAKERS

The future of trust in public health is uncertain. Hearne and Pollack Porter (p. 47) provide public health leaders and professionals a path forward for engaging with policymakers with intention and genuine commitment. Building trust with policymakers requires humility and meaningful relationships. Training opportunities are needed to build political engagement and advocacy skills among public health workers.

The current federal administration has weakened federal advisory committees, leaving gaps in public health policymaking infrastructure. Taylor and Caplan (p. 51) discuss how public health leaders in state governments and in the private sector are taking actions to expand their roles and generate capacity elsewhere to fill in the gaps. Such decentralized stopgap measures, however, remain as incomplete replacements for federal actions and

HISTORY CORNER

21 YEARS AGO

In Their Own Words: Lessons Learned from Those Exposed to Anthrax

A basic goal of public health communication is to provide accurate, accessible information that establishes a bond of trust between those in a position of responsibility and those potentially exposed to a bioterrorist agent. This trust depends on perceptions of competence, objectivity, fairness, and consistency and on the general belief in the good will of those responsible for communication. . . . The events surrounding the anthrax exposures required communication by various public health entities to a highly diverse audience during a period of sustained uncertainty. Screening and treatment recommendations changed as knowledge about the infection and its treatment evolved. . . . In our sample, many reported an initial favorable or neutral opinion of public health agencies, indicating that during the emergency, trust eroded. This problem could potentially have been avoided with more effective communication from the start. . . . Consistency of messages across all groups affected is paramount to encouraging trust.

From *AJPH*, March 2005, pp. 489–494

will face challenges ahead, including efforts to regain the public's trust.

As funding for federal data systems is being cut, great reliance is placed on private and commercial entities to apply innovation and efficiency to collect data and generate information about health. To build public trust and promote innovation, Dasgupta et al. (p. 57) argue that privately held health data need to fit the intended use, be transparent in their methods and selection bias, and be reliable over time.

MINIMAL INFLUENCES AND BIASES

Freedom from undue influence, or independence, enables governmental agencies to make impartial decisions based on facts and laws, thereby strengthening public confidence in the system's fairness and integrity. Lau and Schoendorf (p. 4) discuss how shielding public health institutions from political, ideological, or commercial interference (i.e., scientific independence) is critical for ensuring evidence-based decisions to remain objective and rigorous, and maintaining public trust and cooperation with public health measures.

Government science advisory panels evaluate evidence to issue recommendations to protect the public's health. Chartres et al. (p. 62) discuss how the development of evidence-based guidelines must be safeguarded to minimize financial conflicts of interest and commercial bias to ensure that the public can trust government public health policy and guidance.

COMMUNICATION: CONTENT, AUDIENCE, AND TRAINING

Confusing uncertainty with unreliability can lead the public to mistakenly think that scientists may be dishonest, advocating political ideologies, or simply incompetent. McCain (p. 35) discusses how understanding the nature of science and its inherent uncertainty can help the public better understand what is and is not sound public health advice and why that advice can be trusted even though it can change over time.

Public health researchers are discussing effective communication strategies to improve the credibility of research findings and the effectiveness of those findings in driving policy decisions. Landers and Fiala (p. 67) discuss how the principles of the "Ensuring Quality in Scientific Publication Through Inclusivity and Transparency" guidelines previously published in *AJPH*[8] can help rebuild public trust in the publication of scientific research through transparency, accountability, inclusivity, and community engagement.

Critics cast public health as ideological rather than scientific and as elitist rather than equitable, thereby eroding trust, especially among political conservatives. Castrucci et al. (p. 70) propose a four-part framework—clarity, consistency, cultural competence, and community presence—to improve communication with a particular focus on rural areas and conservative Americans.

Kelly and Bass (p. 74) discuss the imperative of preparing the future public health workforce so that it can effectively navigate the rising mis- and disinformation that is eroding trust. They call for an integration of crisis communication and media relations training in schools and programs of public health.

COMMUNITY ENGAGEMENT AND PRACTICE

Remediating mistrust in public health for marginalized communities begins with acknowledging the history of and ongoing systems of oppression. Padamsee and Allen (p. 79) propose that the key to repairing the relationship between the public health enterprise and communities of color lies in being honest about the historical lack of reliable commitment to communities of color. The focus should be reframing trust as striving for trustworthiness and nurturing case-by-case trust among communities.

Nnaji and Bowleg (p. 82) further emphasize the importance of community engagement and leadership and of shifting the burden onto the public health enterprise to demonstrate its trustworthiness. Along the same theme, Alberti et al. (p. 86) describe the early stages of developing the Principles of Trustworthiness Toolkit that is designed to help institutions demonstrate their trustworthiness to their communities by focusing on respect, transparency, intentionality, commitment, humility, and authenticity.

Ravi et al. (p. 90) describe the Community Engagement Alliance Against COVID-19 that was implemented in South Central Texas to address disparities and misinformation surrounding the pandemic. Through community engagement, community-driven data gathering, and health information dissemination via trusted partners, this initiative fostered trusting partnership among community organizations and developed culturally tailored health messaging.

CONCLUSION

Instead of spurring coordinated responses to assess public health deficiencies and improve our nation's preparedness for future emergencies, the COVID-19 pandemic unfortunately has engendered public mistrusts, antiscience sentiments, and misinformation.[9] This *AJPH* special section aims to promote continued discourse on strategies to restore and expand trust in public health and medical sciences.

Building trust in public health takes time and requires a multipronged strategy that addresses historical inequities and improves institutional practices. Articles published in this section propose fostering partnership with policymakers, minimizing external influences, improving communication, and increasing community engagement.

Forging robust partnerships with policymakers of different political parties would help ensure that health priorities are integrated into policy decisions. In addition, meaningful partnerships between state and local public health leaders and the private sector would help fill the federal gaps in public health policymaking and cultivate their own authority and trustworthiness.

Public health institutions would need to minimize conflicts of interest and external influences by preserving scientific independence, relying on unbiased external scientific experts, implementing transparent policies, and disclosing potential influences, thereby protecting the integrity of scientific guidance.

Regaining trust in public health necessitates a formal apology for previous mistakes and acknowledgment of scientific uncertainty and potential changes over time because of emerging new knowledge. Communication about scientific content requires messages to be clear, consistent, and tailored for diverse audiences, especially across the geo-political spectrum (e.g., marginalized communities, political conservatives and liberals alike, and those in rural areas). Public health professionals also would need to build their competencies in effective communication and be vigilant in correcting misinformation and building scientific literacy.

Finally, engaging communities through shared decision-making and even co-ownership of the research enterprise could be considered, putting the responsibility on public health institutions to demonstrate their trustworthiness. More tools would help institutions effectively build their trustworthiness with the communities they serve.

AJPH welcomes evidence-based research that evaluates these and other approaches to foster public trust across communities, promote trustworthiness in our public health institutions, improve population health outcomes and health equity, and increase the preparedness of our nation's public health enterprise to effectively respond to future crises. AJPH

CORRESPONDENCE

Correspondence should be sent to Denys T. Lau, 800 I St NW, Washington, DC 20001 (e-mail: denys.lau@apha.org). Reprints can be ordered at https://www.ajph.org by clicking the "Reprints" link.

PUBLICATION INFORMATION

Full Citation: Lau DT. Restoring and expanding public trust in public health. *Am J Public Health*. 2026;116(1):31–34.

Acceptance Date: October 20, 2025.

DOI: https://doi.org/10.2105/AJPH.2025.308339

CONFLICTS OF INTEREST

The author has no conflicts of interest to declare.

REFERENCES

1. Perlis RH, Ognyanova K, Uslu A, et al. Trust in physicians and hospitals during the COVID-19 pandemic in a 50-state survey of US adults. *JAMA Netw Open*. 2024;7(7):e2424984. https://doi.org/10.1001/jamanetworkopen.2024.24984
2. Montero A, Sparks G, Mulugeta M, et al. KFF Tracking Poll on Health Information and Trust: Tylenol–autism link and vaccine policies. October 9, 2025. Available at: https://www.kff.org/public-opinion/kff-tracking-poll-on-health-information-and-trust-tylenol-autism-link-and-vaccine-policies. Accessed October 14, 2025.
3. Nanaw J, Sherchan JS, Fernandez JR, Strassle PD, Powell W, Forde AT. Racial/ethnic differences in the associations between trust in the US healthcare system and willingness to test for and vaccinate against COVID-19. *BMC Public Health*. 2024;24(1):1084. https://doi.org/10.1186/s12889-024-18526-6
4. Green J, Long SK. Racial, ethnic, and income-based disparities in health care–related trust. *J Gen Intern Med*. 2021;36(4):1126–1128. https://doi.org/10.1007/s11606-020-06568-6
5. Brownstein M. Poll: Many Americans say they will lose trust in public health recommendations under federal leadership changes. April 29, 2025. Available at: https://hsph.harvard.edu/news/poll-many-americans-say-they-will-lose-trust-in-public-health-recommendations-under-federal-leadership-changes. Accessed October 14, 2025.
6. SteelFisher GK, Findling MG, Caporello HL, et al. Trust in US federal, state, and local public health agencies during COVID-19: responses and policy implications. *Health Aff (Millwood)*. 2023;42(3):328–337. https://doi.org/10.1377/hlthaff.2022.01204
7. Fridman I, Lucas N, Henke D, Zigler C. Association between public knowledge about COVID-19, trust in information sources, and adherence to social distancing: cross-sectional survey. *JMIR Public Health Surveill*. 2020;6(3):e22060. https://doi.org/10.2196/22060
8. Loui M, Morabia A. Ensuring quality in scientific publication through inclusivity and transparency. *Am J Public Health*. 2025;115(7):966–967. https://doi.org/10.2105/AJPH.2025.308174
9. McMurtry CL, Cheu R. Political polarization during disease outbreaks: a meta-analysis of archival survey data from polio to COVID-19. *Am J Public Health*. 2025; epub ahead of print August 28, 2025:e1–e13. https://doi.org/10.2105/AJPH.2025.308226

The Role of Uncertainty in Rebuilding Trust in Science

Kevin McCain, PhD

ABOUT THE AUTHOR

Kevin McCain is professor and chair of the Department of Philosophy, University of Alabama at Birmingham.

See also Trust in Public Health, pp. 31–94.

Editor's Note: With this issue of AJPH, *we are introducing a new editorial offering where I will be inviting deans of schools of public health and public health program directors to provide an academic perspective on that month's special issue focus. For this inaugural column, rather than attempting to provide my own perspective as dean on rebuilding trust in science, I turned to my colleague, Kevin McCain, chair of the Department of Philosophy at the University of Alabama at Birmingham. What would a philosopher have to say about trust in science, especially one who has written books such as* How Science Explains the World *and* Uncertainty: How It Makes Science Advance? *I'm fairly certain his piece will resonate with* AJPH *readers.*

—Paul C. Erwin, Associate Editor, AJPH

A casual peek at the news or, heaven forbid, social media, and one comes away with a clear sense that we face a crisis of public distrust in science. Nevertheless, while there is consensus that trust in science is down, there is some dissent. A recent study hailed as challenging the "low public trust" narrative contends that overall, in the United States and 67 other countries, "trust in scientists is moderately high."[1(p714)]

DISTRUST IN INSTITUTIONS

Additional evidence gives credence to the idea that the narrative of a crisis of public distrust in science is mistaken. For instance, a recent Pew Research Center study found that 76% of people in the United States expressed a great deal or fair amount of confidence in scientists to act in the public's interest.[2] While this is lower than the prepandemic confidence level of 87%, it is still relatively high. Similarly, a recent study by the Annenberg Public Policy Center found that 86% of respondents expressed confidence in their own "doctor, nurse, or other primary health care provider."[3] If one were to just focus on the trust that is reported for scientists or individual health care providers, it would be tempting to think that there is no crisis of public distrust.

Unfortunately, while there is quite a bit of trust in individual scientists and health care providers, trust in scientific institutions has dropped considerably recently. For instance, only 64% of respondents in the Annenberg study were confident that the Centers for Disease Control and Prevention will provide trustworthy information concerning public health (this is down from 72% in September 2024). And confidence in trustworthiness is even lower for the Food and Drug Administration (FDA) and National Institutes of Health (NIH), being only 63% and 62%, respectively. These confidence levels amount to a 10% decrease in confidence in the FDA and a 12% decrease in confidence in the NIH since September 2024. Similar results were found for both National Aeronautics and Space Administration (NASA) and the Environmental Protection Agency (EPA) when respondents were asked about their confidence in these institutions to provide trustworthy information about the public health effects of climate change: 65% expressed confidence in NASA (down from 77% in July 2024), and only 57% expressed confidence in the EPA to provide trustworthy information (down from 70% in July 2024). Hence, although most people still trust these institutions, things are certainly trending toward distrust.

Given the profound impact that distrusting scientific institutions can have on our well-being, just consider the rise in measles outbreaks in the United States[4] brought about at least in part because of suspicion of vaccines, it is important to figure out what can be done to reverse the trend. There are myriad reasons why distrust in science is on the rise. Many would point to the various mistakes in how the COVID-19 pandemic was handled both in terms of measures taken and especially in terms of messaging.[5] Of course, governmental leaders expressing distrust in various areas of science, particularly those related to vaccines and the climate, does not help.[6,7] Neither does the fact that some of our major public health institutions are under the leadership of a Department of Health and

AJPH January 2026, Vol. 116, No. 1

Human Services secretary with an overall confidence rating of 39%, with 37% of Americans being not at all confident in him providing trustworthy public health information.[3] These are all likely contributing factors. However, a factor that is not often given its due is uncertainty. Not uncertainty in terms of being unsure of whether individuals or institutions are trustworthy but, rather, uncertainty in science itself.

UNCERTAINTY

One of the things that scientists do is make clear their level of uncertainty by reporting things like confidence intervals. Nevertheless, the public does not often understand uncertainty or its presence in science. This may lead to unrealistic expectations, which can undermine other efforts to reestablish trust. For instance, many have noted that scientists do not always communicate well with the public.[5,8] In fact, the Pew Center study found that 52% of respondents think that scientists are not good communicators. If efforts are made to help scientists, and official communicators for scientific institutions, better communicate with the public, that may exacerbate public distrust if uncertainty is not properly understood. Honest and clear communication of scientific findings will explain the level of certainty and, thus, just how uncertain the results drawn from the findings are. But the average person may have the mistaken view that genuine science is certain.[9] When they hear scientists claiming that their results are uncertain but should still guide health policy or an individual's health decisions, for example, they are apt to be perplexed. Worse than that, the average person may be inclined to think that the scientist is either lying about the results or merely presenting some nonscientific agenda. Public misunderstanding of uncertainty in science makes the task of balancing the need for giving the public answers quickly and the need to provide the most accurate information even more difficult.

Benjamin Franklin famously said, "in this world, nothing is certain except death and taxes."[10] He may have been wrong about the latter—some sure seem to be able to find ways to avoid taxes—but he is exactly right in the main. Uncertainty is unavoidable in our lives. We are always working with limited information and going with what is most likely given that information. This is true whether we are deciding which college football team we think will win on a given Saturday or deciding that wearing masks is a good way to prevent the spread of COVID-19. One key for rebuilding trust in science is helping the public to see that science does not lie outside the purview of Franklin's dictum.

REBUILDING TRUST

Critically, the public needs to understand that even when our best scientific theories are uncertain, that does not mean that any theory is as good as any other. We have better reasons to trust clinically tested treatments than home remedies that are only supported by anecdotal evidence, even if both treatments are uncertain to some extent. When people realize that science is uncertain but still trustworthy, they can better appreciate honest communication from scientists.

Although many reasons for the increase in distrust of science have been discussed, the role of uncertainty has received relatively little attention. Confusion arising from equating uncertainty with unreliability can lead to mistakenly taking scientists to be lying, pushing political agendas, or simply incompetent. Helping the public better understand the nature of science and the role that uncertainty plays in it can help them better understand what is (and is not) sound public health advice, and why that advice can be trusted, despite the fact that it can (and should be expected to) change over time.

Consequently, if we want to rebuild trust in science, we must first help people better understand what it is that we want them to trust and the uncertainty inherent in that enterprise. Along with this, we must report scientific findings with the appropriate level of humility by being willing to forthrightly acknowledge our level of uncertainty, and even at times apologize for past misleading communications. Of course, it is not certain that educating the public on the uncertainty of science will help solve the problem, but it is quite probable based on the evidence that we have at present. AJPH

CORRESPONDENCE

Correspondence should be sent to Kevin McCain, 5002 University Hall, 1402 10th Ave S, Birmingham, AL 35294 (e-mail: mccain@uab.edu). Reprints can be ordered at https://ajph.org by clicking the "Reprints" link.

PUBLICATION INFORMATION

Full Citation: McCain K. The role of uncertainty in rebuilding trust in science. *Am J Public Health*. 2026;116(1):35–37.

Acceptance Date: October 10, 2025.

DOI: https://doi.org/10.2105/AJPH.2025.308317

ORCID iD:
Kevin McCain https://orcid.org/0000-0002-2447-4046

ACKNOWLEDGMENTS

Many thanks to Paul Erwin, Denys Lau, and Josh May for helpful comments on earlier drafts.

CONFLICTS OF INTEREST

The author reports no conflicts of interest.

REFERENCES

1. Cologna V, Mede NG, Berger S, et al. Trust in scientists and their role in society across 68 countries. *Nat Hum Behav.* 2025;9(4):713–730. https://doi.org/10.1038/s41562-024-02090-5
2. Tyson A, Kennedy B. Public trust in scientists and views on their role in policymaking. Pew Research Center. November 14, 2024. Available at: https://www.pewresearch.org/science/2024/11/14/public-trust-in-scientists-and-views-on-their-role-in-policymaking. Accessed September 23, 2025.
3. Adams S. Public confidence in US health agencies slides, fueled by declines among Democrats. The Annenberg Public Policy Center of the University of Pennsylvania. September 18, 2025. Available at: https://www.annenbergpublicpolicycenter.org/public-confidence-in-u-s-health-agencies-slides-fueled-by-declines-among-democrats. Accessed September 23, 2025.
4. Centers for Disease Control and Prevention. Measles cases and outbreaks. April 25, 2025. Available at: https://www.cdc.gov/measles/data-research/index.html. Accessed September 23, 2025.
5. Pence GE. *What Went Wrong.* New York, NY: Rowman & Littlefield Publishers; 2025.
6. Conger K. How misinformation, medical mistrust fuel vaccine hesitancy. Stanford Medicine News Center. September 2, 2021. Available at: https://med.stanford.edu/news/all-news/2021/09/infodemic-covid-19.html. Accessed October 1, 2025.
7. Schweitzer K. Amid Texas measles outbreak, clinicians struggle to offset increasing vaccine hesitancy. *JAMA.* 2025;333(15):1278–1281. https://doi.org/10.1001/jama.2025.2932
8. Kampourakis K. *Trusting Science.* New York, NY: Oxford University Press; 2025.
9. Kampourakis K, McCain K. *Uncertainty: How It Makes Science Advance.* New York, NY: Oxford University Press; 2020.
10. National Constitution Center. Benjamin Franklin's last great quote and the Constitution. November 13, 2023. Available at: https://constitutioncenter.org/blog/benjamin-franklins-last-great-quote-and-the-constitution. Accessed September 23, 2025.

Public Health, Science, and the Public's Trust

Kenneth Rochel de Camargo, MD, PhD

ABOUT THE AUTHOR

Kenneth Rochel de Camargo is a professor at the Instituto de Medicina Social, Universidade do Estado do Rio de Janeiro, Brazil, and an associate editor of AJPH.

See also Trust in Public Health, pp. 31–94.

As public health researchers and practitioners, we tell people to do certain things, like exercising or vaccinating, and to avoid others, such as smoking or eating ultraprocessed foods. We advocate laws to protect the environment and make workplaces safe. Our actions are grounded on a scientific basis; for our recommendations to take hold, it is necessary that the general population accepts them and, indirectly, the science from which they derive.

Although ideally this would mean a society-wide consensus based on rational appraisal of the evidence, in reality, this is not so easily achieved. Given the complexity and scope of modern science, no matter how much one is invested in learning about its developments, any given individual will be a layperson in far more fields than those in which (s)he can be an expert. This means that for most issues in the public arena in which science has a relevant role, one has to trust experts' work and opinions as a basis for their own positioning.[1,2]

Trust in public health and its underpinning knowledge is, therefore, a keystone for the acceptance and implementation of proposed measures and legislation. While opinion polls show that the majority of society trusts science and scientists, this trust showed an important decline in recent years, especially during the pandemic, with almost a quarter of respondents to a US survey claiming little to no confidence in scientists.[3] To further compound the problem, despite having overall confidence from a majority, when it comes to specific issues such as the aforementioned COVID-19 pandemic or anthropogenic climate change, mistrust seems to dominate, at least in parts of the population, cleaved along political affiliation lines.[4] Similar results have been observed in global surveys.[5]

SCIENCE IN THE MAKING AND MISCONCEPTIONS ABOUT ITS RIGOR

To a certain extent, the way the response to the COVID-19 pandemic took place is paradoxically responsible for this. As is usual in cases where highly specialized knowledge plays a central role, general audiences lacked specific expertise to correctly assess the magnitude of the task at hand. Identifying an emerging infectious disease, determining how it progresses in human populations, and isolating its causal agent was no mean feat, especially in the relatively short time this was achieved. The need to quickly respond to a planetary public health emergency exposed science in the making, with unavoidable hesitations and dead ends as it progresses. This resulted at times in proposing measures that were not yet solidly backed by evidence, which eventually had to be revised. Over time, the scientific community converged to a consensus, as usually happens in the history of science, but the timing to reach this consensus is not necessarily the same that policymaking requires.

Although this is in the end how science works, the public perception was not necessarily that researchers were learning more and adapting to the new circumstances, but, for some people, it was interpreted as if they were being misled.[6] A variety of conspiracy theories, at the same time stemming from distrust in authorities, antiestablishmentarianism, and propagation by political authorities and health care professionals who should have known better,[7,8] took hold of a considerable part of the world population.

Similar processes were observed along the construction of a response to the HIV and AIDS epidemics: incorrect initial assumptions based on incomplete data, such as ascribing the new disease exclusively to gay men or Haitians, contributed to creating stigmas—that unfortunately still echo to this date—and to sowing mistrust among those communities. Conspiracy theories about the origin of the virus or malignant intentions behind the proposed antiviral therapies also proliferated on a global scale, although not with the same intensity, dissemination, and persistency of COVID-19–related disinformation, possibly because of the fact that social media did not exist at that point in time.

At the same time, however, the mobilization of those same communities became a major factor in designing a response to the challenge of the HIV and AIDS epidemics. This included devising novel preventive strategies (such as safe sex), direct engagement with scientists,[9] and organized political pressure against governments who refused to implement proper policies because of a denialist approach. The development of the Brazilian HIV and AIDS program[10] and the Treatment Action Campaign that forced the South African president Thabo Mbeki to provide antiretroviral treatments[11] are successful examples of community responses to public health challenges.

Presenting correct, scientifically sound information that would demonstrate how public measures actually work might seem the logical strategy to combat this problem. Alas, the solution is far from simple. Although undoubtedly producing and disseminating solid knowledge is a necessary condition, it is far from sufficient for a number of reasons. This rather naive approach, dubbed the "deficit model"—that is, the idea that popular opinion adheres to wrongful positions because of lacking correct information and thus can be guided to a rightful path simply by being exposed to scientific findings—fails to take into account a complex network of contextual factors and has been shown to be ineffective.[12,13]

THE DELIBERATE MANIPULATION OF SCIENTIFIC FACTS

This is not to say that science should be blindly trusted. On the one hand, thorough skepticism is a core value of science itself and a key foundation of its trustworthiness; on the other, errors and wrongdoings in the history of public health show that rigorous, systematic criticism is fundamental when health and human lives are involved. That was the case, for instance, of the infamous Tuskegee and subsequent Guatemala syphilis studies, the Cutter incident that led to the production of vaccines that contained live unattenuated polio viruses, the manipulation of clinical trials that hid the health hazards of rofecoxib, and the illegal testing of antibiotics for meningitis in Nigeria. Justified skepticism, however, is not to be confused with the outright muddling of facts that intends to undermine solid scientific consensus, manufacturing doubt in the court of public opinion.[14] This rhetoric gambit characterizes denialism, "the employment of rhetorical arguments to give the appearance of legitimate debate where there is none, an approach that has the ultimate goal of rejecting a proposition on which a scientific consensus exists."[15(p2)]

The paradigmatic example of this kind of maneuver in public health is the decades-long effort by the tobacco industry to undermine the mounting evidence of the health risk its products represent.[16] It took an equally long struggle by epidemiologists and public health officials and a successful lawsuit to finally put an end to such campaigns—although there are signals that similar tactics are being used with regard to the marketing of e-cigarettes and vaping.[17]

Similarly, recent public pronouncements by the US Department of Health and Human Services linking autism with acetaminophen usage during pregnancy muddied the waters of the public debate about a complex issue. Despite relying on flimsy evidence and going against actual experts on the subject, this has created another wave of distrust that will not go away anytime soon.

Misinformation plays a central role in eroding the public trust, to the extent that the World Health Organization Director-General remarked in 2019 that in regard to the COVID-19 pandemic "we're not just battling the virus; we're also battling the trolls and conspiracy theorists that push misinformation and undermine the outbreak response."[18]

THE ROLE OF SOCIAL MEDIA

Social media, with instant and widespread communication over the Internet, is not just a support for the spreading of misinformation but a participant that plays a major role in the process. The business model that became known as the attention economy[19] favors the creation of bubbles that encapsulate communities in an informational environment that only exposes users to the same messages.

As Nguyen[20] pointed out, this can happen by accident; although the algorithms that run those platforms are designed to produce that effect, there is not necessarily an intentionality that specific ideas would be privileged. That author differentiates this situation (dubbed epistemic bubbles) from echo chambers, deliberately produced through the exclusion and discredit of dissenting voices. In the latter case, distrust in outside sources is actively produced, making even harder for participants to be swayed by contrary arguments. To further compound this problem, for people who become heavily invested in such contrarian views, adherence to specific points of view or conspiracy theories is more than just a cognitive matter. This becomes part of their very identity and sociability, markers of being part of specific social groups, which makes it much harder to dispel their lack of trust in science in public policy.[21] (Re)establishing trust in public health requires acknowledging that there are interested agents that work against it.

This configuration became particularly relevant in the emergence of the modern antivaccine movement.[22] Social networks made possible for a relatively small number of actors to have a disproportionate effect on the public debate about health issues; a 2021 study showed that only 12 individuals were responsible for almost two thirds of the misinformation about vaccines on social media platforms,[23] among those the current US Secretary of Health and Human Services. Furthermore, there is evidence that foreign agents deliberately fanned the flames, crafting posts on both sides of the argument as a strategy to sow discord among the population.[24]

(RE)GAINING PUBLIC TRUST

This discussion does not mean that (re)gaining people's trust in public health is impossible, just that it requires more work than simply presenting the facts, especially when faced with challenges by actors interested in undermining it. Although in the past most examples of such actions had an economic motivation, currently, ideological biases have become equally relevant, especially in deeply politically divided societies such as in the United States.

Rebuilding trust was achieved with regard to tobacco control; researchers, public health officials, legislators, and community activists managed to denormalize smoking in public as a socially acceptable act, a key part in reducing the consumption of tobacco products. As for vaccines, there is evidence that community-based initiatives and the direct engagement of parents by health care personnel can be successful in countering antivaccine activism and thus improving vaccine coverage.[25] Community engagement was key not only to overcome distrust but also to actually build responses and even scientific knowledge itself in the case of HIV and AIDS. If concerted efforts can sway the public opinion away from trusting public health, our community working together can counteract those. AJPH

CORRESPONDENCE

Correspondence should be sent to Kenneth Rochel de Camargo, Professor, Universidade do Estado do Rio de Janeiro, Instituto de Medicina Social, CEP 20550-013 Rua São Francisco Xavier, 524/7° andar/Bloco D – Maracanã, Rio de Janeiro - Brazil (e-mail: kenneth@uerj.br). Reprints can be ordered at https://www.ajph.org by clicking the "Reprints" link.

PUBLICATION INFORMATION

Full Citation: Rochel de Camargo K. Public health, science, and the public's trust. *Am J Public Health*. 2026;116(1):38–41.

Acceptance Date: October 14, 2025.

DOI: https://doi.org/10.2105/AJPH.2025.308326

ORCID iD:

Kenneth Rochel de Camargo https://orcid.org/0000-0003-3606-5853

ACKNOWLEDGMENTS

The author is a recipient of research grants from the Brazilian Conselho Nacional de Pesquisa e Desenvolvimento and the Universidade do Estado do Rio de Janeiro.

CONFLICTS OF INTEREST

The author has no conflicts of interest to report.

REFERENCES

1. Collins H, Evans R. *Rethinking Expertise.* Chicago, IL: University of Chicago Press; 2008.
2. Barrotta P, Gronda R. Epistemic inequality and the grounds of trust in scientific experts. In: Fabris A. *Trust: A Philosophical Approach.* Cham, Switzerland: Springer Nature; 2020:81–94.
3. Tyson A, Kennedy B. Public trust in scientists and views on their role in policymaking. Washington, DC: Pew Research Center; 2024:35.
4. Milkoreit M, Smith EK. Rapidly diverging public trust in science in the United States. *Public Underst Sci.* 2025;34(5):616–627. https://doi.org/10.1177/09636625241302970
5. Cologna V, Mede NG, Berger S, et al. Trust in scientists and their role in society across 68 countries. *Nat Hum Behav.* 2025;9(4):713–730. https://doi.org/10.1038/s41562-024-02090-5
6. Abdool Karim SS. Public understanding of science: communicating in the midst of a pandemic. *Public Underst Sci.* 2022;31(3):282–287. https://doi.org/10.1177/09636625221089391
7. Rochel De Camargo K. Disputed expertise and chaotic disinformation: COVID-19 and denialist physicians in Brazil. *Transcult Psychiatry.* 2024;61(5):714–723. https://doi.org/10.1177/13634615231213835
8. Rochel de Camargo K. Trying to make sense out of chaos: science, politics and the COVID-19 pandemic. *Cad Saúde Pública.* 2020;36(4):e00088120. https://doi.org/10.1590/0102-311x00088120
9. Epstein S. *Impure Science: AIDS, Activism, and the Politics of Knowledge.* Berkeley, CA: University of California Press; 1997.
10. Berkman A, Garcia J, Muñoz-Laboy M, Paiva V, Parker R. A critical analysis of the Brazilian response to HIV/AIDS: lessons learned for controlling and mitigating the epidemic in developing countries. *Am J Public Health.* 2005;95(7):1162–1172. https://doi.org/10.2105/AJPH.2004.054593
11. Sabi SC, Rieker M. The role of civil society in health policy making in South Africa: a review of the strategies adopted by the Treatment Action Campaign. *Afr J AIDS Res.* 2017;16(1):57–64. https://doi.org/10.2989/16085906.2017.1296874
12. Sturgis P, Allum N. Science in society: re-evaluating the deficit model of public attitudes. *Public Underst Sci.* 2004;13(1):55–74. https://doi.org/10.1177/0963662504042690
13. Wang VMY. Dismantling the deficit model of science communication using Ludwik Fleck's theory of thinking collectives. In: Tsou JY, Shaw J, Fehr C, eds. *Values, Pluralism, and Pragmatism: Themes from the Work of Matthew J. Brown.* Cham, Switzerland: Springer; 2025:117–137.
14. McGarity TO. *Bending Science: How Special Interests Corrupt Public Health Research.* Cambridge, MA: Harvard University Press; 2012.
15. Diethelm P, McKee M. Denialism: what is it and how should scientists respond? *Eur J Public Health.* 2009;19(1):2–4. https://doi.org/10.1093/eurpub/ckn139
16. Brandt A. *The Cigarette Century: The Rise, Fall, and Deadly Persistence of the Product That Defined America.* Reprint ed. New York, NY: Basic Books; 2009.
17. Tran L. Tobacco industry tactics seek to undermine efforts to protect health. World Health Organization. November 20, 2024. Available at: https://www.who.int/vietnam/news/detail/20-11-2024-tobacco-industry-tactics-seek-to-undermine-efforts-to-protect-health. Accessed August 13, 2025.
18. Ghebreyesus TA. Director-General's remarks at the media briefing on 2019 novel coronavirus on 8 February 2020. World Health Organization. 2020. Available at: https://www.who.int/director-general/speeches/detail/who-director-general-s-remarks-at-the-media-briefing-on-2019-ncov-on-11-february-2020. Accessed June 9, 2022.
19. Bueno CC. *The Attention Economy: Labour, Time and Power in Cognitive Capitalism.* New York, NY: Rowman & Littlefield; 2016.

20. Nguyen CT. Echo chambers and epistemic bubbles. *Episteme.* 2020;17(2):141–161. https://doi.org/10.1017/epi.2018.32
21. McIntyre L. *How to Talk to a Science Denier: Conversations with Flat Earthers, Climate Deniers, and Others Who Defy Reason.* Cambridge, MA: MIT Press; 2021.
22. Westhoff MA, Posovszky C, Debatin KM. How to respond to misinformation from the anti-vaccine movement. *Inquiry.* 2023;60:469580231155723. https://doi.org/10.1177/00469580231155723
23. Center for Countering Digital Hate. *The Disinformation Dozen.* 2021:40. Available at: https://counterhate.com/research/the-disinformation-dozen. Accessed July 18, 2025.
24. Broniatowski DA, Jamison AM, Qi S, et al. Weaponized health communication: Twitter bots and Russian trolls amplify the vaccine debate. *Am J Public Health.* 2018;108(10):1378–1384. https://doi.org/10.2105/AJPH.2018.304567
25. Kaushik A, Fomicheva J, Boonstra N, Faber E, Gupta S, Kest H. Pediatric vaccine hesitancy in the United States—the growing problem and strategies for management including motivational interviewing. *Vaccines (Basel).* 2025;13(2):115. https://doi.org/10.3390/vaccines13020115

Lessons Learned From the COVID-19 Pandemic: "Those Who Cannot Remember the Past Are Condemned to Repeat It"

Robert J. Kim-Farley, MD, MPH

ABOUT THE AUTHOR

Robert J. Kim-Farley is with the Departments of Epidemiology and Community Health Sciences, Fielding School of Public Health, University of California, Los Angeles, and is an associate editor of AJPH.

See also Trust in Public Health, pp. 31–94.

AJPH January 2026, Vol. 116, No. 1

"Ingenuity, knowledge, and organization alter but cannot cancel humanity's vulnerability to invasion by parasitic forms of life. Infectious disease which antedated the emergence of humankind will last as long as humanity itself, and will surely remain, as it has been hitherto, one of the fundamental parameters and determinants of human history."

—*William H. McNeill, Plagues and Peoples*[1]

The COVID-19 pandemic, an unprecedented public health crisis in modern times, laid bare both the strengths and vulnerabilities in preparedness and response to disease threats in the United States and our global society. Despite significant advancements in science, technology, and public health, the world experienced the staggering consequences of unpreparedness, communication failures, and social division. As we look to the future, it is essential to critically examine the "lessons learned," both positive and negative, and to chart a path to a more resilient, equitable, and unified response to future public health emergencies. Such analysis and actions will help promote the public's trust in the integrity of public health science, policy, and actions.

FORGETTING PAST LESSONS IMPERILS FUTURE PREPARATIONS

Public health preparedness—or often the lack thereof—was a defining theme of the COVID-19 pandemic's early months. After the 9/11 attacks and the subsequent anthrax attacks, billions of dollars in federal, state, and local funds were used to strengthen preparedness and response capabilities. This included funds made available to stockpile personal protective equipment, portable field hospitals and treatment centers, vaccines and medical countermeasures; develop pandemic and all-hazards preparedness and response plans; and train and drill personnel to implement such plans.

However, over time as the memory of these attacks faded, the 2008 economic recession ensued, and the pressures of competing priorities intervened, and these preparedness funds began to dwindle at all levels. The state of California, for example, had created a robust public health emergency stockpile. Yet in 2011 the government decided to do away with the stockpile, given the $5.8 million per year cost to maintain it, and Governor Jerry Brown said the programs had been set up to counter "a potential influenza pandemic which did not occur."[2] Then when the COVID-19 pandemic occurred, California, like many other jurisdictions, found that the "the cupboard was bare."

The erosion of strategic stockpiles is a cautionary tale about the dangers of short-term thinking and cost containment at the expense of public safety in the long term. Although sometimes infrequent, the lessons learned from highly impactful events (such as pandemics) need to remain in the collective memory, especially in the minds of elected leaders and decision-makers, to help prevent the dismantling of preparedness measures. These measures are not merely expenditures; they need to be considered a vital "insurance policy" that society must pay the premium for to keep vigilant.

FOLLOWING THE SCIENCE

One oft-heard phrase is "follow the science." A major lesson learned is that there are at least three sciences that needed to be followed in the COVID-19 pandemic. Typically, medical and public health experts dwell more on the biological science when advising the public to follow the science. This includes such factors as modes of transmission, the nature of the virus, and the best approaches to interrupting transmission. However, we also need to take more cognizance of behavioral science: what cultural practices affect a person's behavior and their willingness to change behaviors. Greater use of the behavioral sciences (including experts versed in social marketing) is helpful in crafting messages in ways that resonate with the public and promote greater adherence to recommendations tailored and modified in an appropriate balance between the biological and behavioral sciences. The third science, political science, regarding how decisions are made by governments and how power is exercised in societies, may help to more clearly articulate to the public and policymakers how control measures are implemented under a consistent national policy. Achieving policy consistency may be more difficult in the United States, a federal system with substantial state and local autonomy, compared to a unitary state like China, which has centralized administrative authority.

Appropriately developing policies and strategies that incorporate all three of these sciences—especially in the face of economic pressures, individual rights, antiscience sentiments, and political influences—can result in more nuanced recommendations, guidelines, and health officer orders that may reduce some of the reactions and polarization in society.

COMMUNICATING CLEARLY AND CONSISTENTLY

Mixed messaging from different parts and levels of government may result in confusion in the public's mind. For example, the messaging regarding vaccination was sometimes conflicting between the White House, the Food and Drug Administration, and the Centers for Disease Control and Prevention. In August 2025, for example, the Food and Drug Administration restricted its COVID-19 vaccine official authorization to high-risk groups and seniors, whereas in September 2025 the Centers for Disease Control and Prevention allowed broader, discretionary use by healthy individuals after consulting with a health care provider.

Recommendations in one state or local jurisdiction for masking, as another example, frequently were different from those in other jurisdictions with the same rates of disease. This was often the result of a lack of consultation, reaching consensus, and making a unified decision. It also reflected an increasing polarization and partisan divide on the pandemic.

Additionally, the public received little preparation for evolving guidance over time. Such changes were attributable to continued improvements in the understanding of the behavior of a virus that had never been seen before as well as to the virus itself changing over time, with variants having different characteristics. One specific example of the evolving understanding of severe acute respiratory syndrome coronavirus 2 (SARS-CoV-2) was the shift from the early focus on handwashing and surface disinfection to the later emphasis on airborne transmission and the role of masking—with the concomitant change in recommendations often misconstrued as incompetence or duplicity.

To optimize trust, government officials should have mentioned to the public from the outset that as more information about this novel virus was gained, recommendations might change. Without such proper preparation, the public often took changes in official guidance as "flip-flopping" rather than being based on new emerging scientific knowledge.

INNOVATION AND RAPID SCIENTIFIC RESPONSE

A positive lesson learned was that the scientific community, when confronted with the challenges of a new viral pandemic and provided with the necessary resources, can rise to the occasion and has a remarkable ability to invent. Examples of innovation include the development of advanced diagnostic tests (e.g., highly sensitive laboratory-based PCR [polymerase chain reaction] tests for early detection of SARS-CoV-2 virus and at-home antigen tests for rapid detection of a person's infectiousness), new effective treatment modalities (e.g., nirmatrelvir/ritonavir, remdesivir, and molnupiravir antiviral medications), and novel vaccines (e.g., Comirnaty, Spikevax, and Nuvaxovid). An example of resource mobilization is the US government's Operation Warp Speed, a public–private partnership launched in May 2020 and initially funded with about $10 billion from the CARES Act (Coronavirus Aid, Relief, and Economic Security Act, Pub L No. 116-136 [March 27, 2020]) to accelerate COVID-19 vaccine development.[3]

BALANCING SAFETY, FREEDOM, AND SOCIETAL VALUES

The less than 1% infection fatality rate of COVID-19 itself created controversy. Some people, noting this rate, questioned the need to shut down businesses and schools, whereas others pointed out that this still meant millions were affected and that "every life is precious." The response would likely have been different had the infection fatality rate been 10 times less, say 0.1% (like some seasonal influenzas). Even though public health officials would certainly have been concerned and followed the virus closely, they would not have recommended major changes and disruptions in the operation of businesses and schools. However, had the infection fatality rate been 10 times more, say 10% (as seen in the 2002–2004 SARS [severe acute respiratory syndrome] outbreak), even the general public and elected officials would have been clamoring for public health guidance as their family and friends were dying in large numbers.

Further complicating the situation was the skewed age distribution for severe illness and death: primarily toward the elderly. Young people often could not understand why they were not able to go to school or were losing jobs when this disease primarily affected the elderly. Had the pandemic primarily affected children, with high numbers of child deaths, the societal response may have also been quite different, recognizing the tremendous years of potential life lost in that group. Geographic, racial, socioeconomic, and occupational disparities were also noted. This controversy highlights the importance of recognizing that all policy decisions are ultimately value choices. Striking the balance between the values of safety and security, on the one hand, and personal choice and freedom, on the other, is a challenge that needs to be explicitly addressed and appropriately communicated.

COLLABORATION AMONG THE PROTAGONISTS

Another lesson learned was that the three protagonists—governments and their public health institutions; the community, businesses, and schools; and individuals—all needed to work together in greater synchrony.

Governments and their public health institutions have the roles of monitoring the progress of the pandemic, devising recommendations (in consultation with all sectors of society), and promoting the development of vaccines, medicines, treatment modalities, testing, and ensuring availability of personal protective equipment such as masks. Communities, businesses, and schools have the roles of adapting and implementing these recommendations to the unique circumstances of their settings. Finally, individuals have the roles of taking responsibility for their own preventive measures as well as recognizing the measures that they can take to help protect more vulnerable people with whom they are in contact (e.g., infants, the elderly, and immunocompromised individuals).

Greater dialogue and collaboration among these protagonists fostered through such mechanisms as town hall meetings, outreach to chambers of commerce, and parent–teacher association conferences may facilitate better understanding and finding solutions. These, in turn, may reduce the resentment and lack of trust in public health professionals (based on perceptions of working in isolation, using draconian control methods, and conspiracy theories) because of economic losses from business shutdowns and school closures. A specific example during the pandemic was when some local governments helped restaurants stay in business by altering zoning laws to facilitate outdoor dining.

COMBATING MISINFORMATION

One of the most challenging issues during the COVID-19 pandemic was not only misinformation (false information spread without the intent to harm) but also the proliferation of disinformation (false information spread with the intent to deceive or harm) and malinformation (factual information, often out of context, spread with the intent to cause harm), which were often peddled for profit (e.g., "clicks to be lured" for money on the Internet), political gain (e.g., votes to be attracted), or to promote conspiracy theories.

Disinformation about mRNA COVID-19 vaccine safety, for instance, gained significant traction because of widespread fears regarding the rapid pace of its development. However, the mRNA vaccine technology was not an overnight creation. It rested on decades of foundational research, and the swift development of a COVID-19 vaccine was made possible by rapid genome sequencing of the virus and years of groundwork in vaccine technology. This fact should have been more clearly communicated to the public.

Another lesson learned is that the failure to communicate the anticipated evolutionary nature of scientific guidance further eroded public trust. As new guidance emerged, the lack of clear, unified communication from public health authorities and political leaders fostered confusion and, at times, open rebellion against life-saving interventions (or even advocacy for unproven, and potentially harmful, approaches, such as the use of ivermectin and hydroxychloroquine). The scientific community must learn the lesson to communicate not only facts but also the iterative, self-correcting nature of scientific inquiry.

GLOBAL INTERDEPENDENCE

We are now living in an age of global interdependency with rapid and far-reaching modes of transportation that have truly created a "global village" in which a virus or bacteria that affects a village in Africa can quickly become a problem anywhere. Nobel laureate Joshua Lederberg stated this well:

> The microbe that felled one child in a distant continent yesterday can reach yours today and seed a global pandemic tomorrow. How can we procrastinate any further, or have any reservations, about a common cause—one that responds to every outbreak of disease anywhere as a challenge to us all.[4]

Whereas in more developed countries it is possible to implement stronger social safety net strategies that allow lockdowns and stay at home policies, the least developed countries may not have the resources to do so—and not working can mean starvation. Even in developed countries, the poor are often working in "essential" jobs (e.g., service industries, farming, and food processing plants), placing them at higher risk for exposure because of inadequate physical-distancing measures. Compounding that, the poor, who have less access to medical care and preventive services, are at higher risk for severe illness and death owing to higher levels of preexisting medical conditions.

Developing countries end up not receiving sufficient supplies of vaccines, medicines, and personal protective equipment, whereas wealthy nations develop and often hold on to scarce supplies. Wealthier nations need to be more supportive of developing countries in transferring technology and know-how for vaccine production, surveillance systems, and control measures. Without such support, developing countries may have high levels of disease transmission that sets the stage for variants to emerge and, ultimately, come back and affect the more developed world. An example of a positive effort to address equitable access to COVID-19 vaccines is the COVID-19 Vaccines Global Access initiative—a partnership between the Gavi vaccine alliance, the Coalition for Epidemic Preparedness Innovations, the World Health Organization, and the United Nations Children's Fund.

The pandemic underscored that scientific achievement alone cannot guarantee equitable or just outcomes. Without a robust framework of ethics, even the most effective interventions can perpetuate inequity and mistrust. Addressing these inequities is not only a moral imperative but also a practical necessity.

CONCLUSION

As the world has transitioned to an endemic phase of COVID-19, the lessons learned of vigilance, adaptation, and resilience must remain at the forefront. Although the evolutionary path of the virus may continue to lead to less severe outcomes, akin to the respiratory viruses of the common cold (four strains of which are human coronaviruses "estimated to cause between 15%–30% of common colds in adults"[5(p6)]), complacency is not an option. Our collective ability to respond effectively to future threats will depend on the maturity of our global society and our willingness to recognize that interdependence is an operational necessity. An analogy of the world as a human body is particularly apt: just as the health of one part affects the whole, the well-being of every nation and community affects global stability. This will require an organic transformation of societal structures, placing justice and empathy at the center of public health policy.

The COVID-19 pandemic was, and continues to be, a profound challenge. Yet it also offered an opportunity for transformative growth. By learning from past mistakes and successes—in preparedness, response, communication, and equity—and by integrating ethical principles into the very fabric of scientific and public health endeavors, we can build a more resilient and just society as well as promote trust and integrity in public health.

Let us seize this moment to forge a future in which science and ethics walk hand in hand, communication is clear and inclusive, and the health of every individual is recognized as vital to the health of all. AJPH

CORRESPONDENCE

Correspondence should be sent to Robert J. Kim-Farley, MD, MPH, UCLA Department of Epidemiology, Room 71-279A CHS, 650 Charles E. Young Dr South, Los Angeles, CA 90095 (e-mail: robert@kimfarley.org). Reprints can be ordered at https://www.ajph.org by clicking the "Reprints" link.

PUBLICATION INFORMATION

Full Citation: Kim-Farley RJ. Lessons learned from the COVID-19 pandemic: "those who cannot remember the past are condemned to repeat it". *Am J Public Health*. 2026;116(1):42–46.

Acceptance Date: October 9, 2025.

DOI: https://doi.org/10.2105/AJPH.2025.308318
ORCID iD:
Robert J. Kim-Farley https://orcid.org/0000-0003-3022-6548

ACKNOWLEDGMENTS

I acknowledge that these "lessons learned" have been gleaned and refined from previous talks and lectures that I have given at the University of California, Los Angeles; a presentation on August 2, 2025 for the 49th Annual Conference of the Association of Bahá'í Studies; and numerous interviews that I have given on COVID-19 for television, radio, and printed media during the pandemic as a representative of the UCLA Fielding School of Public Health.

CONFLICTS OF INTEREST

The author reports no conflicts of interest.

REFERENCES

1. McNeill WH. *Plagues and Peoples*. Garden City, NY: Anchor Press/Doubleday; 1976.
2. Williams L, Evans W, Carless W. California once had mobile hospitals and a ventilator stockpile, but it dismantled them. *Los Angeles Times*. March 27, 2020. Available at: https://www.latimes.com/california/story/2020-03-27/coronavirus-california-mobile-hospitals-ventilators. Accessed August 7, 2025.
3. Van Norman GA. "Warp Speed" operations in the COVID-19 pandemic: moving too quickly? *JACC Basic Transl Sci*. 2020;5(7):730–734. https://doi.org/10.1016/j.jacbts.2020.06.001
4. Lederberg JJ. Medical science, infectious disease, and the unity of humankind. January 1988. Available at: https://profiles.nlm.nih.gov/spotlight/bb/catalog/nlm:nlmuid-101584906X19440-doc. Accessed August 7, 2025.
5. Coerdt KM, Khachemoune A. Corona viruses: reaching far beyond the common cold. *Afr Health Sci*. 2021;21(1):207–213. https://doi.org/10.4314/ahs.v21i1.27

Relationships Matter: Rebuilding Policymaker Trust in Public Health Leadership

Shelley A. Hearne, DrPH, MPH, and Keshia M. Pollack Porter, PhD, MPH

ABOUT THE AUTHORS

Both authors are with the Johns Hopkins Bloomberg School of Public Health, Baltimore, MD.

See also Trust in Public Health, pp. 31–94.

"I worry about the future of trust in public health," said former Centers for Disease Control and Prevention (CDC) director Susan Monarez, PhD, during a recent Senate oversight hearing. She had been dismissed from her position for holding the line on scientific integrity.[1] She is not alone. Politicians and some in the public have harassed, threatened, and politically undermined public health officials, eroding their credibility and authority.[2] Hundreds of bullets hit CDC's building in Atlanta, Georgia, in 2025, underscoring how the public health profession is figuratively and literally under fire.

These attacks jeopardize funding, staffing, and the essential programs and policies that protect and save lives. This hostile climate also inflicts a personal toll on our profession and its allies, while undermining trust, weakening our public health institutions, and hindering progress toward achieving the goals of public health practice.

We provide public health professionals a path forward for building policymakers' support and trust by emphasizing humility and relationships.

THE ROOTS OF MISTRUST

It is important to recognize that we live in highly polarized times and that trust in government has steadily declined over the last several decades. In 1958, when Dwight Eisenhower was president, approximately 75% of Americans said they trusted the federal government to do what was right most of the time.[3] Today, that number consistently hovers around 20%, regardless of which party holds office.[3]

Public health agencies are no longer immune to facing mistrust. According to the KFF, public confidence in the CDC has plummeted from 85% at the beginning of the pandemic in March 2020 to a low of 57% in July 2025. Political affiliation further differentiates these trends, with Republicans showing greater trust in the Trump administration and Democrats having had more confidence in the Biden administration.[4] The bottom line is that trust is universally in short supply—a reality that the public health field must directly address.

PRINCIPLES FOR REBUILDING

To earn trust, we must start by acknowledging that it is difficult to trust someone you do not know. We all know what it takes to trust a partner, a friend, or a colleague. We look for someone with integrity, consistency, and authenticity; someone who can find a way to be truthful with us, even if painful; someone who listens and understands our needs and concerns and can speak to us in a way that is fathomable and empathetic.

Policymakers are no different. They are people and face a complex series of trade-offs, powerful interests, and constituent or regulatory demands. One study of former regulators from the Environmental Protection Agency indicated their high preference for substantive engagement through in-person meetings and written materials. Although technical information was valuable, communication style mattered: most respondents viewed compelling arguments and storytelling as effective.[5] Research over time has shown that policymakers prefer to receive information via trusted intermediaries and that they value personal relationships.[6,7]

In "Fighting for Public Health," the Network for Public Health Law reports that policymakers often have not met their local public health constituents.[8] The public health field has long struggled with visibility, leaving it less present than it needs to be. The 2024 documentary *The Invisible Shield* captured this well by emphasizing that "public health saved your life today and you probably don't even know it."[9]

AJPH January 2026, Vol. 116, No. 1

For example, think about the airbags in your vehicle. The life-saving power of this intervention is often not realized until one is in an automobile crash. Public health professionals can fix this invisibility by sharing stories about the power of the public health system and establishing sustained engagement with policymakers.

Back in 1998, the Pew Commission on Environmental Health funded public opinion research to explore how to build greater policymaker support for public health agencies—specifically the CDC and its loose network of state health agencies charged with health protection and promotion. Surveys with registered voters revealed that most Americans did not understand the public health system. Most thought it was health insurance for the poor. When given an actual definition, 57% of the respondents provided negative evaluations of the public health system.[10]

Interestingly, that same survey indicated that the vast majority believed the United States should do more to protect health and ranked public health funding as more deserving than many favorite issues, including tax cuts.[10] The US public remains concerned about their health, as evidenced by recent surveys and the rise of the Make America Healthy Again movement. As is true today, there was work to be done to connect the dots, engage policymakers and the public on health concerns, and find common ground on how to make it better. Legendary House of Representatives speaker Tip O'Neill popularized the phrase "All politics is local."[11] Applying this insight to public health practice requires recognizing that health policies must be approached locally and relationally.

Trust building is at the heart of the recommendations in our book *Policy Engagement*, which offers actionable guidance for public health professionals on how to be effectively relational with decision-makers.[12] The principles are straightforward and mirror what we already knew about creating lasting partnerships:

- *Lead with empathy.* Public health leaders must approach policymakers with both facts and an understanding of the pressures they face, for example, constituent demands, fiscal constraints, and the country's political mood.[13] Policymakers are people too, with different interests, values, and relationships. Understanding them and the forces influencing their decisions creates greater receptivity. Stories offer a powerful means of translating an issue and tying it to what matters to the policymaker, not just you.[14]
- *Engage relationally, not transactionally.* Authentic engagement requires listening, relationship building, and reciprocity. Policymakers, like everyone else, respond to genuine interest and mutual respect. Public health leaders cannot limit their presence to crises or moments when they want something. In her first months as the new dean of Johns Hopkins Bloomberg School of Public Health, one of the authors of this article (K. M. P. P.) participated in the Association of Schools and Programs of Public Health's Virtual Hill Day to support academic public health efforts and open the doors of the school to be a trusted resource for all decision-makers. These visits were about listening to policymakers' priorities and inviting them into a relationship.
- *Be present consistently.* One of the most trusted leaders of the environmental field, Gene Karpinski, recently retired CEO of the League of Conservation Voters, had a basic practice: always show up. Elected officials and other organizations could count on him at town halls, events, coalitions, and fundraisers and to answer telephone calls at any hour. Engagement is an ongoing commitment, not episodic. Building trust involves being present and showing up consistently.
- *Stay grounded in facts.* Trust requires a steadfast commitment to accuracy and evidence. The public health field's greatest strength is its data and science. Policymakers may not always agree with our conclusions, but consistency in fact-based communication builds credibility. So does acknowledging what you do not know (and always following up with information or sources that can answer policymakers' questions).
- *Engage broadly and work constructively with perceived opposition.* The public health field's agenda is strongest and most sustainable when it transcends politics. We acknowledge that this can be difficult, especially when shared goals or values with those who hold different viewpoints seem out of reach. However, by building bridges, the field can maintain credibility and strengthen support from a wide array of stakeholders. Start by seeking to understand their priorities, political pressures, and the constituencies they represent. Look for overlapping values—such as children's health, economic opportunity, or national and community security—and frame health initiatives in shared terms. When public health professionals demonstrate openness and reliability, even those who

were initially skeptical can become unexpected allies on issues of mutual concern. As another Tip O'Neill-ism goes, "Today's adversary may be tomorrow's ally."[10]

HOPE IN THIS MOMENT—A CALL TO ACTION

In a time of societal disconnection and deep mistrust in our civic institutions, there are positive signs. Although they may have taken a hit during the COVID-19 pandemic, most Americans (78%) remain confident that medical scientists act in the public's best interest.[15] All scientists, including those who are health based, rank higher in trust than other respected professions, for example, public school principals and police officers.[15]

Further good news is that our workforce increasingly views policy engagement as a necessary and needed skill. The most recent national public health workforce survey showed public engagement to be the second most important skill for governmental professionals at all job levels in all jurisdictions.[16] The Council on Education for Public Health, which accredits public health schools and programs, requires advocacy to be taught to master of public health students. Now, it is time to put those skills into practice.

In addition, public health professionals should consider how policymakers and their influential constituents obtain the information that shapes their views and trust levels. According to the September 2025 Carnegie Endowment article "For Expertise to Matter, Nonpartisan Institutions Need New Communications Strategies," fact-based institutions can no longer rely on prestige, credentials, or traditional platforms to influence decision-makers.[17] Although traditional reports and op-eds can be valuable in elite circles, their influence is shrinking and must be supported by social media networks. The authors urge nonpartisan institutions to adopt new strategies that engage with digital platforms, collaborate with trusted community voices, and craft narratives and stories that highlight lived experiences as valuable data.[17]

We recommend these action steps to enhance trust and engagement capabilities:

- *Repair and restore relationships.* Acknowledging mistakes and making amends is foundational to rebuilding trust. Public health professionals can learn from restorative practices, which include reflecting on missteps, accepting accountability, naming harms, and moving from harm to healing through dialogue, humility, and partnership.[18] Saying, "I was wrong" or "I supported this action based on what I knew at the time" enhances credibility, lays a foundation to help rebuild trust, and builds strong support for the future fixes needed to advance public health practice.
- *Create professional policy engagement training and support.* Public health professionals are in widely dispersed occupations, such as industrial hygienists and governmental officials. Trade associations and governmental agencies should provide opportunities to learn skills for rebuilding trust: advocacy, political engagement, and recognizing and analyzing power. The Society of Public Health Educators and the American Public Health Association have been leaders, hosting basic advocacy training and providing policymaker outreach events. The Lerner Center for Public Health Advocacy has created in-person and online skill-building programs that provide continuing education credits. Few governmental agencies offer advocacy training, but one emerging model is the Baltimore City Health Department's pilot program, which provides policy engagement fundamentals to staff at all levels. In the six-week initiative created in collaboration with the Lerner Center for Public Health Advocacy, participants received training in agency policy positions, communications, and distinctions between advocacy and lobbying. Participants reported increased knowledge, confidence, and practice in advocacy (Sadiya Muqueeth, DrPH, and Meghan Ames, DrPH, e-mail communication, October 2025).
- *Embrace new ways of engaging to rebuild trust.* Although data and credentials remain valuable in legacy media such as newspapers and television, they carry diminishing weight among many policymakers and their influential constituents. To strengthen our reach, public health professionals must cultivate storytelling skills, forge and sustain authentic community partnerships, and activate trusted voices across social media platforms—where credibility is earned through connection, not just expertise. Public health leaders have never been afraid to take on tough work, although many in the field are wary of advocacy. At this critical moment for the public's health, we must be willing to advocate strategies that are informed by both science and community voices.[18]

Public health professionals must intentionally and consistently invest in genuine relationships with the policymakers who shape our policies and systems and the communities that public health professionals serve. Rebuilding trust requires more than data; it demands presence. Public health leaders must show up, stay grounded in facts, listen with humility, share stories, and engage with authenticity and empathy; they are essential to restoring confidence in our profession, our purpose, and our promise. Together, they form the foundation for achieving health equity and creating a healthier, safer, and fairer world for all. AJPH

CORRESPONDENCE

Correspondence should be sent to Shelley A. Hearne, Lerner Center for Public Health Advocacy, 615 N. Wolfe St., W3041, Baltimore, MD 21215, shearne1@jhu.edu). Reprints can be ordered at https://www.ajph.org by clicking the "Reprints" link.

PUBLICATION INFORMATION

Full Citation: Hearne SA, Pollack Porter KM. Relationships matter: rebuilding policymaker trust in public health leadership. *Am J Public Health*. 2026;116(1):47–50.

Acceptance Date: October 15, 2025.

DOI: https://doi.org/10.2105/AJPH.2025.308330

ORCID iDs:

Shelley A. Hearne https://orcid.org/0009-0003-5155-4468

Keshia M. Pollack Porter https://orcid.org/0000-0001-5363-5462

CONTRIBUTORS

Both authors made substantial contributions to the conception or design of the work; drafted the work, including revised it critically for important intellectual content; and provided final approval of the version to be published. Both authors agree to be accountable for all aspects of the work.

ACKNOWLEDGMENTS

The authors would like to thank Lois Dankwa-Branche for her review and support with references and Tesfa Alexander, Lymari Morales, and Diane Coraggio for their reviews of an earlier draft.

CONFLICTS OF INTEREST

The authors have no real or potential conflicts of interest to declare.

REFERENCES

1. US Senate Committee on Health, Education, Labor & Pensions. Restoring trust through radical transparency: reviewing recent events at the Centers for Disease Control and Prevention and implications for children's health. Available at: https://www.help.senate.gov/hearings/restoring-trust-through-radical-transparency-reviewing-recent-events-at-the-centers-for-disease-control-and-prevention-and-implications-for-childrens-health. Accessed September 24, 2025.
2. Ward JA, Stone EM, Mui P, Resnick B. Pandemic-related workplace violence and its impact on public health officials, March 2020–January 2021. *Am J Public Health.* 2022;112(5):736–746. https://doi.org/10.2105/AJPH.2021.306649
3. Bell P. Public trust in government: 1958–2024. June 2024. Available at: https://www.pewresearch.org/politics/2024/06/24/public-trust-in-government-1958-2024. Accessed September 10, 2025.
4. Hamel L. Challenges for rebuilding trust in the CDC. Available at: https://www.kff.org/quick-take/challenges-for-rebuilding-trust-in-the-cdc. Accessed September 24, 2025.
5. Topazian RJ, McGinty EE, Hearne SA. Understanding the factors that impact federal rulemaking: a survey of former EPA regulators. *Health Aff Scholar.* 2024;2(10):qxae125. https://doi.org/10.1093/haschl/qxae125
6. Oliver K, Innvar S, Lorenc T, Woodman J, Thomas J. A systematic review of barriers to and facilitators of the use of evidence by policymakers. *BMC Health Serv Res.* 2014;14(1):2. https://doi.org/10.1186/1472-6963-14-2
7. Feldman PH, Nadash P, Gursen M. Improving communication between researchers and policy makers in long-term care: or, researchers are from Mars; policy makers are from Venus. *Policy Brief (Cent Home Care Policy Res).* 2001;41(5):1–6.
8. Katz M, Matthews G, Frey M. Fighting for public health: Network for Public Health Law. September 2022. Available at: https://www.networkforphl.org/news-insights/fighting-for-public-health. Accessed September 24, 2025.
9. PBS. *The Invisible Shield.* Available at: https://www.pbs.org/show/the-invisible-shield. Accessed October 13, 2025.
10. Hearne S, Locke P, Mellman M, et al. Public opinion about public health—United States, 1999. *MMWR Morb Mortal Wkly Rep.* 2000;49(12):258–260. [Erratum in: *MMWR Morb Mortal Wkly Rep.* 2000; 49(13):286.]
11. O'Neill T, Hymel G. *All Politics Is Local, and Other Rules of the Game.* Holbrook, MA: Adams Media; 1994.
12. Hearne S, Pollack Porter KM, Forrest KS. *Policy Engagement.* Washington, DC: APHA Press; 2023. Available at: https://ajph.aphapublications.org/doi/book/10.2105/9780875533391. Accessed November 8, 2025.
13. Kingdon JW. *Agendas, Alternatives, and Public Policies.* 2nd ed. Harlow, UK: Pearson; 2014. Available at: https://questanbridge.com/wp-content/uploads/2024/11/Agendas-Alternatives-and-Public-Policies.pdf. Accessed November 8, 2025.
14. Storr W. *The Science of Storytelling: Why Stories Make Us Human and How to Tell Them Better.* New York, NY: Abrams; 2020. Available at: http://ebookcentral.proquest.com/lib/jhu/detail.action?docID=6119479. Accessed September 24, 2025.
15. Tyson A, Kennedy B. Public trust in scientists and views on their role in policymaking. November 2024. Available at: https://www.pewresearch.org/science/2024/11/14/public-trust-in-scientists-and-views-on-their-role-in-policymaking. Accessed September 4, 2025.
16. de Beaumont Foundation. Public health workforce interests and needs survey (PH WINS). 2024 findings. Available at: https://debeaumont.org/phwins/2024-survey. Accessed September 24, 2025.
17. DiResta R, Kleinfeld R. For expertise to matter, nonpartisan institutions need new communications strategies. September 2025. Available at: https://carnegie-production-assets.s3.amazonaws.com/static/files/Kleinfeld_DiResta_New%20Comms.pdf. Accessed November 8, 2025.
18. Head LJT, Koller CF. From shame and trauma to hope and healing: an act of reconciliation and restorative justice for the Tuskegee syphilis study. *Health Aff Forefront.* November 29, 2022. https://doi.org/10.1377/forefront.20221128.277996. Available at: https://www.healthaffairs.org/content/forefront/shame-and-trauma-hope-and-healing-act-reconciliation-and-restorative-justice-tuskegee. Accessed November 8, 2025.

Public Health Policymaking Outside of the Federal Government: Reflections on Authority and Trust-Building Challenges

Lauren A. Taylor, PhD, MDiv, and Arthur L. Caplan, PhD

ABOUT THE AUTHORS

Lauren A. Taylor and Arthur L. Caplan are with the Department of Population Health, NYU Grossman School of Medicine, New York, NY.

See also Trust in Public Health, pp. 31–94.

Many in public health communities are rightly concerned about the recent federal actions to dissolve or otherwise undermine important, scientific advisory bodies. Box 1 outlines several examples. The committees discussed in Box 1 have played a range of roles but can broadly be understood as part of the public health policymaking infrastructure. Although none authored legislation directly, each was formed to inform the policies promulgated by the Department of Health and Human Services (HHS).

Although several of the committee titles indicate advisory roles, frequently their impact is more direct. For example, the Advisory Committee on Immunization Practices (ACIP) of the Centers for Disease Control and Prevention (CDC) made vaccine coverage recommendations that were statutorily required to be followed in the Vaccines for Children program.[1] In some cases, the role these committees have played in policymaking has been so instrumental that it raised fears that the committee members might be insufficiently accountable to the public in light of their policymaking power. The Supreme Court recently ruled on this issue and found that in the case of the US Prevention Services Task Force, there was sufficient oversight by federal employees to warrant no further legal action.[2]

The injury to these advisory committees has varied to date. In some cases, such as the Secretary's Advisory Committee on Human Research Protections (SACHRP), all committee members were terminated and the committee effectively disbanded. In other cases, such as ACIP, all members of the committee were terminated and replaced by new members chosen by HHS secretary Robert F. Kennedy Jr., many of whom have professional track records of vaccine skepticism. At the Federal Trade Commission, from which Chairwoman Lina Khan and then other Democratic members were dismissed, research and legal strategies designed to combat public health threats to children and youths on social media have been put in jeopardy. We anticipate that additional changes to federal policymaking landscape are likely to continue as Secretary Kennedy attempts to "dramatically reduce the size of the federal government"[3] and sever accountability relationships between federal agencies and the scientific community, which he views as left leaning,[4] corrupt, and financially conflicted.[5]

These changes raise an important question for the public health community about how to fill the policymaking gaps left by the changes at the federal level. Two strategies are emerging. The first strategy is to move some of the policymaking work that the federal advisory committees had previously done to the state level or, in some cases, to multistate coalitions that can promulgate state-level policies as regional blocs. The second strategy is to move the policymaking work to private, nonprofit organizations that can issue guidance, recommendations, and even industry regulations from outside government. Both strategies face challenges in establishing authority and earning trust in a political landscape defined by polarization and mistrust of institutions.

STATES EXPANDING THEIR ROLES

The states have a long underappreciated track record of handling many matters of national public health concern on their own, including Medicaid program design, clean air and water regulations, quarantine and isolation mandates, and vaccine policy. States have been especially active in stepping up to fill the gap created by recent and anticipated changes to federal vaccine policy.

These changes include the removal of COVID-19 vaccination from the list of

AJPH January 2026, Vol. 116, No. 1

BOX 1— Recent Changes to Federal Scientific Advisory Bodies: United States, 2025

Federal Change	Role of Federal Body	Who Was Advised	Who Is Stepping In
ACIP: All 17 members were abruptly removed by RFK Jr. in June 2025 and swiftly replaced with eight new members who were more aligned with the MAHA movement.	Housed in the CDC, ACIP provides guidance for creating and approving vaccine schedules, as well as discussing the safety and efficacy of new vaccines. The committee also influences insurers, who then decide which vaccines to provide coverage for.	HHS, CDC, state and local health departments, health care providers, and the public	State alliances, e.g., the West Coast Health Alliance (of WA, CA, OR); states revising regulations to amplify guidance from their own state health departments; privately funded endeavors, e.g., VIP (hosted at the University of Minnesota); medical societies, e.g., the AAFP accepting guidance from the VIP; lawsuits from various medical societies against HHS.
USPSTF: In July 2025, potential plans to remove all members were unveiled but have not yet been enacted.	Creates guidance on preventive services (e.g., HIV PrEP) that are required to be covered by insurers under the Affordable Care Act.	HHS, insurers, health care providers, and the public	The proposed dissolution has not yet occurred, but medical associations are releasing statements warning of public health consequences if the changes ultimately go through.
SACHRP: The committee was abruptly disbanded in March 2025.	Provided expert guidance to the secretary of HHS on human research protections and informed policy for the OHRP, which implements regulations for IRBs.	HHS, OHRP, and IRBs	Former SACHRP members have independently formed the NACHRP, and they plan to continue to post their guidance for research institutions to use.
FTC: Chairwoman Lina Khan and two Democratic commissioners were abruptly removed by President Trump, and their roles have not been filled.[6]	Enforces antitrust and consumer protection laws and creates policy recommendations, many of which affect public health. Most notable are recommendations for public health concerns regarding social media and youths.[7]	State governments, federal government, businesses, and the public	It is unclear whether and how the FTC will continue its policy recommendation work, although states are taking the initiative specifically on social media's risks to children. Texas's attorney general launched an inquiry into Meta (Menlo Park, CA) in August 2025 regarding its mental health effects, and California signed the LEAD Children's Act October 2025 to protect children from chatbots that provide harmful or sexually explicit content.

Note. AAFP = American Academy of Family Physicians; ACIP = Advisory Committee on Immunization Practices; CDC = Centers for Disease Control and Prevention; FTC = Federal Trade Commission; HHS = US Department of Health and Human Services; IRB = institutional review board; MAHA = Make America Healthy Again; NACHRP = National Advisory Committee on Human Research Protections; OHRP = Office of Human Research Protections; PrEP = preexposure prophylaxis; SACHRP = Secretary's Advisory Committee on Human Research Protections; USPSTF = US Preventive Services Task Force; VIP = Vaccine Integrity Project. LEAD Children's Act = Leading Ethical AI Development (LEAD) for Kids Act, California AB 1064 (vetoed October 13, 2025; https://legiscan.com/CA/text/AB1064/id/3227472).

CDC-recommended vaccines for pregnant women and healthy children in May 2025.[8] And in September 2025, the newly appointed ACIP removed the measles, mumps, rubella, and varicella combination vaccine from its recommended vaccine schedule for children younger than four years.[9] Additional recommendations for vaccines may well be rescinded. Federal officials have suggested that their changes are not intended as a recommendation against vaccines but rather an allowance for parents to make their own decisions. Unfortunately, by reversing previous recommendations for long-available and endorsed vaccines, the federal government has left many parents without a clear signal about what they should pursue while jeopardizing the benefits of coordinated action, such as herd immunity and vaccine availability.

At least two state consortiums appear to be stepping into this vacuum to communicate with pediatricians and parents about evidence-based vaccination. In September, the governors of California, Washington, and Oregon jointly announced the creation of the West Coast Health Alliance.[10] The alliance will coordinate health guidelines by aligning immunization recommendations informed by national medical organizations. Importantly, public communications about the alliance noted an interest in providing residents with consistent, science-based recommendations on which they can rely "regardless of shifting federal actions."[11] In the Northeast, a similar alliance was formed when health officials from eight states met in summer 2025 to discuss not only coordinated vaccine recommendations but also disease tracking and emergency response management in light of recent changes to the federal government's policymaking and funding footprint.[12]

PRIVATE, NONPROFIT ORGANIZATIONS STEPPING UP

Some policymaking work previously undertaken by the federal government also appears to be moving across the public–private boundary into the domain of private nonprofits. Although this may seem to signal a diminution of policymaking power, there are several examples of extremely durable regulatory functions that emanate from outside government. Consider the Joint Commission (formerly the Joint Commission on Accreditation of Healthcare Organizations), which is among the most powerful regulators of US hospitals.[13] The Joint Commission promulgates accreditation standards that must be met for a hospital to maintain accreditation and subsequently participate in Medicare and Medicaid.

The dissolution of SACHRP and its reconstitution as NACHRP provides the clearest move of policymaking activity across the public–private boundary to date. SACHRP had directly advised the secretary of HHS and the Office of Human Research Protections on research ethics policy, including standards for institutional review boards within and beyond academic institutions.[14] The committee was deactivated in 2025 after 49 years of service with little rationale apart from a downsizing of the federal bureaucracy. Several members of the committee and former Office of Human Research Protections appointees volunteered to continue serving in an advisory capacity. They quickly put up a new website to communicate their reconstitution as the "National" rather than "Secretary's" Advisory Committee on Human Research Protections, making clear that the committee was not part of government, although they intend to collaborate "with regulators." To this end, NACHRP plans to publish annual advisory reports, create educational resources for the public and the research community, and give presentations at national conferences.

Given President Donald Trump and Secretary Kennedy's actions to date, it is likely that the federal government will continue to withdraw from other matters of public health policymaking, which at best leaves policymaking gaps and at worst serve as implicit recommendations against key public health practices. We offer three insights that may inform how the public health community understands and responds to these changes.

SOME POLICYMAKING ROLES ARE MORE PORTABLE THAN OTHERS

It is important to recognize that some policymaking roles are more portable out of the federal government than others. In other words, some can be packed up and transported elsewhere with limited losses to effectiveness; others simply cannot. Advisory bodies that have the primary purpose of advising the public, for instance, may be easiest to rehome in states or nonprofits, although there are still losses to consider. Being part of the federal government has historically lent an important source of authority to advisory bodies designed to shape public behavior, and that authority will have to be rebuilt outside the state apparatus.

Advisory bodies assembled to advise industry or create recommendations or standards for practice have frequently been filled by private nonprofits in the public health and health care space. Medical specialty societies and the Accreditation Council for Graduate Medical Education come to mind, although it is notable that many of the credentials awarded by these entities have been endorsed by government through licensure and insurance policies. Finally, advisory bodies whose primary function is to create forceful recommendations for a government official or body are difficult to recreate by states or nonprofits. This is why epidemiologist Michael Osterholm has said that even laudable new efforts such as the Vaccine Integrity Project cannot replace ACIP.[15] States and nonprofits can and do influence federal policy without serving as a standing advisory body—this is lobbying—but they do so without the imprimatur of having been convened in a transparent and accountable manner for the express purpose of providing scientific advice.

PREPARE FOR MORE INEQUITY

Whether the policymaking role goes to states or private sector actors, we should brace ourselves for exacerbated inequality in the domains of policy that the federal government steps back from. Widening inequalities may manifest in mortality rates of children younger than five, life expectancies, and disability rates. Political scientist Jamila Michener incisively describes how a federalist approach to health policy, which purposefully allows variation in state approaches, also delivers inequality:

> Federalism has historically conferred an abundance of policy options and the choices made in the face of those possibilities have bred deep spatial inequalities.[16(p38)]

In some policy arenas, state-level variation may be morally defensible—or even appropriate—given the considerable diversity of the country. This defensibility rests on several assumptions: (1) all states have the capacity to make equally sound policy, (2) states are democratically accountable to their citizens, and (3) people can exit a state without significant hardship. All three assumptions may reasonably invite skepticism in today's political environment, in which case the resulting public health inequities will be very difficult to justify in a country premised on equality of opportunity.

Inequities can also be expected to play out if traditional roles for government policy are taken up by multiple nonprofit organizations. Whereas state variation in policymaking breeds spatial inequality, nonprofit variation in policymaking may breed inequalities based on other characteristics, such as political party, education status, and social media participation. The result will be unequal guidance and policies, with Americans subject to different expectations depending on their jurisdiction.

BUILDING AUTHORITY IN NEW POLICY SOURCES

Whether the formerly federal advisory roles are taken up by states or private actors, the key challenge going forward is building authority in new sources of health policy. Authority is frequently discussed as roughly belonging to one of three types: (1) authority over, meaning formal authority to make and enforce rules; (2) authority on, meaning expertise on a subject; and (3) authority with, meaning readily accepted influence on the basis of virtue or demonstrated leadership. Federal and state governments have primary claims to public health policymaking authority, which is granted by legal and regulatory systems to which people generally submit. This authority has been bolstered by a historical perception that governments, by eliciting expert service and volunteerism, also have authority on the public health topics at hand. But the public's views of who can claim to be an authority on scientific matters has been deeply challenged, with the result that even government's previously held authority over the public on matters of health is in question.

A small number of strongly Democratic states may be able to claim new types of formal authority over public health policy by passing legislation that delinks their policymaking from that of the federal government.[17] However, for most states and all new nonprofits, the challenge of building authority will largely rest on the cultivation of informal authority—meaning the authority on public health topics and authority with communities. Both efforts are inextricably tied to cultivating a perception of trustworthiness in a political landscape marked by mistrust of institutions believed to be nontransparent and financially conflicted. Rather than relying on institutions as sources of guidance, many Americans have chosen to distribute their trust over broad swaths of social media personas and effectively crowdsource advice from people with "lived experience."[18] Any new source of policy looking to build a reputation for trustworthiness and authority must grapple squarely with this reality.

Nonprofits face particular authority hurdles, particularly in achieving sufficient authority to issue guidance that will be taken seriously by broad political segments of Americans. In some cases, it may be strategic for existing entities, such as medical societies, to expand their roles rather than create new entities and in so doing draw on the authority they have built in an established domain to make public health recommendations.

New organizations may similarly seek to "borrow" existing authorities by recruiting people who previously held government positions (as in the case of NACHRP and the Vaccine Integrity Project) or people who have other professional affiliations with authoritative institutions (e.g., the military, the Department of Veterans Affairs, and the National Academies of Sciences, Engineering, and Medicine). Nonprofits seeking to build authority to make public health recommendations may seek to do so by mimicking the kind of political accountability that makes governments credibly authoritative. This may include the creation of outlets for communication between nonprofit leaders and the public, opportunities for public comment, and transparent bases for decision making. Most critical is that in any given policymaking space, public health leaders quickly consolidate their support for and activities in a single nonprofit.

The degree of political polarization the United States currently faces exacerbates the difficulty of building authority in new sources of public health policymaking. Republicans and Democrats ascribe authority to different people and institutions. The overlap is shrinking, risking a scenario where states held by governors and legislative houses of one party are dismissed as untrustworthy and therefore unauthoritative by the most extreme factions of the other political party. Even nonprofits are quick to be labeled as biased to the right or left.

NEXT STEPS

In conclusion, the privatization and localization of public health expertise is not ideal, but it is a legitimate response to the assault on scientifically grounded public health advice and policy being undertaken by the current federal administration. Whoever takes up the mantle of public health policymaking should seek to cultivate their own authority—and trustworthiness—by making and keeping several commitments:

1. Policymakers must avoid even perceived conflicts of interest whenever possible. When one or the other side of the political spectrum is looking for a reason to dismiss scientific guidance on ideological grounds, policymakers should not miss an opportunity to demonstrate independence.
2. Policymakers must make a clear and accountable commitment to the scientific method. Even in a hyperpoliticized environment, few (if any) are willing to clearly state that they do not believe in or do not support the scientific method. Gold standard science is frequently invoked by Secretary Kennedy, the US Food and Drug Administration commissioner Marty Makary, and others seeking to diminish the previous federal role in public health.
3. Policymaking bodies should seek to be as inclusive and transparent in their policymaking process as feasible. For example, in creating advisory committees or boards, transparency in the selection of members and the opportunity to offer feedback and commentary are crucial for cementing trust.
4. Perhaps most counterintuitively, scientific policymakers must be willing to trust the public to win their trust. The natural instinct of many scientific authorities is to withdraw in the face of a public that appears hostile to expertise—but sustained engagement is key. The more that the public sees science as isolated and obfuscated, the harder it will be to rebuild the authority needed to effectively carry out public health policymaking. AJPH

CORRESPONDENCE

Correspondence should be sent to Lauren A Taylor, PhD, MDiv, Translational Research Building, 227 E 30th St, Department of Population Health, NYU Grossman School of Medicine, New York, NY 10016 (e-mail: lauren.taylor@nyulangone.org). Reprints can be ordered at https://www.ajph.org by clicking the "Reprints" link.

PUBLICATION INFORMATION

Full Citation: Taylor LA, Caplan AL. Public health policymaking outside of the federal government: reflections on authority and trust-building challenges. *Am J Public Health*. 2026;116(1):51–56.

Acceptance Date: October 15, 2025.

DOI: https://doi.org/10.2105/AJPH.2025.308331

ORCID iDs:

Lauren A. Taylor https://orcid.org/0000-0002-9608-6878

Arthur L. Caplan https://orcid.org/0000-0002-4061-8011

CONTRIBUTORS

The authors contributed equally to this work.

ACKNOWLEDGMENTS

The authors would like to acknowledge two fantastic research assistants, Ria Dharnidharka and Caroline Shore, for their support.

CONFLICTS OF INTEREST

The authors have no conflicts of interest to disclose.

REFERENCES

1. Schwartz JL. Evaluating and deploying COVID-19 vaccines—the importance of transparency, scientific integrity, and public trust. *N Engl J Med*. 2020;383(18):1703–1705. https://doi.org/10.1056/NEJMp2026393
2. *Kennedy, Secretary of Health and Human Services, et al. v. Braidwood Management, Inc., et al.*, No. 24–316, slip op. at 10 (U.S. June 27, 2025).
3. White House. Commencing the reduction of the federal bureaucracy. February 19, 2025. Available at: https://www.whitehouse.gov/presidential-actions/2025/02/commencing-the-reduction-of-the-federal-bureaucracy. Accessed November 9, 2025.
4. White House. Restoring gold standard science. May 23, 2025. Available at: https://www.whitehouse.gov/presidential-actions/2025/05/restoring-gold-standard-science. Accessed November 9, 2025.
5. Kennedy RF Jr. RFK Jr.: HHS moves to restore public trust in vaccines. *Wall Street Journal*. June 9, 2025. Available at: https://www.wsj.com/opinion/rfk-jr-hhs-moves-to-restore-public-trust-in-vaccines-45495112. Accessed November 9, 2025.
6. McCabe D, Kang C. Trump fires Democrats on Federal Trade Commission. *New York Times*. March 18, 2025. Available at: https://www.nytimes.com/2025/03/18/technology/trump-ftc-fires-democrats.html?searchResultPosition=2. Accessed November 9, 2025.
7. Federal Trade Commission. The attention economy: how big tech firms exploit children and hurt families. June 4, 2025. Available at: https://www.ftc.gov/news-events/events/2025/06/attention-economy-tech-firms-exploit-children. Accessed November 9, 2025.
8. Schwartz JL. Revised recommendations for COVID-19 vaccines—US vaccination policy under threat. *N Engl J Med*. 2025;393(5):417–419. https://doi.org/10.1056/NEJMp2507766
9. Stone W, Stein R, Huang P, Wroth C. CDC advisers punt on hepatitis B vaccine vote, after changing guidance on MMRV. 2025. Available at: https://www.npr.org/2025/09/18/nx-s1-5542082/cdc-acip-vaccine-hepatitis-b-mmrv. Accessed November 9, 2025.
10. Madani D. West Coast states band together to provide vaccine recommendation after RFK Jr. replaces CDC panel. September 3, 2025. Available at: https://www.nbcnews.com/health/health-news/california-oregon-washington-vaccine-cdc-rfk-jr-rcna228800. Accessed November 9, 2025.
11. Office of Governor Gavin Newsom. California, Oregon, and Washington to launch new West Coast Health Alliance to uphold scientific integrity in public health as Trump destroys CDC's credibility. September 3, 2025. Available at: https://www.gov.ca.gov/2025/09/03/california-oregon-and-washington-to-launch-new-west-coast-health-alliance-to-uphold-scientific-integrity-in-public-health-as-trump-destroys-cdcs-credibility. Accessed November 9, 2025.
12. Laughlin J. Eight states, including Mass., met this week in a step toward public health independence from the federal government. *The Boston Globe*. August 22, 2025. Available at: https://www.bostonglobe.com/2025/08/22/metro/vaccine-public-health-massachusetts-pennsylvania-rhode-island-vermont-connecticut-maine-kennedy-trump. Accessed November 9, 2025.
13. Joint Commission. The new standard. Accreditation 360. Available at: https://www.jointcommission.org/en-us. Accessed November 9, 2025.
14. US Government Accountability Office. Institutional review boards: actions needed to improve federal oversight and examine effectiveness. January 2023. Available at: https://www.gao.gov/assets/gao-23-104721.pdf. Accessed November 9, 2025.

15. Osterholm MT. The U.S. government is failing on vaccine policy: the Vaccine Integrity Project is here to help. July 3, 2025. Available at: https://www.statnews.com/2025/07/03/vaccine-integrity-project-michael-osterholm-cidrap-rsv-flu-covid. Accessed November 9, 2025.
16. Michener JD. *Fragmented Democracy: Medicaid, Federalism, and Unequal Politics.* Cambridge, UK: Cambridge University Press; 2018.
17. Healey M, Driscoll K. Governor Healey announces immediate steps to ensure vaccine availability in Massachusetts amid Trump, RFK rollbacks. September 4, 2025. Available at: https://www.mass.gov/news/governor-healey-announces-immediate-steps-to-ensure-vaccine-availability-in-massachusetts-amid-trump-rfk-rollbacks. Accessed November 9, 2025.
18. Felsenthal E. An expert on trust says we're thinking about it all wrong. *Time.* March 17, 2024. Available at: https://time.com/6957741/rachel-botsman-trust-interview. Accessed November 9, 2025.

Public Trust, Private Data: Four Considerations for the Future of Health

Nabarun Dasgupta, MPH, PhD, Jennifer D. Schoendorf, PhD, Denys T. Lau, PhD, and Lorna Thorpe, PhD

ABOUT THE AUTHORS

All authors are editors of AJPH. *Nabarun Dasgupta is with the Gillings School of Global Public Health, University of North Carolina, Chapel Hill. Jennifer D. Schoendorf is with the School of Public Health, University of Maryland, College Park. Denys T. Lau is with Johns Hopkins University, Baltimore, MD. Lorna Thorpe is with the Department of Population Health, NYU Grossman School of Medicine, New York, NY.*

See also Trust in Public Health, pp. 31–94.

The current political movement toward deregulation[1] is explicitly intended to increase the presence of private and commercial entities in American health. Information technology is one area in which the private sector can potentially achieve gains that elude government. We posit that publicly held governmental data systems are better suited to answer questions of prevalence and incidence. In contrast, privately held data can often provide better in-depth detail on causes and consequences. As funding for federal data systems is cut, there is an assumption that private-sector innovations will automatically deliver more trustworthy data. We fear disappointment.

While the coming transformation of health data systems affords opportunity for genuine innovation, privatization may also decrement trust. Drawing on examples from across public health, we highlight four domains: (1) data being fit for purpose, (2) methods transparency, (3) selection bias, and (4) long-term reliability. The throughline is independent data quality assessment to build public trust and promote innovation.

EXAMPLES OF PRIVATELY AND PUBLICLY HELD DATA

To orient readers, we provide the following definitions.

Privately Held Data

We use the term privately held data to refer to the wide range of nonpublic data sources generated by nongovernmental organizations, whether corporations and nonprofits. Privately held data encompass commercial laboratory testing, electronic health records, and field reports from humanitarian relief agencies during natural disasters.

Data collected during the process of nonresearch activity, like delivering clinical care, are also called secondary data. Quality is optimized for operations or transactions, so information may not be as complete or accurate as researchers would like. We use the broader term privately held data instead. We emphasize that modern commercial systems are often designed to monetize delivery of services *and* sale of data simultaneously: biometric data from consumer smartwatches inform public perception of health when released in aggregate by the company or via external researchers. In an information-hungry environment, the speedy availability of privately held data can drive public and scientific consensus. Based on the impulse to envision the breadth of future possibilities, examples from Mpox, coronavirus, and other "infodemics" have been studied.[2] Careful studies with nuanced results may be published later, but by then, attention has waned, and beliefs have settled. That rigorous studies are overlooked by the public in favor of less formal data is persistently frustrating.

In the field of public health monitoring or surveillance, these informal information sources are used for situational awareness: news and social media, school closures, hospital bed capacity, air quality indices, 911 calls, and mobile phone movement data. If considered in isolation, these sources are insufficient to base immediate population health decisions, but when triangulated provide context for more established, but limited, sources. Fast-moving data also shape trust in short-term government responses because they are timely and have inherent real-world simplicity, such as quantifying opioids and cocaine in wastewater[3] by a private company. These types of metrics grain immediate traction because they leverage our preconception of what should be possible. Simple metrics are often preferred by journalists and influencers, allowing them to quickly build a narrative around a straightforward data point.

Publicly Held Data

We now contrast publicly held data. These are data sources funded and, or, produced by government where the intent is for the information to be widely accessible. (We further differentiate "publicly held data" from "public data" meaning data sets accessed for free without restriction.) Examples of publicly held data include open mapping data sets from municipalities, large federally managed representative surveys, vital statistics of births and deaths, claims from government benefits, and public housing data. Based on standards of government accountability and intended use, these data sets have detailed documentation, but there are time lags. With taxpayer investment, methods and governance emphasize generalizability and strong privacy protections.

Communities of practice develop, with users sharing code and experiences while uncovering limitations. This process is imbued with transparency and marked by communal desire to improve knowledge yet can be dependent on technical training, limiting who participates. The ability of government agencies to provide user support differs by resources and priorities.

FITNESS OF PURPOSE

The first question of any data source is whether it contains information to answer the specific question. In federal statistics[4,5] the concept is called fitness of purpose: to what purposes are the data best suited? We offer a simple rubric: publicly held data are better suited to answer "How many?" and "Where?" Privately held data can answer "Why?" and "So what?"

Human cognition is tuned to crave novelty, and clever repurposing of tools at hand is a widely celebrated cultural value. If new data sources cannot answer actual questions, they become an expensive distraction. Therefore, assessing fitness should precede investment to obtain and develop new data sets.

We offer an example from nutrition.[6] Public governmental surveys have been the established measure of food insecurity, providing estimates that are nationally representative. By contrast, data from subsidized benefits utilization offer localized granularity yet are distinctly different because only certain households access benefits. In contrast, privately held data sources illuminate underlying causes and dynamics: weekly fluctuations in food pantry demand elucidate acute local scarcity; grocery receipt data track changes in dietary preferences; and food outlet mapping reveals areas of limited access. Ironic then that the large federal survey was terminated in September 2025 by the US Department of Agriculture for being "redundant."[7]

Usability design principles make it easy to start using a new tool, but when applied superficially, the metric of commercial success becomes uptake, not appropriateness. Possible solutions include showing appropriate use cases, having guidelines in licensing agreements, and tempering promotion with humility. We gain proficiency in the data system we use most or for which we are responsible. Yet, there is space to mingle, requiring researchers to become familiar with adjacent data sets. In turn, this requires data holders to be explicit about methods.

THE OPACITY PROBLEM

Methods to collect and process privately held data are often undisclosed. Sampling can be a closely held competitive secret, such as sales of medications. Commercial data vendors withhold geographically precise locations from researchers to protect the identity of individuals and medical facilities they have contracted, limiting spatial granularity. Producing and maintaining documentation can also be costly.

However, many privately held data systems are critical because there are no governmental correlates. For example, the US Food and Drug Administration (FDA) relies on commercial vendors for drug sales data because medical product utilization is not recorded with precision in national surveys. Validation studies can foster confidence in privately held data. An example is fast-reporting private data from pharmacy sales of cancer medications, compared with what can be gleaned from slower-but-more-comprehensive government-sponsored cancer registries.[8]

Beyond sampling, algorithms created by commercial entities often lack basic methodology disclosure. For example, clinical decision support tools for opioid prescribing "risk" have been criticized[9] for having arbitrary scores generated by a black box algorithm. During the early stages of the coronavirus pandemic, public scandal erupted when a data vendor grossly imputed patient-level missing data on therapies.[10] While we do not automatically ascribe malicious intent by commercial data vendors, these examples offer cautions.

Systematic assessment of data quality is not often found in journal guidelines or presented in academic search engines, and existing checklists focus on disclosure of analytical processes. As proprietary methods resist external scrutiny, we wonder if there is need for standardized and self-reportable data quality metrics[11] that simultaneously protect intellectual property.

The solution to the opacity problem is methods transparency and independent validation. This can be bolstered by incentives for internal and external assessments and validation studies, or appropriate use demonstrations.

Independent validation is therefore a lubricant to acceptability of private sector–led innovation, and the disappearance of validation studies will be detrimental to public health and commercial success. A resource-intensive alternative is the FDA's preparatory work for Advisory Committee meetings. The same data sets are analyzed by federal scientists and industry sponsors, with results presented publicly in tandem. Scaling back support for regulatory science and methods research hampers scientific progress and leads to public distrust.

SELECTION BIAS IN MARKET DATA

Corporations are answerable primarily to shareholders, not the public health community. In contrast, public agencies are mandated to serve all. State health department reports include *all* counties, not only populous ones. Seeking data volume, commercial data often follow population patterns; the absolute number of people will be considerably higher from urban areas. The experiences of Americans in rural areas may be systematically excluded. Returning to the smartwatch example, residents where cellular or Wi-Fi connectivity is spotty will be less inclined to purchase the gadget. Those who do purchase might have outsized benefits. One study in Kentucky found that mobile devices improved inclusivity for some cancer patients, but participation was also dependent on digital literacy.[12] We must ask how much of their community these individuals are being asked to stand in for, to represent as part of the broader whole.

An employee benefits company released a report that purported to identify the top 25 locations with the worst opioid abuse problems nationwide, but locations seemed to cluster in the southeastern United States.[13] The company did not disclose that its clients were largely limited to urban areas of the South. The report was cited by health professionals, news organizations, and government officials, without critical examination of selection bias. Publicly held data would have been preferable for a question of prevalence.

Every ingenious new sampling strategy (e.g., untapped customer market) also confers selection bias.[14] The central questions center around what public health questions to apply these to, and what the bounds of appropriate inference are. Again, the role of independent assessors is central to commercialization success *and* public trust. To be fair, traditional large cohort-based studies with purposeful sampling can also be plagued[15] by biases, and plummeting response rates[16] are a major concern for long-term viability of large probability-sampled governmental surveys.

With investment in assessing data quality, these biases can rise to the surface and methods can be developed to account for them collaboratively. Yet cuts in biomedical funding paradoxically threaten public inclusivity, trust, and accuracy that assist innovation adoption.

PITFALLS OF THE PIVOT

The key to commercial innovation is the pivot: the ability for companies to change offerings when existing business models are not delivering returns. Similarly, service organizations will shift to providing services where they are needed. A major gain from private-led innovation is rapid development of new technology and products to fill underserved niches, because governmental surveys can take years to evaluate, test, and adopt new questions; meanwhile, report generation and maintenance in high-accountability settings can make results irrelevant.

Time trend graphs are a mainstay of public health reports; a tangible benefit of publicly held data is constancy. Longitudinal trends are possible with consistent measurement, and public discourse often centers around whether disease is increasing or decreasing. Consistently collected publicly held data satisfies a major societal need.

Another kind of pivot with commercial entities involves acquisitions. Recently a major direct-to-consumer genetic testing company whose data had been used in research filed for bankruptcy[17] after experiencing a major data breach. The court ordered the company to be sold immediately to pay back investors. The future of immense detailed genetic information hangs in limbo. While publicly held data systems are also sunset, government accountability standards are more likely to result in orderly phase-out.

Solutions are limited. When companies pivot, it may be conceivable that they make historical data public. Instead of abandoning projects completely, it may also be possible for end-of-life planning to include handoffs. Contractual commitments to longer-term service could also be achieved with public–private incentivization.

BUILDING ON SUCCESS

Public health domains with strong historical collaboration between private

AJPH January 2026, Vol. 116, No. 1

data holders and researchers can be found in occupational epidemiology, environmental health, pharmacoepidemiology, military health, and sports medicine.

Data from the National Basketball Association[18] and National Football League[19] during the 2020 season were some of the earliest quantifications of coronavirus transmissibility and testing accuracy. In these instances, the need for accurate data aligned with the commercial imperative to keep professional athletes, vendors, coaches, and support staff healthy. They consented to wearing biosensors and regular blood draws, with the shared goal of keeping their sports alive at a time when other forms of civic engagement were curtailed. By collaborating with qualified scientists, the sampling methodology and measurements were reliable for inference by design. Researchers took advantage of isolation "bubbles," deployed novel biosensing devices, made public presentations, conducted validation, and published methods in high-quality journals. Their effort was not intended to be permanent but, rather, a cleverly focused effort to address a major public need.

Private entities complement traditional public sources by rapidly integrating novel data streams, creating previously impossible linkages that reveal hidden population health patterns. Technology platforms enable businesses to synthesize information across multiple sources with unprecedented speed, generating insights that would require years to achieve through conventional governmental processes. Industry's operational flexibility allows for rapid pilot testing and iterative refinement, providing valuable proof-of-concept models that government agencies can adapt and scale. While government agencies operate under necessary privacy protections and data-sharing restrictions that ensure accountability, these same constraints limit their ability to experiment with emerging technology and higher-volume data sharing.

LIMITATIONS

This examination of trust in health data is not intended to be exhaustive. "Public trust" is a broad concept,[20] oft discussed but understudied. We leave open the question of who should be involved in quality assessment and minimum levels of human competency. There are more potential data sets than formally qualified epidemiologists and data scientists; perhaps automation and citizen science have roles. We also find that while researchers are customers, they are often in thrall to monopolistic vendors and cannot effectively demand methods transparency. Simple frameworks for quality assessment require private-sector participation. These open issues demonstrate the difficulties.

CONCLUSIONS

As trusted government sources disappear, it will be human nature to search for alternatives. Commercial entities with privately held data are engines of ingenuity. We should welcome new ideas and well-validated tools in public health, especially as the pace of technology development accelerates.

But corporations should be ready to embrace scrutiny to monetize their data products responsibly. For outputs to be trusted across the public health community and by the general public, candor would be appreciated as to which questions their data can and cannot answer. Publicly held data are likely the bedrock of knowledge-making for the immediate future, but privately held data are an indelible part of the broader information landscape, and we ignore them to our detriment.

When it comes to trust, industry has obligations. Explicitly stating conflicts of interest is a spotty practice. In the United States, individual-level privacy is not guaranteed. Protecting private-sector data from malicious actors requires more than passive reliance on encryption. We are one data breach away from a public trust catastrophe.

In the free market of health knowledge, at the nexus of public and private data, are the independent evaluators. Paradoxically, health methods research is being cut concurrently with deregulation, just as long-heralded advances in artificial intelligence and portable devices are coming to fruition. This is shortsighted and harms both public trust and commercial viability. AJPH

CORRESPONDENCE

Correspondence should be sent to Nabarun Dasgupta, 725 MLK Jr Blvd, CB 7505, University of North Carolina, Chapel Hill, NC 27599 (e-mail: nab@unc.edu). Reprints can be ordered at https://www.ajph.org by clicking the "Reprints" link.

PUBLICATION INFORMATION

Full Citation: Dasgupta N, Schoendorf JD, Lau DT, Thorpe L. Public trust, private data: four considerations for the future of health. *Am J Public Health*. 2026;116(1):57–63.

Acceptance Date: October 14, 2025.

DOI: https://doi.org/10.2105/AJPH.2025.308328

ORCID iDs:

Nabarun Dasgupta https://orcid.org/0000-0002-4098-605X

Lorna Thorpe https://orcid.org/0000-0002-5535-2674

CONTRIBUTORS

All authors contributed equally to this article.

CONFLICTS OF INTEREST

The authors report no conflicts of interest.

REFERENCES

1. Department of Health and Human Services, Office of the Secretary. Request for Information (RFI): Ensuring Lawful Regulation and Unleashing Innovation to Make American Healthy Again. *Federal Register* 2025;90 FR 20478(2025-08384). Available at: https://www.federalregister.gov/documents/2025/05/14/2025-08384/request-for-information-rfi-ensuring-lawful-regulation-and-unleashing-innovation-to-make-american. Accessed October 1, 2025.
2. Kirk J. Infodemic, ignorance, or imagination? The problem of misinformation in health emergencies. *Int Polit Sociol.* 2024;18(4):olae036. https://doi.org/10.1093/ips/olae036
3. Endo N, Ghaeli N, Duvallet C, et al. Rapid assessment of opioid exposure and treatment in cities through robotic collection and chemical analysis of wastewater. *J Med Toxicol.* 2020;16(2):195–203. https://doi.org/10.1007/s13181-019-00756-5
4. Federal Committee on Statistical Methodology. *A Framework for Data Quality*. September 2020. Available at: https://nces.ed.gov/fcsm/pdf/FCSM.20.04_A_Framework_for_Data_Quality.pdf. Accessed October 1, 2025.
5. US Department of Health and Human Services. HHS announces crackdown on health data blocking. September 3, 2025. Available at: https://www.hhs.gov/press-room/hhs-crackdown-health-data-blocking.html. Accessed October 1, 2025.
6. Arteaga I, Wilde PE. Measuring food security in the United States for more than 25 years: history, methods, findings, and opportunities. *J Acad Nutr Diet.* 2023;123(10S):S5–S19. https://doi.org/10.1016/j.jand.2023.01.007
7. US Department of Agriculture. USDA terminates redundant food insecurity survey. September 20, 2025. Available at: https://www.usda.gov/about-usda/news/press-releases/2025/09/20/usda-terminates-redundant-food-insecurity-survey. Accessed October 1, 2025.
8. Tran Q, Warren JL, Barrett MJ, et al. An evaluation of the utility of Big Data to supplement cancer treatment information: linkage between IQVIA pharmacy database and the Surveillance, Epidemiology, and End Results Program. *J Natl Cancer Inst Monogr.* 2020;2020(55):72–81. https://doi.org/10.1093/jncimonographs/lgz036
9. Buonora MJ, Axson SA, Cohen SM, Becker WC. Paths forward for clinicians amidst the rise of unregulated clinical decision support software: our perspective on NarxCare. *J Gen Intern Med.* 2024;39(5):858–862. https://doi.org/10.1007/s11606-023-08528-2
10. Servick K, Enserink M. The pandemic's first major research scandal erupts. *Science.* 2020;368(6495):1041–1042. https://doi.org/10.1126/science.368.6495.1041
11. Parker JD, Mirel LB, Lee P, Mintz R, Tungate A, Vaidyanathan A. Evaluating data quality for blended data using a data quality framework. *Stat J IAOS.* 2024;40(1):125–136. https://doi.org/10.3233/SJI-230125
12. Donawa A, Powell C, Wang R, et al. Designing survey-based mobile interfaces for rural patients with cancer using Apple's ResearchKit and CareKit: usability study. *JMIR Form Res.* 2024;8:e57801. https://doi.org/10.2196/57801
13. Knopf T. Four North Carolina cities make top 25 list for opioid abuse. *North Carolina Health News.* July 27, 2017. Available at: https://www.northcarolinahealthnews.org/2017/07/27/four-north-carolina-cities-make-top-25-list-opioid-abuse. Accessed October 1, 2025.
14. Kundu R, Shi X, Morrison J, Barrett J, Mukherjee B. A framework for understanding selection bias in real-world healthcare data. *J R Stat Soc Ser A Stat Soc.* 2024;187(3):606–635. https://doi.org/10.1093/jrsssa/qnae039
15. Fry A, Littlejohns TJ, Sudlow C, et al. Comparison of sociodemographic and health-related characteristics of UK Biobank participants with those of the general population. *Am J Epidemiol.* 2017;186(9):1026–1034. https://doi.org/10.1093/aje/kwx246
16. Czajka JL, Beyler A. Declining response rates in federal surveys: trends and implications. Mathematica Policy Research. 2016. Available at: https://aspe.hhs.gov/sites/default/files/private/pdf/255531/Decliningresponserates.pdf. Accessed October 1, 2025.
17. Gerke S, Jacoby MB, Cohen IG. 23andMe's bankruptcy raises concerns about privacy in the era of big data. *BMJ.* 2025;389:r1071. https://doi.org/10.1136/bmj.r1071
18. Mack CD, DiFiori J, Tai CG, et al. SARS-CoV-2 transmission risk among National Basketball Association players, staff, and vendors exposed to individuals with positive test results after COVID-19 recovery during the 2020 regular and postseason. *JAMA Intern Med.* 2021;181(7):960–966. https://doi.org/10.1001/jamainternmed.2021.2114
19. Lopez MJ, Mack C, Bliss T, et al. Observed versus expected COVID-19 infections among National Football League players during the 2020 season. *Epidemiology.* 2022;33(2):193–199. https://doi.org/10.1097/EDE.0000000000001416
20. Gille F, Smith S, Mays N. What is public trust in the healthcare system? A new conceptual framework developed from qualitative data in England. *Soc Theory Health.* 2021;19(1):1–20. https://doi.org/10.1057/s41285-020-00129-x

Restoring Trust in Public Health by Preventing Financial Conflicts of Interest in the Scientific Literature and Government Decision-Making

Nicholas Chartres, PhD, MHum Nutr, Tracey J. Woodruff, PhD, MPH, and Lisa A. Bero, PhD

ABOUT THE AUTHORS

Nicholas Chartres is with the School of Pharmacy, Faculty of Medicine & Health, The University of Sydney, Australia, and The Center to End Corporate Harm, University of California, San Francisco. Tracey J. Woodruff is with the Program on Reproductive Health and the Environment, Department of Obstetrics, Gynecology, and Reproductive Sciences, and The Center to End Corporate Harm, University of California, San Francisco. Lisa A. Bero is with the Center for Bioethics and Humanities, School of Medicine and Colorado School of Public Health, University of Colorado Anschutz Medical Campus, Denver.

AJPH January 2026, Vol. 116, No. 1

See also Trust in Public Health, pp. 31–94.

Government decisions dictate the health of populations. For example, the PFAS (per and poly fluoroalkyl substances) National Primary Drinking Water Regulation set by the US Environmental Protection Agency (EPA) is expected to prevent more than 9600 deaths, including infant mortality, and reduce approximately 30 000 serious illnesses, including cardiovascular disease, with $1.5 billion per year in cost savings.[1] In addition, the Clean Air Act by EPA has lowered air pollution levels (i.e., particulate matter of 2.5 micrometers or smaller [$PM_{2.5}$] & Ozone), resulting in approximately 237 000 fewer early deaths and 2 400 000 fewer cases of asthma exacerbation in 2020, with $2 trillion in benefits, exceeding costs by a factor of more than 30 to 1.[2]

Government health-related decisions, such as those for PFAS and air pollutant–related health effects, and the development of public health guidelines, including *The Dietary Guidelines for Americans* and those produced by the US Preventive Services Task Force, are based on evaluating the available science. Thus, the rules or methods that are used to identify and evaluate the science have profound consequences for people's health. As a consequence, it is critical that government decision-making be based on transparent, consistent methods that reduce bias. High-quality systematic reviews are increasingly being used as the evidence base for decision-making as this method reduces bias in evidence evaluation. In addition, the science review panels that peer review government science-based documents and decisions influence the scientific basis of decision-making. Therefore, rigorous financial conflict of interest (COI) policies are required to protect the integrity of government recommendations.

Industry involvement in government public health processes can distort the evidence-based decision-making process and harm the integrity of government recommendations or regulations. For example, nine out of 20 members of the 2025 Dietary Guidelines Advisory Committee had a COI either from research collaborations or consultancy with food, pharmaceutical, or weight-loss companies.[3] This committee did not issue recommendations limiting the consumption of ultra-processed foods in the 2025 Dietary Guidelines Advisory Committee report, despite evidence from rigorous systematic reviews establishing that ultra-processed food consumption is associated with numerous adverse health effects.[4] In addition, the American Academy of Pediatrics (AAP) guidelines for prescribing antiobesity drugs (including GLP-1 agonists such as Ozempic) concluded that pediatricians "should offer adolescents 12 y and older with obesity [weight] loss pharmacotherapy" and "may" offer these drugs to children aged 8 to 11 years.[5] AAP has received approximately $2 million sponsorship from GLP-1 drug companies, with payments also to AAP's national leaders and members of its guideline committee, leading to potentially harmful drug prescribing to children.[5]

In this editorial, we review two critical parts of developing guidelines or regulations (collectively called "government decision-making") where bias can be introduced: (1) the methods, particularly the systematic review methods (or lack thereof), used to evaluate the evidence to inform them; and (2) the scientific review committees or guideline panelists that review science and formulate recommendations based on science.[6] We then provide actionable examples of necessary safeguards to protect scientific integrity to inform guideline recommendations and regulations and models for developing guideline panels and government scientific committees that should be adopted globally to restore trust in public health.

SYSTEMATIC REVIEW METHODS

Systematic review is a key method for reducing bias in guideline development and regulations. Systematic reviews use transparent, consistent, and valid methods to identify, evaluate, and summarize all available data to answer a specific research question and are considered the gold standard in clinical medicine and in environmental health, and have been recommended by multiple US National Academies of Sciences, Engineering, and Medicine (NASEM) committees.[7,8] Systematic reviews result in evaluation of the scientific data that has less bias and error and thus increases the reliability and trust in the results and conclusions drawn from the review.[7] For example, the EPA used systematic reviews to evaluate the evidence on the human health effects of PFAS chemicals to develop the National Primary Drinking Water Regulations for PFAS, and EPA was able to identify more health effects than previously would have been possible, including developmental effects such as reduced fetal growth and resultant infant mortality.[9] These methods were advanced over several years by the Office of Research and Development as part of EPA's Integrated Risk Information System Process following feedback from the NASEM, with several critical NASEM recommendations still yet to be adopted.[8] However, systematic reviews are of variable quality and there has been an increase in the misappropriation of the term, with many failing to comply with best-practice methods that minimize bias and error.[10,11] Bias in systematic reviews can result either from how bias is assessed in the individual studies included within the review or from the conduct of the review itself.

FINANCIAL CONFLICTS OF INTEREST IN SYSTEMATIC REVIEWS

Financial COIs must be systematically evaluated and eliminated as a bias from systematic reviews used to inform guidelines and regulations. Financial COIs can influence study outcomes independent of other methods, and thus, it is recommended to be accounted for in the evaluation of the study quality in the evidence review. To identify the most reliable studies, a key step in conducting a systematic review is to assess the internal validity or "risk of bias" of the individual studies included in the review. Bias in an individual study can be attributable to its methodological or design features, including how the participants were enrolled into a study, leading to differences in baseline characteristics between groups that may influence the effect of an intervention or exposure in one direction (e.g., different age characteristics or health status) or how the exposure and outcomes were assessed (e.g., whether comparable validated and reliable approaches were used across all study participants to measure them). Assessment of the risk of bias across studies can help categorize studies as being lower or higher risk when synthesizing study results all together—for example, when conducting a meta-analysis (the quantitative combining of individual study results). If all the included studies have many biases, there will be lower overall confidence in the results drawn from the evidence than if they have none.

However, bias in studies included in systematic reviews can also arise because of nonmethodological factors, such whether the study is funded by an industry (corporation) that makes the product under evaluation (e.g., chemical, drug, food) or whether the study authors have a financial COI.[12] Evidence across multiple disciplines, including pharmaceuticals, chemicals, tobacco, and nutrition, has shown that even when accounting for differences in the methodological biases across studies, studies with either industry sponsorship or authors with a financial COI (collectively known as financial COI) are more likely to report results that are favorable toward the sponsor's product under evaluation (e.g., drugs are more efficacious, chemicals are less harmful).[13–15] This research also demonstrates that disclosures of financial COIs are insufficient to mitigate this bias. If this empirically established bias is not evaluated and accounted for when synthesizing individual studies, it can skew the evidence and distort the results on the product under evaluation. Thus, the recommendations that are made in guidelines or regulations that have used systematic reviews to inform them could be at best misleading and at worst harmful to human health. Furthermore, the findings of systematic reviews can be influenced by industry sponsorship or author financial COIs of the review itself and should also be prevented.[13,14,16]

ASSESSMENT FOR POTENTIAL RISK OF BIAS

Financial COIs should be assessed as a potential risk of bias and used to test the influence of these studies on guideline recommendations and regulations. Current approaches and tools to assess the risk of bias of studies included in systematic reviews do not routinely assess whether a study has a financial COI. It is argued that biases that may be introduced into a study by a financial COI would be detected by assessing the design and conduct of the study. However, there are multiple ways financial COIs can bias research including the types of study questions asked, study design and conduct (e.g., unfair comparisons), coding of the data, incomplete reporting of the data, or misleading presentation of study conclusions ("spin").[17] Investigating the sources of bias requires different methods. For example, internal industry document analyses can determine if a study has intentionally incompletely reported data to introduce a bias. Therefore, these potential mechanisms cannot be feasibly identified and accounted for using current risk of bias approaches.[12]

One of the simplest and most important ways to systematically evaluate and eliminate financial COIs from the evidentiary base used in systematic reviews is to include financial COIs as part of the risk of bias assessment when conducting a systematic review. The NASEM have recommended in multiple reports that funding sources and funding bias should be assessed in EPA's assessments,[18] including in the conduct of risk of bias assessments of individual studies.[8] Including financial COIs as a risk of bias does not automatically exclude a study from consideration. Rather, it means documenting it as one of several domains that may potentially bias a study result. Additional analysis can then be conducted to see if the results of studies differ by the presence of financial COIs. If they do not, all the evidence is recommended to be considered together.

SAFEGUARDING SCIENTIFIC INTEGRITY TO INFORM GUIDELINES

Such assessments of financial COIs, however, can only be conducted if there are full disclosures of funding source and author financial COIs. One solution to prevent fragmented disclosures across journals could be the creation of a central registry of payments from various industries to scientists and academic institutions, similar to the Physicians Payments Sunshine Act of 2013.[19]

Journals could also play an important role in ensuring all authors disclose any financial COIs. If study authors are found not to disclose a financial COI according to the International Committee of Medical Journal Editors' recommendations, penalties for noncompliance may be necessary, including prohibiting authors from publishing across journals that register to implement a disclosure policy. Journals could also restrict the influence of industry-funded research further by implementing policies that prohibit the publication of such research. A number of journals already refuse to publish tobacco industry–funded research.[20,21] Similar policies should be considered for other industries that produce health-harming products, including chemical, fossil fuel, alcohol, ultra-processed foods, gambling, firearms, and pharmaceuticals. Restrictions on authors with a financial COI should also be considered that would ensure the first and last authors along with the majority of authors are free from financial COIs.[21] In addition, systematic review teams should also be free of financial COIs, and reviews should not be sponsored by an industry whose product is included in the review to minimize bias in the conduct of systematic reviews used to inform guidelines and regulations.[21]

A key mechanism to fully ameliorate the impact of financial COIs on the evidence that is used in systematic reviews to inform public health guidelines and regulations is through alternative funding models that remove any commercial interest from the research process. These mechanisms and structures include an increase in government funding for public health research or alternative sources (e.g., from tax on corporate marketing).[19] Such an approach would eliminate researchers' reliance on industry sponsorship and remove any direct contact or involvement with commercial funders.

FINANCIAL CONFLICTS OF INTEREST IN GOVERNMENT DECISION-MAKING

Evaluating the scientific evidence is one part in the development of government decision-making, including public health guidelines and regulations. Government science advisory boards or other government commissioned entities will peer review government scientific products. In other cases, scientific guideline panels will formulate recommendations based on a range of scientific information and other important considerations. It has been well established that financial COIs of guideline panels and scientific recommendations result in recommendations that favor the interests of the entities from which they receive financial benefits.[22]

Disclosure of financial COIs of guideline panel members is often recommended as a way to "manage" COIs in the guideline process. However, disclosure does not eliminate or reduce bias. It has been identified that, paradoxically, members of panels who disclose their COIs provide more biased advice based on the belief they have provided sufficient warning about their conflicts or to compensate in the belief that the opinion and advice they offer will likely be disregarded because of the disclosure.[23] In addition, as discussed previously, evidence from several systematic reviews has demonstrated that disclosures do not reduce bias, as financial COI is associated with research outcomes biased toward the sponsor's product.[13–15] Therefore, financial COIs should be disclosed, identified, and prevented from influencing the decision-making process so that those with financial COIs are disqualified when identifying candidates for scientific committees and guideline panels.[24] An exception process could be defined that, for specific circumstances, such conflicts will be allowed (e.g., unusually specific expertise), but the member should not be included in the interpretation and evaluation of any scientific data or in formulating a committee's conclusions on what is known about the topic or product under evaluation.[6]

A government scientific committee's and guideline panel's definition of what constitutes a financial COI should include receiving financial compensation from companies or their trade associations for performing a range of science-related tasks, including research, or providing advice on the interpretation of scientific studies. Where the work performed relates directly to the product under review by a committee or panel, the financial relationship between the prospective committee or panel member and the company should be treated as evidence of bias, and the member should be disqualified.

GUIDELINE PANEL AND GOVERNMENT SCIENTIFIC COMMITTEE MODELS

All federal agencies that develop public health guidelines and regulations could adhere to the model implemented by the International Agency for Research on Cancer (IARC) for selecting scientific experts in developing Monographs that assess the evidence of carcinogenicity. Working Group members of IARC Monographs are selected based on consideration of subject matter expertise, relevant methodologies, and "absence of conflicts of interest."[25(p4)] "Invited specialists . . . who have critical knowledge and experience but who also have a conflict of interest that warrants exclusion from developing or influencing the evaluations of carcinogenicity"[25(p5)] are permitted. Invited specialists do not participate in key elements of the Monographs process, including drafting sections of the Monograph related to the description or interpretation of cancer data or participating in the evaluations. Critically, only limited numbers of experts are invited to be part of the Monographs to contribute their knowledge and expertise to the discussions in circumstances when it is determined necessary to assist the Working Group.[25] Thus, this strict process safeguards against reduced scientific quality of the Monographs as they are developed by independent experts free of any financial COIs, while ensuring input from all the best-qualified experts.

CONCLUSION

To increase trust and integrity in public health guidelines, regulations, and government decision-making, the systematic reviews used to inform them, the scientific review committees responsible for evaluating the science, and the guideline panels responsible for developing recommendations must be free of financial COIs. AJPH

CORRESPONDENCE

Correspondence should be sent to Nicholas Chartres, School of Pharmacy, Faculty of Medicine & Health, The University of Sydney, Sydney 2006, Australia (e-mail: nicholas.chartres@sydney.edu.au). Reprints can be ordered at https://www.ajph.org by clicking the "Reprints" link.

PUBLICATION INFORMATION

Full Citation: Chartres N, Woodruff TJ, Bero LA. Restoring trust in public health by preventing financial conflicts of interest in the scientific literature and government decision-making. *Am J Public Health*. 2026;116(1):62–66.

Acceptance Date: October 21, 2025.

DOI: https://doi.org/10.2105/AJPH.2025.308338

ORCID iDs:

Nicholas Chartres https://orcid.org/0000-0002-9659-6739

Tracey J. Woodruff https://orcid.org/0000-0003-3622-1297

Lisa A. Bero https://orcid.org/0000-0003-1893-6651

CONTRIBUTORS

All authors contributed equally to the conceptualization, drafting, and final approval of the article.

CONFLICTS OF INTEREST

The authors have no conflicts of interest to disclose.

REFERENCES

1. US Environmental Protection Agency. Final PFAS National Primary Drinking Water Regulation. Available at: https://www.epa.gov/system/files/documents/2024-04/drinking-water-utilities-and-professionals-technical-overview-of-pfas-npdwr.pdf. Accessed September 10, 2025.

2. US Environmental Protection Agency. Clean Air Act overview. Progress cleaning the air and improving people's health. Available at: https://www.epa.gov/clean-air-act-overview/progress-cleaning-air-and-improving-peoples-health. Accessed September 9, 2025.
3. Mahase E. US dietary committee is plagued with "high risk conflicts of interest," report finds. *BMJ.* 2023;383:2313. https://doi.org/10.1136/bmj.p2313
4. Lane MM, Gamage E, Du S, et al. Ultra-processed food exposure and adverse health outcomes: umbrella review of epidemiological meta-analyses. *BMJ.* 2024;384:e077310. https://doi.org/10.1136/bmj-2023-077310
5. Hagenaars LL, Bero LA, van der Voorn B, Schmidt LA. Caution is prescribed for American Academy of Paediatrics' guidelines on weight loss medications for childhood obesity. *BMJ.* 2025;390:e084760. https://doi.org/10.1136/bmj-2025-084760
6. Parker L, Bero L. Managing risk from conflicts of interest in guideline development committees. *BMJ.* 2022;379:e072252. https://doi.org/10.1136/bmj-2022-072252
7. Woodruff TJ, Sutton P. The Navigation Guide systematic review methodology: a rigorous and transparent method for translating environmental health science into better health outcomes. *Environ Health Perspect.* 2014;122(10):1007–1014. https://doi.org/10.1289/ehp.1307175
8. National Research Council. *Review of EPA's Integrated Risk Information System (IRIS) Process.* Washington, DC: The National Academies Press; 2014:170.
9. US Environmental Protection Agency Office of Water Health and Ecological Criteria Division. FINAL Human Health Toxicity Assessment for Perfluorooctanoic Acid (PFOA) and Related Salts. Available at: https://www.epa.gov/system/files/documents/2024-05/final-human-health-toxicity-assessment-pfoa.pdf. Accessed September 8, 2025.
10. Rayasam SDG, Koman PD, Axelrad DA, Woodruff TJ, Chartres N. Toxic Substances Control Act (TSCA) implementation: how the amended law has failed to protect vulnerable populations from toxic chemicals in the United States. *Environ Sci Technol.* 2022;56(17):11969–11982. https://doi.org/10.1021/acs.est.2c02079
11. Bero L. Systematic review: a method at risk for being corrupted. *Am J Public Health.* 2017;107(1):93–96. https://doi.org/10.2105/ajph.2016.303518
12. Bero LA. Why the Cochrane risk of bias tool should include funding source as a standard item. *Cochrane Database Syst Rev.* 2013;2013(12):ED000075. https://doi.org/10.1002/14651858.Ed000075
13. Lundh A, Lexchin J, Mintzes B, Schroll JB, Bero L. Industry sponsorship and research outcome. *Cochrane Database Syst Rev.* 2017;2(2):MR000033. https://doi.org/10.1002/14651858.MR000033.pub3
14. Barnes DE, Bero LA. Industry-funded research and conflict of interest: an analysis of research sponsored by the tobacco industry through the Center for Indoor Air Research. *J Health Polit Policy Law.* 1996;21(3):515–542. https://doi.org/10.1215/03616878-21-3-515
15. Chartres N, Fabbri A, McDonald S, Diong J, McKenzie JE, Bero L. Association of food industry ties with findings of studies examining the effect of dairy food intake on cardiovascular disease and mortality: systematic review and meta-analysis. *BMJ Open.* 2020;10(12):e039036. https://doi.org/10.1136/bmjopen-2020-039036
16. Yank V, Rennie D, Bero LA. Financial ties and concordance between results and conclusions in meta-analyses: retrospective cohort study. *BMJ.* Dec 8 2007;335(7631):1202–1205. https://doi.org/10.1136/bmj.39376.447211.BE
17. Odierna DH, Forsyth SR, White J, Bero LA. The cycle of bias in health research: a framework and toolbox for critical appraisal training. *Account Res.* 2013;20(2):127–141. https://doi.org/10.1080/08989621.2013.768931
18. National Academies of Sciences, Engineering, and Medicine. *Review of US EPA's ORD Staff Handbook for Developing IRIS Assessments: 2020 Version.* 2022. https://doi.org/10.17226/26289
19. Lexchin J, Bero LA, Davis C, Gagnon MA. Achieving greater independence from commercial influence in research. *BMJ.* 2021;372:n370. https://doi.org/10.1136/bmj.n370
20. Godlee F, Malone R, Timmis A, et al. Journal policy on research funded by the tobacco industry. *BMJ.* 2013;347:f5193. https://doi.org/10.1136/bmj.f5193
21. Cochrane Library. Cochrane Database of Systematic Reviews: editorial policies. Conflict of interest policy for Cochrane Library content. 2020. Available at: https://www.cochranelibrary.com/cdsr/editorial-policies#coi. Accessed September 8, 2025.
22. Nejstgaard CH, Bero L, Hróbjartsson A, et al. Association between conflicts of interest and favourable recommendations in clinical guidelines, advisory committee reports, opinion pieces, and narrative reviews: systematic review. *BMJ.* 2020;371:m4234. https://doi.org/10.1136/bmj.m4234
23. Loewenstein G, Sah S, Cain DM. The unintended consequences of conflict of interest disclosure. *JAMA.* 2012;307(7):669–670. https://doi.org/10.1001/jama.2012.154
24. World Health Organization. *WHO Handbook for Guideline Development.* 2nd ed. 2014. Available at: https://www.who.int/publications/i/item/9789241548960. Accessed September 8, 2025.
25. International Agency for Research on Cancer. IARC Monographs on the Identification of Carcinogenic Hazards to Humans. Preamble. World Health Organization. Available at: https://monographs.iarc.who.int/wp-content/uploads/2019/07/Preamble-2019.pdf. Accessed September, 8, 2025.

Building Trust in Public Health Information Through Transparency, Inclusivity, and Community Engagement

Stewart Landers, JD, MCP, and Steven C. Fiala, PhD, MPH

ABOUT THE AUTHORS

Stewart Landers is an editor emeritus of AJPH. *Steven C. Fiala is with the Oregon Public Health Division, Portland, and is the* AJPH *deputy editor for open access supplements.*

See also Trust in Public Health, pp. 31–94.

The COVID-19 pandemic marked a turning point with respect to trust in public health decision-makers across the United States. Faced with a novel and deadly virus, public health leaders sought to protect the public from infection and severe illness or death while navigating rapidly changing information with respect to transmission modalities, screening tests, isolation and social distancing, and protective equipment, including masks, treatment, and vaccination.

Assessing the effectiveness of these activities was challenging because of limited use of rigorous methods like randomized controlled trials. Most available data came from natural experiments, such as comparing outcomes (hospitalizations, mortality) across states with different policies or between vaccinated and unvaccinated patients. The economic and social impact of restrictive policies, especially vaccine mandates, created a backlash against and especially a loss of trust in public health authorities, which has continued to grow in the aftermath of the pandemic and whose impact extends beyond COVID-19 to many facets of public health including COVID-19 and other vaccines, fluoridation, autism causes and treatment, and more.

As skepticism toward the scientific community, including public health decision-makers, increases, public health researchers and leaders have launched broad discussions about effective communication strategies and channels in a changed environment. This includes strategies to improve the effectiveness and credibility of evidence-based research findings and how those findings are utilized to drive policy decisions.

Public trust in the scientific method is an essential ingredient for the "theory-to-practice" loop to be effective, informing the acceptability of evidence-based policy interventions by the public. A set of guidelines published in *AJPH* in June 2025, the Guidance for Ensuring Quality in Scientific Publication Through Inclusivity and Transparency or EQSPI, offers strategies to ensure the quality of scientific publications through more equitable editorial practices.[1] While trust is only briefly mentioned as an outcome of the EQSPI strategies, it is worth unpacking how the implementation of these recommended practices will help build or rebuild the public's trust in the publication of scientific research through promotion of transparency, inclusivity, and community engagement.

TRANSPARENCY

Transparency is increasingly emphasized as a method to foster trust in the dissemination and application of public health information. The EQSPI guidance emphasizes that transparency in scientific publication "can be advanced through collecting stakeholder feedback, analyzing editorial and peer review disparities, publishing data on review timelines and acceptance rates, and conducting internal audits aimed at improving the peer review process."[1(p966)] The EQSPI guidance pulls back the curtain on journal processes like peer review and spotlights whose research is getting published and whose is not, linking that information to principles of accountability, which is essential for trust building.

Practices to systematically collect and publish the demographic characteristics of journal staff, editorial board members, authors, and reviewers (especially when measured against benchmarks for improvement) hold journals accountable to promised changes in potentially inequitable processes over which they have control.

Increasingly, journals may require reflexivity statements from authors to investigate potential bias and appropriateness of authorship depending on the topic. This may include statements attesting to the inclusion of people with lived experience in authorship when research is conducted with minoritized communities. Researchers are also providing information in their articles that describes their personal characteristics that may create an unintended bias in the work that they do. Such disclosures are also important to compare research staff and author characteristics to the characteristics of the population that they are studying. While study participants may want to ensure they have a voice in developing research tools and processes, there is increasing interest that the research team also reflects those voices.

Building trust through transparency and accountability is an essential endeavor given the role that academic journals have played in privileging the research of certain communities and excluding the perspectives and research of people with minoritized identities. Similarly, public health practitioners can center transparency in decision-making processes to foster public trust in resulting policy and program recommendations. Indeed, models of collaborative governance, in which public agencies and nonstate parties engage in collective decision-making, emphasize that opportunities for public participation must have clear ground rules and process transparency to ensure legitimacy of the process and trust in the outcomes.[2]

EQSPI identifies conflicts of interest (COIs) as another aspect of transparency. Every COI does not necessarily disqualify individuals from participation in developing public health information through publishing or positions in public health practice. Rather, disclosure of COIs, such as receiving money from a commercial interest, needs to be disclosed. For authors of scientific papers, this may raise questions about the independence of any research. For practitioners, including policymakers, disclosure of conflicts of interest can lead to recusal from certain activities or decisions. This, in turn, can increase trust in that information or the decisions of policymakers.

Recently, Robert F. Kennedy Jr, US Secretary of Health and Human Services, dismissed all members of the Centers for Disease Control and Prevention Advisory Committee on Immunization Practices (ACIP) claiming that COIs were rampant and impairing the judgment of its members. However, a recent study found that COIs among ACIP members were quite low with only an average of 6.2% reporting a COI at recent meetings.[3] New members replacing those dismissed by the secretary are also required to disclose their COIs at the start of each ACIP meeting. These COIs are posted on the ACIP website to further support transparency.

INCLUSIVITY AND COMMUNITY ENGAGEMENT

Trusted public health information builds upon a foundation of relationships. When researchers, policymakers, coalitions, public health departments, and community-based organizations have built reputations as reliable partners, the likelihood that information and policies will be received with an open mind increases.

Part of this reputation is an organization that emphasizes inclusivity and community engagement. In the EQSPI guidelines, inclusivity refers to both the topics and perspectives covered by journals, as well as the use of inclusive language. Expanding the perspectives reflected in the published science could be supported through outreach to groups often excluded from publishing, like community-based organizations, or through the direct solicitation of oft-missing perspectives through dedicated calls for papers and invited editorials. The peer review process would also benefit from a community orientation, including inviting peer reviewers with lived experience who may fall outside typical professional and practice networks.

The EQSPI guidelines suggest that journals can foster inclusive language by helping "authors use respectful, inclusive, and precise terminology that reflects diverse human experiences."[1(p967)] Inclusivity may also be fostered through efforts to make the science more accessible to the public, such as plain-language summaries of articles or video or visual abstracts that tell the story of the science. Inclusivity fosters trust in the research enterprise and published science by ensuring that more people see the issues they care about and may be experiencing represented and delivered by researchers and practitioners with similar backgrounds and perspectives.

A similar focus on inclusivity across the public health enterprise continues to be essential to ensure that all communities within a population are welcome, respected, and engaged.

This is the crux, of course, of meaningful community engagement. The World Health Organization defines "meaningful community engagement" as "a process of developing relationships that enable stakeholders to work together to address health-related issues and promote well-being to achieve positive health impact and outcomes."[4(p1)]

Strategies to build trust through community engagement must also look at larger structural changes that need to be made. Ojikutu et al., exploring the roots of medical mistrust, describe how medical mistrust spans a continuum from skepticism to belief in unproven conspiracy theories. While this spectrum may seem spurious, it is often the result of real harms that have been perpetrated, especially with respect to disadvantaged, often racial minorities. In seeking potential solutions, they conclude that "promoting resilience and empowerment require that we acknowledge the root cause of mistrust and support the development of community-led solutions that confront systemic inequity."[5(p403)]

CONCLUSION

The EQSPI guidelines published in *AJPH* seek to improve the quality of publications and build trust in its content through transparency and inclusivity. Building upon those strategies, community engagement is similarly a way to increase trust among individuals and organizations at all levels of public health policy and practice. Consistent and faithful adherence to these principles will support greater trust in public health information through publishing as well as in the development and implementation of programs and policies. AJPH

CORRESPONDENCE

Correspondence should be sent to Stewart Landers, 156 Porter St, Unit 425, Boston, MA 02128 (e-mail: stewartjaylanders@gmail.com). Reprints can be ordered at https://www.ajph.org by clicking the "Reprints" link.

PUBLICATION INFORMATION

Full Citation: Landers S, Fiala SC. Building trust in public health information through transparency, inclusivity, and community engagement. *Am J Public Health*. 2026;116(1):67–69.

Acceptance Date: October 16, 2025.

DOI: https://doi.org/10.2105/AJPH.2025.308335

ORCID iDs:

Stewart Landers https://orcid.org/0009-0005-5101-4108

Steven C. Fiala https://orcid.org/0000-0001-8881-5762

CONTRIBUTORS

S. Landers originated and wrote the first draft of the editorial, worked on subsequent edits, provided final approval of the editorial, and attests to the integrity of the work. S. C. Fiala provided initial input to help shape the writing of the first draft, participated in all subsequent rounds of editing including significant writing of new material, provided final approval of the editorial, and attests to the integrity of the work.

CONFLICTS OF INTEREST

The authors report no conflicts of interest.

REFERENCES

1. Loui M, Morabia A. Ensuring quality in scientific publication through inclusivity and transparency. *Am J Public Health*. 2025;115(7):966–967. https://doi.org/10.2105/AJPH.2025.308174
2. Ansell C, Gash A. Collaborative governance in theory and practice. *J Public Adm Res Theory*. 2008;18(4):543–571. https://doi.org/10.1093/jopart/mum032
3. Kanter GP, Mankowitz T, Lurie P. Conflicts of interest in federal vaccine advisory committees. *JAMA*. 2025;334(14):1295–1297. https://doi.org/10.1001/jama.2025.13245
4. World Health Organization. Community engagement: a health promotion guide for universal health coverage in the hands of the people. October 5, 2020. Available at: https://www.who.int/publications/i/item/9789240010529. Accessed October 12, 2025.
5. Ojikutu BO, Bogart LM, Dong L. Mistrust, empowerment, and structural change: lessons we should be learning from COVID-19. *Am J Public Health*. 2022;112(3):401–404. https://doi.org/10.2105/AJPH.2021.306604

Freedom, Fairness, and Trust: Speaking the Language of Public Health Across the Political Divide

Brian C. Castrucci, DrPH, Jessica Malaty Rivera, MS, and Amanda Kwong, MPH

ABOUT THE AUTHORS

Brian C. Castrucci and Jessica Malaty Rivera are with the de Beaumont Foundation, Bethesda, MD. Amanda Kwong is with the Public Health Communications Collaborative, Bethesda, MD.

See also Trust in Public Health, pp. 31–94.

AJPH January 2026, Vol. 116, No. 1

Public health practice is not broken, but its communication is and that failure magnifies the risk of the next emergency. During the COVID-19 pandemic, public health institutions became a political proxy—alternately celebrated and vilified—until trust was badly eroded, particularly among conservatives and rural communities.[1–3] If communication does not improve, the response to the next crisis will fail before it begins—not because of science but because of silence, mixed messages, and mistrust.

COVID-19 guidance landed in a culture primed for polarization. Accepting or rejecting masks, school closures, and vaccines became signals of identity and partisanship.[4–6] Often missing from this discussion was the recognition that public health practice is an iterative, deeply human process. At times, messaging was delivered with premature certainty about evolving science. Technical accuracy was prioritized over public understanding. And guidance appeared inconsistent in ways that fueled perceptions of political bias. These missteps allowed opponents to cast public health authority as ideological rather than scientific, eroding trust that will take years to rebuild—especially among conservatives.

Yet conservatives are not unreachable. In a recent Harvard–de Beaumont Foundation poll, 48% of Republicans reported mostly positive views of the Centers for Disease Control and Prevention, and majorities hold somewhat positive views of state and local health departments.[7] Roughly half say they "somewhat trust" recommendations from these agencies—a sign that trust is fragile but recoverable.[1] That fragile trust creates an opening, and the shared priorities across party lines define the common ground where rebuilding can begin.

There is broad bipartisan agreement on core public health priorities: preventing chronic disease, preparing for future pandemics, reducing maternal and infant mortality, ensuring safe tap water, addressing mental health, and combating the opioid crisis.[2,7] These shared concerns offer an untapped opportunity to rebuild credibility—if public health messengers can communicate in ways that resonate across ideological lines.

There is no slogan, hashtag, or clever social media post that will solve public health's communication challenge. Effective communication is a long game—one made harder by deepening politicization and polarization. Some physicians, once among the most trusted voices in science,[8] now use social and broadcast media to spread misinformation—sometimes for personal profit.[9] When the very professions and agencies meant to protect health contribute to confusion, the need for clear, consistent communication becomes even more urgent.

But acknowledging that there is no quick fix does not mean there is no fix at all. There may be no magic words, but there are tools: proven approaches for communicating effectively across ideological divides. The path forward requires more than good intentions. It requires disciplined, deliberate communication built on four essential components:

1. Speaking with clarity—defining the purpose of public health's mission simply and consistently, framing it in terms that resonate with values like freedom, stability, and personal responsibility.
2. Being consistent—applying science-based guidance uniformly across scenarios, explaining changes clearly, and avoiding mixed messages that can be perceived as politically motivated.
3. Practicing cultural competence with conservatives—engaging conservative and rural communities with respect and using language, messengers, and framing that

reflect their lived experiences and priorities.

4. Cultivating community presence—maintaining visibility and dialogue between crises, building familiarity so that messages are more likely to be heard and trusted when emergencies arise.

Together, these four components form a communication strategy that speaks to shared values, reduces polarization, and equips public health practitioners to reach conservative audiences effectively—not just in the next crisis but every day.

SPEAKING WITH CLARITY

Do you remember the game Pictionary? One person takes a card, the timer starts, and the challenge is simple: sketch something teammates can recognize. A plane? Easy—a couple of wings and a tail. A hamburger? Two buns, a rectangle for the patty, and a squiggle for lettuce. The answer is shouted in seconds.

Now ask a room full of public health professionals to draw "public health." The pens freeze. People hesitate. A few try: a syringe here, a mask there, maybe a hospital or a jogging stick figure. But no two drawings look alike.

That is more than a party trick; it is a warning sign. When public health's mission cannot be drawn in a way others immediately recognize, it cannot be expected to win funding, inspire public support, or withstand political attack. This "Pictionary problem" leaves the public health field vulnerable to disinformation and easy to dismiss as government overreach or elitism.

The solution starts with clarity—a simple, consistent value proposition that answers the question every audience is silently asking: What's in it for me? Public health professionals too often communicate in institutional terms—budgets, staffing, programs—but the public wants to know what they will gain.

For many conservatives, the "what's in it for me" test often centers on freedom and stability—limited government intrusion and predictable daily life—whereas many progressives emphasize fairness—protecting vulnerable people and reducing inequities. This freedom–fairness contrast is not new: the public health community has long debated "freedom from" preventable harm versus "freedom to" choose (e.g., tobacco and sugary drink policies).[10–12] By stating concrete, personal benefits—not just programs and processes—the public health community can build credibility across the spectrum.

At its core, public health work is freedom infrastructure: freedom from preventable disease, cascading economic disruptions, and avoidable suffering as well as freedom to work, worship, learn, and participate safely in civic life. These are not abstractions; they are measurable outcomes that strong public health systems deliver every day.

BEING CONSISTENT

The events of 2020 illustrate how public health credibility can falter when communication appears politicized.[13,14] The murder of George Floyd and the subsequent protests coincided with guidance urging Americans to avoid large gatherings. When a widely publicized letter from public health practitioners stated, "We do not condemn these gatherings as risky for COVID-19 transmission. We support them as vital to national public health. . . . This should not be confused with a permissive stance on all gatherings, particularly protests against stay-home orders,"[15] many heard a double standard.

This perception was captured by Senator Josh Hawley (R, MO) when he called for a civil rights investigation into COVID-19 prevention restrictions on churches, arguing that jurisdictions were allowing protests over George Floyd's murder but keeping houses of worship closed or severely restricted.[16] This confirmed the fears of religious communities, small business owners, and conservatives that public health leadership had abandoned neutrality.

Future crises demand consistency. Public health messaging must do the following:

- Clearly distinguish scientific facts from value judgments;
- Apply recommendations uniformly across similar scenarios;
- Be transparent about trade-offs, especially when values influence decisions;
- Ensure that key messengers are pulling from the same talking points; and
- Make community touchpoints routine, not reactive.

Consistency may not eliminate controversy, but it prevents avoidable credibility crises and signals that public health guidance is based on evidence, not ideology.

However, consistency does not mean that guidance should remain static. Science is dynamic, evolving as new evidence emerges, and emergencies will always require shifts in guidance and policy; language and messaging must allow for flexibility and updates. Change is both inevitable and appropriate as evidence evolves. Recognizing that new discoveries may alter accepted recommendations, public health practitioners

AJPH January 2026, Vol. 116, No. 1

should avoid issuing guidance and stating the science with absolute certainty. Yet during the COVID-19 pandemic, public health practitioners sometimes communicated early findings with excessive certainty about a novel and rapidly evolving virus. As a result, many Americans remember this as a time of shifting and sometimes contradictory recommendations. These changes—although scientifically justified—were poorly explained, fueling confusion and eroding trust.[17,18]

Without clear, plain language communication about why the science was changing, appeals to "trust the science" rang hollow, leaving some to view reversals as arbitrary or politically driven.[19] In times of emergency, science progresses rapidly and information evolves. When issuing guidance, public health and scientific leaders must commit to being honest with the public, including acknowledging when things change and updates are needed.

PRACTICING CULTURAL COMPETENCE WITH CONSERVATIVES

Public health practitioners are expected to understand the nuances of language, history, culture, and values before engaging with diverse communities. Yet conservative and rural communities are often approached without similar preparation—and sometimes even with open disdain. This blind spot fuels mistrust, makes guidance easier to dismiss, and reinforces the perception that public health work serves only certain groups and ignores others.

Engagement with conservative communities cannot be treated as optional or secondary. It requires the same rigor applied to work with any population: listening first, building trust over time, and framing messages in ways that resonate with core values such as faith, family, personal responsibility, and freedom. It also means making space for conservative voices in the field itself. Recruiting conservatives into and elevating them in public health practice brings perspectives that strengthen policy decisions, broaden coalition support, and enable message crafting that resonates across the ideological spectrum.

The de Beaumont Foundation's partnership with Republican pollster Frank Luntz during the pandemic demonstrates what is possible when public health leadership truly listens to conservative audiences.[20,21] Through focus groups and polling, the project identified language that resonated with conservatives, emphasizing personal freedom, protecting loved ones, and keeping schools and businesses open.

These findings were translated into message briefs, talking points, and public service announcements featuring Republican elected officials. Materials were used to brief members of Congress, governors' offices, and community leaders, equipping them to communicate effectively with conservative audiences. By reframing vaccination as a tool for preserving freedom and normalcy—not as a government mandate—the campaign helped reach hesitant audiences and demonstrated that bipartisan communication can shift behavior.

The public health system is strongest when it reflects the full diversity of the nation it serves. Treating conservative communities as partners rather than opponents is not capitulation: it is strategy. It is the work of creating a shared foundation so that, in the next crisis, guidance is met with collaboration rather than suspicion, action rather than resistance.

CULTIVATING COMMUNITY PRESENCE

Trust cannot be built for the first time during an emergency, especially with audiences who are already skeptical. It must be cultivated in ordinary, noncrisis moments by showing up where conservative and rural communities already gather, for example, school board meetings, church services, veterans halls, business roundtables, and county fairs. Consistent presence in these spaces communicates respect and helps public health representatives become a familiar, approachable part of community life rather than a distant institution that appears only to deliver rules.

Presence must also come through trusted voices. For many conservatives, pastors, veterans, farmers, and small business owners carry far more credibility than government spokespeople. Identifying, training, and equipping these trusted messengers in advance ensures that, when critical information must be shared, it comes from someone who understands and reflects the community's values. Local microinfluencers—individuals with modest but deeply engaged followings—can be particularly powerful in countering rumors, addressing misinformation, and reinforcing accurate information when it matters most.

Embedding public health presence in the everyday fabric of conservative communities reframes it as a protector, not a threat. This approach safeguards what matters most: the freedom to work, worship, educate children, and keep life moving even in times of crisis.

IMPROVING PUBLIC HEALTH COMMUNICATION

Public health does not need a rebrand; it needs a reckoning. Communication failures squandered trust, weakened influence, and cost lives. Rebuilding that trust is not a task for tomorrow—it is the most urgent work of today.

Public health's next great intervention is not a new vaccine or policy but the restoration of credibility that makes every intervention possible. That credibility depends on clarity, consistency, cultural competence, and community presence. It depends on meeting skepticism where it lives—in rural communities, in faith spaces, in small businesses—and showing that public health is not an enemy of freedom but its ally. It depends on humility to acknowledge past missteps, consistency to apply science-based guidance without double standards, and courage to stand firm on facts even when they are unpopular.

The future success of the public health system will not be measured only in the number of vaccines administered or outbreaks contained but in the strength of the relationship between the public health sector and the public itself. That relationship is the infrastructure on which every success depends. Rebuilding it is not optional: it is the most urgent public health intervention of our time. AJPH

CORRESPONDENCE

Correspondence should be sent to Brian C. Castrucci, 7501 Wisconsin Ave, #1310e, Bethesda, MD 20814 (e-mail: Castrucci@debeaumont.org). Reprints can be ordered at https://www.ajph.org by clicking the "Reprints" link.

PUBLICATION INFORMATION

Full Citation: Castrucci BC, Rivera JM, Kwong A. Freedom, fairness, and trust: speaking the language of public health across the political divide. *Am J Public Health*. 2026;116(1):70–73.

Acceptance Date: October 14, 2025.

DOI: https://doi.org/10.2105/AJPH.2025.308327

CONTRIBUTORS

The authors contributed equally to this work.

CONFLICTS OF INTEREST

The authors have no conflicts of interest to disclose.

REFERENCES

1. Kearney A, Sparks G, Liz Hamel L, Montalvo J, III, Valdes I, Kirzinger A. KFF tracking poll on health information and trust. January 28, 2025. Available at: https://www.kff.org/health-information-trust/kff-tracking-poll-on-health-information-and-trust-january-2025?utm_source=chatgpt.com. Accessed October 11, 2025.
2. Pasquini G, Yam E. Americans' views on who influences health policy and which health issues to prioritize. July 10, 2025. Available at: https://www.pewresearch.org/science/2025/07/10/americans-views-on-who-influences-health-policy-and-which-health-issues-to-prioritize. Accessed October 11, 2025.
3. Centers for Disease Control and Prevention. Disparities in COVID-19 vaccination coverage between urban and rural counties—United States, December 14, 2020–April 10, 2021. *MMWR Morb Mortal Wkly Rep*. 2021;70(20):759–764. https://doi.org/10.15585/mmwr.mm7020e3
4. Gollwitzer A, Martel C, Brady WJ, et al. Partisan differences in physical distancing are linked to health outcomes during the COVID-19 pandemic. *Nat Hum Behav*. 2020;4(11):1186–1197. https://doi.org/10.1038/s41562-020-00977-7
5. Young DG, Rasheed H, Bleakley A, Langbaum JB. The politics of mask-wearing: political preferences, reactance, and conflict aversion during COVID. *Soc Sci Med*. 2022;298:114836. https://doi.org/10.1016/j.socscimed.2022.114836
6. Gelfand M, Li R, Stamkou E, et al. Persuading Republicans and Democrats to comply with mask wearing: an intervention tournament. *J Exp Soc Psychol*. 2022;101:104299. https://doi.org/10.1016/j.jesp.2022.104299
7. Harvard T.H. Chan School of Public Health; de Beaumont Foundation. A view from 100 days: public expectations about the changing public health landscape. April 2025. Available at: https://hsph.harvard.edu/wp-content/uploads/2025/04/dBF-HSPH_100DaysPollReport_Apr-29-2025_final.pdf. Accessed September 6, 2025.
8. de Beaumont; No License for Disinformation. Disinformation doctors: licensed to mislead. December 2021. Available at: https://debeaumont.org/wp-content/uploads/2021/12/dBF-NLFD-Disinformation-Doctors-report-vf.pdf. Accessed September 22, 2025.
9. Weber L. Tax records reveal the lucrative world of covid misinformation. February 21, 2024. *The Washington Post*. Available at: https://www.washingtonpost.com/nation/2024/02/21/covid-misinformation-earnings. Accessed November 7, 2025.
10. Berlin I. *Four Essays on Liberty*. Oxford, UK: Oxford University Press; 1969.
11. Friedman LC, Cheyne A, Givelber D, Gottlieb MA, Daynard RA. Tobacco industry use of personal responsibility rhetoric in public relations and litigation: disguising freedom to harm as freedom of choice. *Am J Public Health*. 2015;105(2):250–260. https://doi.org/10.2105/AJPH.2014.302226
12. Véliz C, Maslen H, Essman M, Taillie LS, Savulescu J. Sugar, taxes, & choice. *Hastings Cent Rep*. 2019;49(6):22–31. https://doi.org/10.1002/hast.1067
13. Ramjee D, Pollack CC, Charpignon ML, et al. Evolving face mask guidance during a pandemic and potential harm to public perception: infodemiology study of sentiment and emotion on Twitter. *J Med Internet Res*. 2023;25:e40706. https://doi.org/10.2196/40706
14. Rafkin C, Shreekumar A, Vautrey PL. When guidance changes: government stances and public beliefs. *J Public Econ*. 2021;196:104319. https://doi.org/10.1016/j.jpubeco.2020.104319
15. Friedersdorf C. The protesters deserve the truth about the coronavirus. *The Atlantic*. June 4, 2020. Available at: https://www.theatlantic.com/ideas/archive/2020/06/protests-carry-risk-even-when-theyre-justified/612652. Accessed September 22, 2025.
16. Allassan F. Josh Hawley requests civil rights probe into coronavirus church restrictions. June 9, 2020. Available at: https://www.axios.com/2020/06/09/josh-hawley-coronavirus-churches. Accessed September 22, 2025.
17. Kreps SE, Kriner DL. Model uncertainty, political contestation, and public trust in science: evidence from the COVID-19 pandemic. *Sci Adv*. 2020;6(43):eabd4563. https://doi.org/10.1126/sciadv.abd4563
18. Dries C, McDowell M, Schneider CR, Rebitschek FG. The effect of uncertainty communication on public trust depends on belief–evidence consistency. *PNAS Nexus*. 2025;4(3):pgaf071. https://doi.org/10.1093/pnasnexus/pgaf071
19. SteelFisher GK, Findling MG, Caporello HL, et al. Trust in US federal, state, and local public health agencies during COVID-19: responses and policy implications. *Health Aff (Millwood)*. 2023;42(3):328–337. https://doi.org/10.1377/hlthaff.2022.01204
20. de Beaumont Foundation. Language that works to improve vaccine acceptance. December 2020. Available at: https://debeaumont.org/wp-content/uploads/2021/01/VaccineToolkit_1pger.pdf. Accessed September 22, 2025.
21. de Beaumont Foundation. Changing the COVID conversation. 2025. Available at: https://debeaumont.org/changing-the-covid-conversation. Accessed September 22, 2025.

"What We've Got Here Is Failure to Communicate": The Need for Crisis Communication Skills Training in Public Health Graduate Programs

Patrick J. A. Kelly, MPH, and Sarah Bauerle Bass, PhD, MPH

ABOUT THE AUTHORS

Patrick J. A. Kelly is with the Department of Behavioral and Social Sciences, Brown University School of Public Health, Providence, RI. Sarah Bauerle Bass is with the Department of Social and Behavioral Sciences and the Risk Communication Lab, Temple University College of Public Health, Philadelphia, PA.

See also Trust in Public Health, pp. 31–94.

In the 1967 film *Cool Hand Luke*, the captain declares, "What we've got here is failure to communicate" when the titular character attempts to escape a chain gang. The well-known quotation has endured because of its persistent applicability. It captures the costs of misunderstandings and garbled communication. The relevance to how communication about public health occurs is clear: we have been limited by an outdated curricular system that has not kept up with the critical skills that are needed to communicate the importance of public health, especially during periods of crisis.

Public confidence in science has been high for many decades in the United States.[1] But communication challenges faced during the COVID-19 pandemic eroded trust in public health significantly, with only 29% of US adults expressing a great deal of confidence in medical scientists to act in the best interest of the public.[2] Partly a reflection of contradictory messaging from local and state health departments compared with the federal government, mis- and disinformation about COVID-19 mitigation strategies and treatments spread rapidly. A 2021 survey showed that nearly 80% of US adults believed or were unsure about at least one of eight incorrect statements about COVID-19.[3]

Scientists, who early in the pandemic were platformed to provide the public with information that was evolving as we learned more about transmission, mitigation needs, and treatment, were often unsure how to pivot as messages changed; this caused contradictory messaging that led to heightened media scrutiny, skepticism, and trust erosion.[4] This erosion has continued. For example, amid changes in federal health priorities since January 2025, just half of US adults now have confidence in the Centers for Disease Control and Prevention and the Food and Drug Administration to ensure vaccine safety.[5]

Communication training to combat the ongoing erosion of trust in public health leaders is critical. Although some graduate programs in public health provide health communication training in individual-level health interventions, there is little or no training in how to communicate scientific evidence to the public to address ongoing public health crises in the age of 24–7 news cycles. We argue that accredited public health programs should integrate crisis communication and media relations training into curricula. "Crisis communication" refers to the process of providing factual information to the public about an unexpected emergency that requires a timely response.[6] "Media relations" refers broadly to the process of working with diverse media to provide information to the public about an organization and its messages; for example, public health organizations communicate factual information, often via the media, to promote well-being. Savvy media relations skills are an important aspect of effective crisis communication in public health. Consequently, a reworking of public health communications training to encompass crisis communication and media relations is needed to develop a scientific workforce equipped to restore public trust in science and safeguard the credibility of the public health profession.

THE CURRENT EDUCATIONAL LANDSCAPE

The Council of Education in Public Health, the accrediting body for US schools of public health and public health programs, determines curricular competencies for public health degrees. Educational competencies for the master of public health (MPH) and the doctor of public health (DrPH) degrees focus on rigorous training in theory, research design, and analysis and include subdiscipline-specific competencies.[7] Communication competencies for the MPH degree include selecting communication strategies for diverse audiences, developing written and oral audience-appropriate public health content, and demonstrating cultural competency in public health communication. No competencies are specific to crisis communication or media relations. Similarly, no crisis communication or media relations curricula are required for DrPH degrees, and PhD degree programs have no communication competencies at all.

Although social and behavioral science programs typically include content on health communication relevant for behavioral health interventions, limiting communication training only to the behavioral sciences leaves those in other subdisciplines, such as epidemiology and biostatistics, unprepared to communicate to audiences outside academia using evidence-based strategies. Translating what can be complex or ambiguous statistical results into digestible information for a public that needs simple information to make decisions is challenging but foundational to crisis communication. Yet public health students generally receive little or no training in how to clearly communicate probabilistic information to a general audience—a sorely felt curricular omission that hinders the public's ability to interpret and appreciate scientific evidence.

Understanding how to rigorously and ethically design and conduct human participant research is essential but insufficient public health training. Graduate programs in public health, and in particular doctoral programs, are disproportionately focused on scientific output (e.g., journal articles) relative to the time spent educating students about the translation of science for diverse audiences beyond the academy. Given our current media environment of tailored algorithms, politicized news, and generative artificial intelligence shaping health narratives,[8,9] students should be trained to be nimble communicators of scientific evidence who are capable of adapting to the needs of diverse audiences, especially during a crisis.

The crisis communication and media relations training gaps are glaring when considering the roles that graduate-level public health professionals, and in particular doctoral-level researchers, assume after graduation. Graduates working in academia, industry, government, and nonprofit sectors are frequently called on to speak as public-facing experts about timely public health topics. When health crises occur, scientists are asked to explain, and increasingly defend, evidence-based public health strategies. Yet, because of curricular deficiencies, most graduate-level public health scientists have not practiced how to perform essential communication tasks, such as giving an interview to the press, fielding challenging questions, and, perhaps most importantly, situating scientific evidence in a way that maintains public trust for an increasingly skeptical public. Graduate programs should strongly consider establishing a required course in crisis communication and media relations to ensure that all graduates have foundational training in these highly relevant and urgently needed skills.

MEDIA SHAPES THE MESSAGE

Public health communication during times of crisis is shaped by the media channel through which messages are communicated. Foundational frameworks, such as Coombs's situational crisis communication theory[10] and Benoit's image repair theory,[11] provide widely used models for understanding how to respond to crisis situations. However, as Jong argues,[12] these frameworks treat crises as static events, when they more appropriately should be considered dynamic processes shaped by media amplification and evolving public understanding. Media coverage reshapes messages once communicated by the messenger, influencing what the public is exposed to and believes.

Public health crises are inherently unpredictable, but what is certain is that public health professionals are thrown into situations where they are asked to communicate about public health. When tapped for a recorded interview with a journalist or when speaking at a press conference, those working in public health may find that they are asked to speak for the entire field despite geographic, population, or behavioral differences in large-scale crises. Scientists are also asked to defend evidence that is sometimes misconstrued or not understood by an audience unfamiliar with science. Also critical is to offer reassurance in moments of fear and uncertainty. Thus, the synergy between the content of a message and messaging channels illuminates why media relations training is critical.

It is not that scientists should seek to control headlines. Instead, we must prepare scientists to communicate messages that are clear and accessible to the public so that they are perceived as credible and accurate to prevent or mitigate misinformation. Public health professionals, and by extension public health organizations, who cultivate media relationships and learn how to communicate clearly and transparently can reduce additional erosion of public trust while advancing the core values of public health.

OFF THE DEEP END

One of the key tenets in crisis communication is to establish the credibility of messengers.[13] In past public health crises, the public health sector benefited from federal leadership that supported—not sidelined—the overall mission of the public health enterprise. Public health as a field was not prepared to be out of sync with messages from federal leadership, nor was the field prepared to compete for credibility or airtime during the COVID-19 pandemic. The field also lacked skill in how to communicate rapidly changing science at a time when political rhetoric was hyperfocused on emphasizing that messages were contradictory; what was needed was skill in communicating that science is iterative and builds on precedence, which is why public health messages evolve with time. Another challenge was the urgency of communicating with the public about vaccination as a matter of public health policy. Public health professionals were ill-prepared to share information with audiences who consumed health messages on social media.

The consequences of mismanaged communication during the COVID-19 pandemic have been profound and wide reaching. Garbled messaging discredited the field of public health, allowing misinformation to amplify at the expense of accuracy. During times of crisis, people seek answers from those they trust and need to feel they are being told the truth, even if the truth is unknown or difficult. People want to know what they can do to mitigate a risk and be told if information is not known.[14] There was a failure to clearly acknowledge how much was unknown about COVID-19 and how much would likely change about our understanding of the pandemic. We lost sight of and failed to communicate that science is iterative and balanced when at its best; scientists should be cautious about making definitive claims because evidence will evolve as a crisis unfolds. Scientists need to know how to communicate evolving evidence without undermining the credibility of the profession, but this training is seldom provided, let alone required, in graduate education.

REIMAGINING PUBLIC HEALTH COMMUNICATION

Enhanced training in crisis communication and media relations would complement, not replace, competencies at accredited public health programs. Institutions should retain the curricular freedom to determine how students achieve these essential competencies, but students should be familiar with seminal crisis communication frameworks and understand how to adapt existing theories to the realities of a changing media landscape. Media relations training is also needed so that students know how to stay on message, control quotations through repetition of a central message, and navigate challenging questions.

Importantly, there are opportunities for interdisciplinary partnerships when designing a crisis communication course for the contemporary media landscape. Collaborating with journalists for a guest lecture could help students understand the dynamics that shape a newsroom in a churning news cycle. Relatedly, students should understand how to translate scientific findings and public health messaging clearly and accurately. Communicators must balance simplifying messages with avoiding excessive dilution to ensure that audiences are not overwhelmed by jargon and can clearly understand the core message. To that end, telling the story of the science with accessible analogies that resonate with diverse audiences can frame a core message in a persuasive way. Submitting op-eds and commentaries is another strategic way to translate scientific evidence into compelling arguments.

But clear communication is achieved not only through articulate messages. Scientists should recognize how their own background and institutional role shape the way their messages are perceived by the audiences they are attempting to reach. This is particularly important when speaking to communities who have historically been overlooked in public health. This was acutely seen during the COVID-19 pandemic, especially when it came to vaccination.[15] Scientists who do not share identity or experience with their audience should explore the opportunity for partnership with communities and credible messengers who can deliver core messages to maximize message salience to the audience. Using inclusive language and avoiding message framing that stigmatizes certain behaviors or communities are essential to prevent amplifying stigma and alienating audiences. Leading with respect honors the relationship between scientists and diverse communities, which is essential for maintaining credibility and building back trust in the public health field.

HOW TO MOVE FORWARD

We are aware that graduate curricula in public health are already extensive. Although some may say that current competencies leave no room for additions, we believe that there can be flexible ways to cover this training. Half credit courses, invited seminars, and workshops with attendance requirements through university strategic communication offices could achieve competencies without bloating curricula or unduly burdening students. There are also pragmatic challenges to curricular revisions; for example, programs may lack qualified faculty who can teach these topics. Interdisciplinary course design models, in which public health faculty coteach with journalism, business, or communication sciences scholars is one strategy that would enrich the student experience and fill a gap in institutional capacity to offer this training. It is also important to evaluate the delivery and content of curricular additions to inform evidence-based approaches to teaching crisis communication to public health students in an ever-changing media landscape.

Revisions to Council of Education in Public Health accreditation criteria will take time. Nonetheless, there are steps that can be taken to enrich communications training as broader revitalization is pursued. Faculty can advocate curricular revisions at their institutions, regardless of whether competencies are expanded. Programs could more clearly center a communications focus in existing programming and sponsor seminars and invited lectures on the importance of crisis communication and media relations. Professional societies should promote sessions on topics such as media engagement and translating science to diverse audiences for graduate students and early career researchers. Students could also seek opportunities for enrichment by attending conferences, interning with department of public health professionals working in communications, and using freely available vetted online resources such as the Public Health and Crisis Communications Resource Hub through the Association of State and Territorial Health Officials.[16]

CONCLUSION

Reflecting on the restoration of trust in public health professionals reveals how essential communication is to the path forward. It is not a question of if but when the next public health professional will be called to the microphone to chart us collectively through a crisis. Without the ability to communicate clearly and strategically, a communication void is created that is filled with mis- and disinformation, eroding public trust in science. Building crisis communication and media relations training into public health graduate programs should no longer be considered discipline specific but an urgent priority to modernize the training of our public health workforce.

As the line from *Cool Hand Luke* goes, what we are experiencing in public health is a failure to communicate. But this is not an unalterable reality. Reimaging curricular requirements to better prepare emerging public health scientists to communicate about the challenges of our time can help to see us through crises. Ensuring that public health professionals can connect to others and communicate the importance of public health is an essential skill in our world. As new knowledge is generated of the multidimensionality of health and as media platforms evolve, scientists should be ready to take the microphone as one of many strategies to rebuild trust in public health. AJPH

CORRESPONDENCE

Correspondence should be sent to Patrick J. A. Kelly, MPH, 121 S. Main St, Providence, RI 02903 (e-mail: patrick_kelly@brown.edu). Reprints can be ordered at https://www.ajph.org by clicking the "Reprints" link.

PUBLICATION INFORMATION

Full Citation: Kelly PJA, Bass SB. "What we've got here is failure to communicate": the need for crisis communication skills training in public health graduate programs. *Am J Public Health*. 2026; 116(1):74–78.

Acceptance Date: September 25, 2025.

DOI: https://doi.org/10.2105/AJPH.2025.308303

ORCID iD:
Patrick J. A. Kelly https://orcid.org/0000-0003-1462-1150

CONTRIBUTORS

P. J. A. Kelly wrote the original draft and S. B. Bass revised it. The authors conceptualized this article equally and approved the final version to be published.

CONFLICTS OF INTEREST

The authors have no conflicts of interest to disclose.

REFERENCES

1. US National Science Foundation. Science and technology: public perceptions, awareness, and information sources. February 14, 2024. Available at: https://ncses.nsf.gov/pubs/nsb20244/executive-summary. Accessed September 8, 2025.
2. Kennedy B, Tyson A, Funk C. Americans' trust in scientists, other groups declines. February 15, 2022. Available at: https://www.jstor.org/stable/resrep63558. Accessed September 8, 2025.
3. Palosky C. COVID-19 misinformation is ubiquitous: 78% of the public believes or is unsure about at least one false statement, and nearly a third believe at least four of eight false statements tested. November 8, 2021. Available at: https://www.kff.org/health-information-trust/covid-19-misinformation-is-ubiquitous-78-of-the-public-believes-or-is-unsure-about-at-least-one-false-statement-and-nearly-at-third-believe-at-least-four-of-eight-false-statements-tested. Accessed September 10, 2025.
4. Li H, Chen B, Chen Z, Shi L, Su D. Americans' trust in COVID-19 information from governmental sources in the Trump era: individuals' adoption of preventive measures, and health implications. *Health Commun.* 2022;37(12):1552–1561. https://doi.org/10.1080/10410236.2022.2074776
5. Sparks G, Montalvo J III, Schumacher S, Kirzinger A, Hamel L. KFF tracking poll on health information and trust: COVID-19 vaccine update. August 1, 2025. Available at: https://www.kff.org/health-information-trust/kff-tracking-poll-on-health-information-and-trust-covid-19-vaccine-update. Accessed September 10, 2025.
6. Centers for Disease Control and Prevention. Crisis and emergency risk communication: introduction. 2018. Available at: https://www.cdc.gov/cerc/media/pdfs/CERC_Introduction.pdf. Accessed October 30, 2025.

7. Council on Education for Public Health. About CEPH. Available at: https://ceph.org/about/org-info. Accessed September 10, 2025.
8. Menz BD, Modi ND, Sorich MJ, Hopkins AM. Health disinformation use case highlighting the urgent need for artificial intelligence vigilance: weapons of mass disinformation. *JAMA Intern Med.* 2024;184(1):92–96. https://doi.org/10.1001/jamainternmed.2023.5947
9. Saeidnia HR, Hosseini E, Lund B, Tehrani MA, Zaker S, Molaei S. Artificial intelligence in the battle against disinformation and misinformation: a systematic review of challenges and approaches. *Knowl Inf Syst.* 2025;67(4):3139–3158. https://doi.org/10.1007/s10115-024-02337-7
10. Coombs WT. *Ongoing Crisis Communication: Planning, Managing, and Responding.* Thousand Oaks, CA: SAGE; 2007.
11. Benoit WL. Image repair discourse and crisis communication. *Public Relat Rev.* 1997;23(2):177–186. https://doi.org/10.1016/S0363-8111(97)90023-0
12. Jong W. Beyond the snapshot: rethinking crisis communication theories in dynamic crisis situations. *Public Relat Rev.* 2025;51(3):102586. https://doi.org/10.1016/j.pubrev.2025.102586
13. Spitale G, Germani F, Biller-Andorno N. The PHERCC matrix: an ethical framework for planning, governing, and evaluating risk and crisis communication in the context of public health emergencies. *Am J Bioeth.* 2024;24(4):67–82. https://doi.org/10.1080/15265161.2023.2201191
14. Centers for Disease Control and Prevention. CERC: psychology of a crisis. 2019. Available at: https://www.cdc.gov/cerc/media/pdfs/CERC_Psychology_of_a_Crisis.pdf. Accessed September 8, 2025.
15. Walker RJ, Eisenhauer E, Thompson EL, et al. COVID-19 information, trust, and risk perception across diverse communities in the United States: initial findings from a multistate community engagement alliance (CEAL). *Am J Public Health.* 2024;114(suppl 1):S112–S123. https://doi.org/10.2105/AJPH.2023.307504
16. Association of State and Territorial Health Officials. Public health & crisis communications resource hub. 2025. Available at: https://www.astho.org/topic/crisis-communications. Accessed September 8, 2025.

The Challenge of Trust in Public Health Institutions Among Communities of Color: Where Do We Go From Here?

Tasleem J. Padamsee, PhD, and Johnnie Chip Allen, MPH

ABOUT THE AUTHORS

Tasleem J. Padamsee is with the College of Public Health and the James Comprehensive Cancer Center, The Ohio State University, Columbus, and writes as a private citizen. Johnnie Chip Allen is a health equity subject matter expert and lecturer.

See also Trust in Public Health, pp. 31–94.

Trust is considered a necessary foundation on which public health institutions build programs to protect and improve the health of populations, but it involves a delicate balancing act. Black, Hispanic, and other US communities of color face substantial long-standing and ongoing disparities that profoundly affect health and well-being across the life course, including in life expectancy and infant mortality as well as hypertension, diabetes, asthma, and cancer deaths. National and regional health institutions—such as the National Institutes of Health, the Centers for Disease Control and Prevention, and local public health agencies—have the expertise and resources to understand and ameliorate these disparities but have often struggled to engage communities of color in medical research, prevention activities, and health care interventions. Much of this problem is traceable not to lack of interest—communities of color are intensely driven to protect and nurture their own positive health outcomes—but to lack of trust in public health science and institutions.

Many studies have demonstrated this pairing of prohealth community attitudes with the "trust problem." Black women facing elevated cancer risk, for instance, articulate a strong motivation to educate themselves about those risks and proactively protect their health, but they also describe the need for intense self-advocacy to get cancer-related information and resources from their health care providers.[1] During the COVID-19 pandemic, which caused disproportionately high illness and death rates in their communities, Black Americans reported vaccination intentions comparable to those of White Americans in late 2020 but showed significantly greater increases over the following six months, reflecting growing belief in the need for vaccination to protect themselves and their communities.[2]

We build on the critical, ongoing work of local community leaders, scholars, and practitioners in public health to propose two strategic moves to advance health equity and alleviate the ongoing morbidity and mortality crisis in communities of color.

First, we must reframe the problem from one of trust to one of trustworthiness. This rearticulation shifts our understanding of both the core issue at hand and the responsibility for addressing it. A trustworthiness frame shifts our gaze from the disparities we wish to rectify to the inequities and political determinants that underly them: the social and structural processes that create systematically worse outcomes for communities of color. These underlying processes include the historical abuses through which much distrust of health institutions has been earned—injustices that continue to reverberate: the Tuskegee Syphilis Study, the unauthorized use of Henrietta Lacks's cells for medical research, the forced sterilization of Puerto Rican women, and many more. Critically, however, they also include the widespread contemporary inequities grounded in structural and everyday racism, for example, the undertreatment of pain in Black patients, the misdiagnosis of mental illness and learning disabilities among people of color, and the direct attacks on health equity and diversity, equity, and inclusion initiatives that were specifically designed to support optimal health outcomes for people of color. In this context, the problem is less about community members' feelings of trust and more about the trustworthiness of our governmental and public health institutions, their statements, their representatives, and their actions.

Second, we propose reframing the "ask" from macrolevel trust in institutions to microlevel trust within specific relationships and contexts. Expecting communities to offer blanket trust in governmental agencies, medical researchers, or public health advisers is profoundly unreasonable, particularly given the routine inconsistencies in the commitments those entities express. In some times and places, institutions devote considerable resources to the health of populations of color. In the wake of inequitable COVID-19 rates and the televised murder of George Floyd in 2020, many public health agencies appointed dedicated health equity directors and advisory boards and launched new programs guided by this expertise.[3] The National Institutes of Health has supported efforts to increase the inclusion of people of color in clinical trials and a wide range of health disparities studies and interventions.

However, federal policies and the current political environment have undermined these commitments. Health equity champions have been removed from positions of power and influence, research and prevention programs focused on the needs of communities of color have been canceled and defunded, and the term "health equity" has itself been recast as a political liability. Nor is this the first time in US history that people of color have witnessed the cancellation, reversal, or defunding of programs designed to support their health. We must acknowledge that the commitments and priorities of institutions with respect to the health of people of color will likely continue to waver over time.

Nevertheless, we do not believe that all hope is lost; the underlying commitments of most practicing health researchers and public health practitioners are far less malleable. It may therefore be more realistic to nurture trust on a case-by-case basis: to ask communities of color to trust specific researchers, projects, leaders, and agencies that have a record of serving the legitimate health interests of communities and are willing to invest the resources necessary to convey that trustworthiness. This includes entities that have maintained their strong commitments to diversity, equity, and inclusion efforts in the current political environment.[3] Some communities of color are already aware of such entities in their midst, and these offer immediate opportunities for case-by-case trust.

In a statewide assessment of COVID-19–related needs in socially marginalized groups in Ohio, for instance, Black/African American, Hispanic/Latine, Asian/Asian American, immigrant, and refugee groups identified specific medical, public health, and social service leaders and organizations that could be trusted as entry points for conveying necessary information and resources.[4] Among the key methods for building this microlevel trust are (1) acknowledging the existence of historical and contemporary health inequities and injustices and naming them in specific contexts; (2) grounding our health policy and practice recommendations in science and articulating that evidence honestly, including when it changes or is uncertain; and (3) changing the flavor of health-related interactions by increasing the proportion of leaders and practitioners of color at every level, creating more roles for community-based health workers, and sharing consistently tailored educational materials.[4]

With the integrity of institutions such as the Centers for Disease Control and Prevention and the National Institutes of Health currently in jeopardy, and with expertly trained and highly experienced public experts dismissed, it may be the health of the American people—not only that of our communities of color—that depends on a new approach to trust.

To be clear, mistrust—like trust—is earned, especially over a protracted period of time. In the long term, institutions must find the courage to acknowledge the harmful effects of their inconsistent ability to equitably serve people of color. A series of truth and reconciliation activities would be a step in the right direction. Otherwise, the protective distrust of communities will continue to be nurtured, and health institutions will continue struggling to meet their core mission. This constitutes a no-win situation for everyone.

In the short term, the broad goal of getting communities to trust large-scale health care and public health institutions may be both unfair and unrealistic. Instead, shifting our focus to establishing trustworthiness and nurturing case-by-case trust is a viable way forward. Where they are applied systematically, these priorities can shrink health disparities, reduce inequitable treatment, and offer the promise of slowly building better, more health-protective relationships between communities of color and the health experts and institutions who serve them. AJPH

CORRESPONDENCE

Correspondence should be sent to Tasleem J. Padamsee, 280F Cunz Hall, The Ohio State University College of Public Health, 1841 Neil Ave, Columbus, OH 43210 (e-mail: padamsee.1@osu.edu). Reprints can be ordered at https://www.ajph.org by clicking the "Reprints" link.

PUBLICATION INFORMATION

Full Citation: Padamsee TJ, Allen JC. The challenge of trust in public health institutions among communities of color: where do we go from here? *Am J Public Health*. 2026;116(1):79–81.

Acceptance Date: October 16, 2025.

DOI: https://doi.org/10.2105/AJPH.2025.308334

ORCID iD:

Tasleem J. Padamsee https://orcid.org/0000-0001-6644-8084

CONTRIBUTORS

The authors contributed equally to this work.

CONFLICTS OF INTEREST

The authors have no conflicts of interest to report.

REFERENCES

1. Padamsee TJ, Meadows R, Hils M. Layers of information: interacting constraints on breast cancer risk management by high-risk African American women. *Ethn Health.* 2021;26(6):787–810. https://doi.org/10.1080/13557858.2018.1562053
2. Padamsee TJ, Bond RM, Dixon GN, et al. Changes in COVID-19 vaccine hesitancy among Black and White individuals in the US. *JAMA Netw Open.* 2022;5(1):e2144470. https://doi.org/10.1001/jamanetworkopen.2021.44470
3. Williams KP, Allen JC. Finding the courage and will to achieve health equity: asking the right questions. *Perspectives in Primary Care.* Harvard University. March 4, 2022. Available at: https://info.primarycare.hms.harvard.edu/perspectives/articles/asking-the-right-questions. Accessed October 29, 2025.
4. Nemeth JM, Padamsee TJ; Needs Assessment Writers' Team. *Ohio's COVID-19 Populations Needs Assessment: Minimizing the Disparate Impact of the Pandemic and Building Foundations for Health Equity.* October 2020. Available at: https://bpb-us-w2.wpmucdn.com/u.osu.edu/dist/a/112664/files/2024/02/1-Full-Report-9c055cfc4fb22245.pdf. Accessed October 29, 2025.

Stop Asking Communities to Trust You: Make Public Health Trustworthy

Chioma Nnaji, MPH, MEd, and Lisa Bowleg, PhD, MA

ABOUT THE AUTHORS

The authors are AJPH Associate Editors. Chioma Nnaji is with the Multicultural AIDS Coalition, and Ocha Transformations, Boston, MA. Lisa Bowleg is with the George Washington University, Washington, DC, and the Intersectionality Training Institute, Philadelphia, PA.

See also Trust in Public Health, pp. 31–94.

Distrust in science is rational. In public health, distrust remains an ongoing reality for racialized and marginalized communities in the United States because of historical atrocities such as the US Public Health Service Syphilis Study at Tuskegee[1] and present-day failures like the inequitable COVID-19 response[2] and the Flint water crisis.[3] These harms are not isolated events but are embedded in systems and structures of power that create, sustain, and reinforce multiple and interlocking systems of oppression such as racism, sexism, classism, heterosexism, cisgenderism, and ableism.[4] The current political climate has deepened public distrust by dismantling key public health institutions. In addition, ongoing attacks on science and the deliberate spread of disinformation have further weaponized distrust for political gain.[5] The consequences are likely dire; they portend not only adverse health outcomes but also the public's persistent skepticism and resistance, even when scientific and public health interventions could improve community health.

For racialized and marginalized communities, remediating distrust begins with acknowledging the history of atrocities and their ongoing manifestations. Then it requires restructuring the development of public health science so that community engagement and leadership are essential to building an ethical foundation of trustworthiness. We conceptualize community engagement and community leadership as a compound construct through which trustworthiness can be both established and sustained. As Best et al.[6] rightly argue, the burden is not on communities to demonstrate trust but on institutions to demonstrate trustworthiness. Thus, as public health practitioners in government, academic institutions, philanthropic organizations, public health agencies, and community-based organizations, our question is not "How can communities trust us?" but "Why should communities trust us?" and "How will we become trustworthy?"

COMMUNITY ENGAGEMENT AND LEADERSHIP IN PRAXIS

Praxis, understood as the ongoing cycle of reflection and action directed toward transformation,[7] provides a foundation for embedding community engagement and leadership into public health. In this context, praxis requires systematically integrating theory, practice, and community knowledge into structures and processes to advance equity. When done correctly, it can serve as a route to trustworthiness by grounding public health in community-led praxis.

Many health equity practitioners increasingly recognize community engagement not only as an approach but also as a core value of public health. Community engagement involves "working collaboratively with a group of people with common values, concerns and aspirations, as well as incorporating those common interests into decision-making processes."[8(p3)] This definition aligns with the third edition of the *Principles of Community Engagement*, which explicitly added trustworthiness as a core principle for effective engagement.[9]

Having community engagement and leadership as praxis is a pathway not only to strengthen science but also to confront and repair distrust by embedding transparency, equity, and reciprocity into public health. Being a praxis means community engagement and leadership is a part of everyday work rather than optional. It requires the public health ecosystem to weave equitable practices into its core operation. This is a systems-level approach that shifts structural power, such as redistributing resources and institutionalizing participatory decision-making processes. For example, the Robert Wood Johnson Foundation recently released requests for research proposals that allowed only community-based organizations to serve as the lead.[10] In addition, democratic deliberation, a method in which decisions are made through informed discussion and consensus among community members, has been used to determine health priorities and improve health sector

AJPH January 2026, Vol. 116, No. 1

governance.[11] Both illustrate how institutions can operationalize community engagement and leadership. When practiced daily, it shifts from being a one-time consultation to a sustained commitment that shapes research priorities, program design, policy development, and service delivery. In this way, community engagement and leadership become not only a value but also a standard of practice that ensures public health efforts are responsive and grounded in the lived realities of the communities they aim to serve.

FROM SHARED LEADERSHIP TO COMMUNITY-LED

Understanding community engagement and leadership as praxis also reframes how we think about the continuum of community engagement. Increasingly promoted across research, policy, and practice, different versions of the continuum use varied terms but describe the same core concept. Engagement can range from basic consultation, where community involvement is limited to providing feedback without shared decision-making, to shared leadership, where responsibility and decision-making are equally distributed between communities and institutions. As you move along the continuum, the depth of engagement increases, shifting to cocreation, shared decision-making, and mutual accountability.

Public health practitioners committed to health equity and community engagement often describe shared leadership as the gold standard. However, there is growing advocacy for community-led and community-defined approaches where communities set the agenda, define priorities, and control resources, while institutions such as universities or state governments serve as facilitators or supporters.[12,13] This shift recognizes that even shared leadership models can leave ultimate authority with institutions and perpetuate inequitable practices. Too often, researchers linked to powerful institutions co-opt community engagement to secure funding or fulfill compliance requirements.[14] Frequently, these practices are bolstered by funding agencies that recognize only institutionally based researchers as experts and ignore the histories, wisdom, expertise, and longstanding commitment of communities. When partnering with public health agencies and academic institutions, communities frequently encounter inequities such as inadequate or absent compensation, expectations of unpaid labor, being treated as adjunct rather than integral to the research, exclusion from important decisions, and timelines that clash with their priorities and capacities.

These inequitable practices reflect performative engagement and, in turn, deepen distrust in public health science, especially in communities with histories of exclusion and neglect. Communities feel undervalued and often devalued. Performative engagement also reinforces perceptions that systems, including public health, are self-serving rather than interested in or accountable to the public good. Community-led approaches, by contrast, cultivate leadership and reposition power in ways that align with transparency and accountability to build authentic trust.

COMMUNITY ENGAGEMENT AND LEADERSHIP AS AN ETHIC

The ethics of science have often been narrowly equated with technical metrics such as rigor and systematic and postpositivist criteria such as reproducibility and generalizability.[15,16] These are essential, but insufficient for communities whom public health systems have harmed or excluded. Technical soundness alone does not guarantee ethical or equitable outcomes. A study can be methodologically rigorous but an ethical failure if it marginalizes community voices, reinforces harm, produces findings irrelevant to individuals most impacted by inequities, or benefits only the researcher. Hence, the ethics and integrity of public health science must also be relational and acknowledge that what researchers know is shaped by relationships with and between people, communities, and systems.[17]

Public health already claims values such as equity, accountability, and service to the public good.[18,19] Yet, until these values are translated into enforceable standards, they remain largely aspirational. This is where community engagement and leadership must operate as a criterion for trustworthiness. Community engagement cannot be separated from community leadership. Engagement without prioritizing community leadership, whether by cultivating existing leaders or creating new opportunities, is incomplete and ultimately inauthentic. There is no shifting of power. It risks reducing communities to advisory or consultative roles rather than positioning them as co-decision-makers with authority over priorities, resources, and outcomes. Anything less is performative and undermines both the ethics and legitimacy of public health science. For this reason, community engagement and leadership must be treated as a compound, nonnegotiable criterion of trustworthiness.

As a measurable and nonnegotiable benchmark, community engagement and leadership determine whether public health science can credibly claim to be trustworthy for public good. In their 20-year longitudinal study of community-based participatory research, Wallerstein et al.[20] found that projects with deeper engagement, such as having communities participate in decision-making, agenda-setting, and dissemination, showed stronger outcomes in trust, relevance, sustainability, and uptake. Similarly, Ahmed and Palermo[21] argue that engagement is not an "add-on" but central to scientific quality because it improves cultural appropriateness, ensures data validity, and enhances community capacity.

Beyond research, public health failures highlight the cost of neglecting community engagement and leadership. The Flint water crisis only came to light because community members partnered with independent researchers to challenge official local-level public health data and expose contamination.[3] During COVID-19, the lack of engagement with Black and immigrant communities fueled misinformation and undermined vaccine confidence. In contrast, initiatives that partnered with trusted local organizations[22] or were led by community experts, such as the Black Doctors COVID-19 Consortium,[23] achieved higher vaccination uptake than traditional institutions.

System-level supports are essential for sustaining this practice. Academic institutions, for example, can embed community-engaged work into promotion and tenure guidelines, acknowledge it as a faculty annual review criterion, and provide equitable seed funding for community partnerships. Health departments can institutionalize community engagement and leadership metrics within performance evaluations.

A core barrier to moving toward trustworthiness is that the very institutions and systems that have created and sustained harm have also been the ones to define it. This should not be the case. When powerful institutions define trustworthiness, the definition typically serves their interests, not those of the community. Trustworthiness risks being reduced to a checkbox that does not address the root causes of inequities. True trustworthiness must be defined by communities; they, not researchers, must be the arbiters of whether they deem public health systems to be accountable, equitable, and aligned with community needs, values, and leadership.

To operationalize community engagement and leadership as a criterion for trustworthiness, measurable standards should assess questions such as these:

- Are communities equitably represented in decision-making structures?
- Do communities direct funds and set priorities or simply provide feedback?
- Are communities equitably compensated for their contributions?
- Are outcomes and data shared back and governed by the communities who provided the data?
- Are results shared with communities in the formats they want and need?
- Are community-defined priorities reflected in policies, interventions, and research agendas?
- Are communities acknowledged for their contributions, including with authorship and presenter credits?

By holding public health science to these questions, we create a nonnegotiable benchmark for whether science and the institutions that upheld science can credibly claim trustworthiness.

THE WAY FORWARD: REIMAGINING SYSTEMS

Community engagement and leadership, when equitable, sustained, and structurally embedded, is a critical praxis for shifting power and an essential criterion for evaluating whether communities deem public health science to be trustworthy. Clearly, none of what we have suggested here will be a quick fix. Building trust in public health science is neither linear nor transactional. It is participatory and iterative and requires flexibility. Frameworks such as intersectionality,[4] public health critical race praxis,[24] and liberatory design[25] remind us that communities must be at the center of shaping the questions, defining success, and reimagining systems. If community engagement and leadership is to serve as both a criterion and a praxis for trustworthiness in public health science, then public health scientists and practitioners must operationalize trust. Trust is not built in a single gesture; it is phased, layered, cumulative, and earned. For many racialized and marginalized communities, it is grounded in generational experiences, knowledge, and trauma. Hence, public health must grapple with the questions communities are already asking and, in many cases, demanding answers to, including, "Why, given how public health has historically treated our communities, should we trust public health science?"

To answer this question and other provocative questions like it, we need a well-resourced systems-level process, led by communities, to center communities' understanding of trustwothiness and embed it into the structures of public health science so that community engagement and leadership become both intrinsically how public health operates and a measure to validate public health science. What this looks like and how we get there will require lots of critical reflection, some discomfort, a willingness to shift mindsets and systems, and true commitments to improve the public's health. AJPH

CORRESPONDENCE

Correspondence should be sent to Chioma Nnaji, 7 Palmer St, Roxbury, MA 02119 (e-mail: chioma@ochatransformations.com). Reprints can be ordered at https://www.ajph.org by clicking the "Reprints" link.

PUBLICATION INFORMATION

Full Citation: Nnaji C, Bowleg L. Stop asking communities to trust you: make public health trustworthy. *Am J Public Health*. 2026;116(1): 82–87.

Acceptance Date: October 19, 2025.

DOI: https://doi.org/10.2105/AJPH.2025.308336

ORCID iDs:

Chioma Nnaji https://orcid.org/0000-0001-8512-7913

Lisa Bowleg https://orcid.org/0000-0003-4677-8195

CONTRIBUTORS

C. Nnaji conceptualized this editorial and led the writing, including revisions. L. Bowleg contributed to the conceptual refinement of the article and provided critical review and editing throughout its development. Both authors approved the final version for submission.

CONFLICTS OF INTEREST

The authors have no conflicts of interest to declare.

REFERENCES

1. Gamble VN. Under the shadow of Tuskegee: African Americans and health care. *Am J Public Health*. 1997;87(11):1773–1778. https://doi.org/10.2105/AJPH.87.11.1773
2. Sze S, Pan D, Nevill CR, et al. Ethnicity and clinical outcomes in COVID-19: a systematic review and meta-analysis. *EClinicalMedicine*. 2020;29:100630. https://doi.org/10.1016/j.eclinm.2020.100630
3. Hanna-Attisha M, LaChance J, Sadler RC, Schnepp AC. Elevated blood lead levels in children associated with the Flint drinking water crisis: a spatial analysis of risk and public health response. *Am J Public Health*. 2016;106(2): 283–290. https://doi.org/10.2105/AJPH.2015.303003
4. Bowleg L. The problem with the phrase women and minorities: intersectionality—an important theoretical framework for public health. *Am J Public Health*. 2012;102(7):1267–1273. https://doi.org/10.2105/AJPH.2012.300750
5. Ishizumi A, Kolis J, Abad N, et al. Beyond misinformation: developing a public health prevention framework for managing information ecosystems. *Lancet Public Health*. 2024;9(6):e397–e406. https://doi.org/10.1016/S2468-2667(24)00031-8
6. Best AL, Fletcher FE, Kadono M, Warren RC. Institutional distrust among African Americans and building trustworthiness in the COVID-19 response: implications for ethical public health practice. *J Health Care Poor Underserved*. 2021;32(1):90–98. https://doi.org/10.1353/hpu.2021.0010
7. Freire P. *Pedagogy of the Oppressed*. 30th anniversary ed. New York, NY: Continuum; 2000.
8. Turin TC, Abedin T, Chowdhury N, et al. Community engagement with immigrant communities involving health and wellness research: a systematic review protocol towards developing a taxonomy of community engagement definitions, frameworks, and methods. *BMJ Open*. 2020;10(4):e035649. https://doi.org/10.1136/bmjopen-2019-035649
9. Michener, JL, Williams A, Oto-Kent D, Aguilar-Gaxiola SA. Community engagement: a foundation for health equity and resilience. *Am J Public Health*. 2025;115(suppl 2):S104–S109. https://doi.org/10.2105/AJPH.2025.308029
10. Robert Wood Johnson Foundation. 2025. Research to Advance Racial and Indigenous Health Equity. Call for proposals. Available at: https://www.rwjf.org/en/grants/active-funding-opportunities/2025/research-to-advance-racial-and-indigenous-health-equity.html. Accessed September 30, 2025.
11. Bosché M, Krust R, Fung A, Pawar AS. Exploring democratic deliberation in public health: bridging division and enhancing community engagement. *Am J Public Health*. 2025;115(4):500–505.
12. Key KD, Furr-Holden D, Lewis EY, et al. The continuum of community engagement in research: a roadmap for achieving equity. *Prog Community Health Partnersh*. 2019;13(4):427–434. https://doi.org/10.1353/cpr.2019.0064
13. Nnaji C, Anyango L, Bova C, et al. The Tulumbe! Partnership: a case study in developing a community-led research agenda to address HIV among African immigrants in the United States. *Front Public Health*. 2024;12:1406397. https://doi.org/10.3389/fpubh.2024.1406397
14. Lett E, Adekunle D, McMurray P, et al. Health equity tourism: ravaging the justice landscape. *J Med Syst*. 2022;46(3):17. https://doi.org/10.1007/s10916-022-01803-5
15. Coughlin SS, Barker A, Dawson A. Ethics and scientific integrity in public health, epidemiological, and clinical research. *Public Health Rev*. 2012;34(1): 71–83. https://doi.org/10.1007/BF03391657
16. Diaba-Nuhoho P, Amponsah-Offeh M. Reproducibility and research integrity: the role of scientists and institutions. *BMC Res Notes*. 2021;14(1):342. https://doi.org/10.1186/s13104-021-05875-3
17. Kenny NP, Sherwin S, Baylis F. Re-visioning public health ethics: a relational perspective. *Can J Public Health*. 2010;101(1):9–11. https://doi.org/10.1007/BF03405552
18. American Public Health Association. Public Health Code of Ethics. 2019. Available at: https://apha.org/-/media/Files/PDF/membergroups/ethics/code_of_ethics.ashx. Accessed September 30, 2025.
19. Institute of Medicine. *The Future of the Public's Health in the 21st Century*. Washington, DC: National Academies Press; 2002. https://doi.org/10.17226/10548
20. Wallerstein N, Oetzel JG, Sanchez-Youngman S, et al. Engage for Equity: a long-term study of community-based participatory research and community-engaged research practices and outcomes. *Health Educ Behav*. 2020;47(3):380–390. https://doi.org/10.1177/1090198119897075
21. Ahmed SM, Palermo A-GS. Community engagement in research: frameworks for education and peer review. *Am J Public Health*. 2010;100(8): 1380–1387. Available at: https://doi.org/10.2105/AJPH.2009.178137
22. Auerbach J, Chen AT. Strengthening the partnerships that promote health equity and social justice. *Health Security*. 2023;21(suppl 1):S42–S46. https://doi.org/10.1089/hs.2023.0012
23. Black Doctors COVID-19 Consortium. Center for Health Equity. Available at: https://blackdoctorsconsortium.com/center-for-health-equity. Accessed September 21, 2025.
24. Ford CL, Airhihenbuwa CO. Critical race theory, race equity, and public health: toward antiracism praxis. *Am J Public Health*. 2010;100(suppl 1): S30–S35. https://doi.org/10.2105/ajph.2009.171058
25. Anaissie T, Cary V, Clifford D, Malarkey T, Wise S. 2021. Liberatory design. Available at: http://www.liberatorydesign.com. Accessed September 30, 2025.

To Demonstrate Trustworthiness, Public Health Must Listen, Reflect, Act, and Revisit

Philip M. Alberti, PhD, Jennifer K. Bretsch, MS, Debra Oto-Kent, MPH, and Keyonna M. King, DrPH

ABOUT THE AUTHORS

Philip M. Alberti and Jennifer K. Bretsch are with the Association of American Medical Colleges (AAMC) Center for Health Justice, Washington, DC. Debra Oto-Kent is with the Health Education Council, Sacramento, CA. Keyonna M. King is with the University of Nebraska Medical Center, College of Public Health, Center for Reducing Health Disparities, Health Promotion Department, Omaha, NE.

See also Trust in Public Health, pp. 31–94.

AJPH January 2026, Vol. 116, No. 1

For too long, organizations with power and privilege—from public health departments to hospitals to police departments—have urged communities to "get over" their mis- and distrust. They have asked people to ignore the ripples of past abuses that still wash across their communities' sidewalks, to ignore the flood of mis- and disinformation inundating their screens, and to ignore their very own eyes that saw new injustice and inequity swell after our public health and health care system's response to COVID-19.[1–3] Organizational urging and messaging are not enough to turn this tide. Indeed, over the past four years, there has been a steady decline in US adults' trust in our institutions, with only 79% of adults in 2024 trusting that public health departments "treat everyone in their local community fairly," a 3% decline since 2021.[4] For certain groups—conservative adults and younger adults, specifically—that proportion was even lower: 75% and 73%, respectively.

Instead of giving assurances, organizations should ensure their behavior—through the services they offer, the coalitions they join, the causes they trumpet, the policies and practices they endorse—demonstrates they are worthy of trust. What is seen as trustworthy will differ by sector, context, and population, so centering hyperlocal community wisdom is key: only communities themselves can decide what trustworthy behavior looks like.

The importance of authentic community engagement is true, too, for the development of tools and resources created to rebuild trust or to build it anew. While public health and other researchers have produced an ever-deepening literature on relevant definitions, distinctions, and measurement of trust and trustworthiness,[5–7] there is a paucity of action-oriented tools focused on how trust is built and how trustworthiness is demonstrated.

Almost five years ago, the Association of American Medical Colleges (AAMC) Center for Health Justice (the Center) released its Principles of Trustworthiness Toolkit, a resource originated by and codeveloped with dozens of researchers and multisector community partners from across the United States.[8,9] The Toolkit was designed to help institutions earn the trust of their community by demonstrating they are worthy of it and lifted up community-identified key behaviors on which organizations should focus such as respect, transparency, intentionality, commitment, humility, and authenticity, among others. Through dozens of recorded videos of one-on-one interviews with community members from seven regions across the United States, the Center team, alongside nine researchers from its AAMC Collaborative for Health Equity: Act, Research, Generate Evidence (CHARGE)[10] and the interviewees themselves, partnered to identify themes, translate those themes into the 10 principles, and build complementary tools and resources to operationalize the work of demonstrating trustworthiness. The core innovation of the Toolkit, beyond its focus on action and accountability, was its centering of the lived experience of community members and its reliance on their wisdom to identify and define the behaviors local institutions should take to demonstrate they are worthy of trust.

Despite tens of thousands of views, downloads, and shares, and despite the Toolkit's influence on the addition of "trustworthiness" as a new, tenth principle in the Centers for Disease Control and Prevention's (CDC's) community engagement framework,[11] we did not know what it meant to *use* the tools. We did not know how communities beyond those that originally developed the tools would respond to them. We did not know if the Toolkit worked.

To evaluate outcomes and identify potential improvements, in 2024, the Center launched a pilot of the Toolkit.[12]

Based on the multisector nature of their proposed collaboration, the specific communities and concerns of interest, and the depth (or newness) of their focus on trustworthiness, four diverse and distinct partnerships were selected by the Center team and members of its Multisector Partner Group.[13] The TRUE (Trust, Respect, Unity, and Equity) Together team focused on the Latino and farmworker community in rural Northern California, which faces historic and current injustices in environmental health hazard exposure, economic stress, and housing. Their partnership included a local radio station, a county health and human services agency, and a local health education council among others. An established nonprofit partnership in Atlanta, Georgia, Fathers Matter ATL, sought to address trust between city agencies and Black fathers, including those returning to the community from incarceration. The county board of health, a CDC-funded academic research center, and a managed care plan were among the project collaborators. The Engaging Alton for Equity collaboration based in Alton, Illinois, sought to rebuild trust in the once-thriving Mississippi River commercial center that has since seen trust erode and gun violence, economic disparity, and racial profiling increase. Their team included the local school of medicine, the mayor's office, and the area school district. Finally, the United in Trust team from Omaha, Nebraska, wanted to initiate a long overdue conversation about trust and how the area's medical and government institutions could demonstrate trustworthiness to the Black, Native American, and Bhutanese, Karen, Somali, and other refugee communities in North Omaha. Their team included a university, the county health department, an academic medical center, and local community-based organizations.

The Center did not specify or prescribe an implementation plan, urging the multisector project partners to use the tools in ways that made sense locally. Beyond leadership roles on the pilot communities' core teams, community members were engaged in various ways that aligned with local norms: through listening sessions, community gatherings, one-on-one conversations, and local media. Emergent ideas and themes were captured in an online project discussion board and through monthly "all site" project team meetings. The Center team was also available for individual project team consultation and conversation throughout the year.

Many lessons were learned. One significant lesson developed and endorsed by all four pilot communities was the need for the Toolkit to provide a more formal structure and process. Over the course of our monthly team meetings and based on their own local implementation strategies' successes and challenges, they proposed a four-stage "Listen, Reflect, Act, Revisit" cycle (Figure 1).

Thinking back on the yearlong pilot and our own "Listen, Reflect, Act, and Revisit" journey, the Center and the collaborative learned crucial lessons about how public health departments, health care systems, and other powerful organizations can evolve and deepen their community engagement efforts in ways that lay the foundation for trust and effective action. The lessons learned also apply to the development of tools and resources such organizations can use to build bridges and forge trusting partnerships.

LISTEN

Engaging communities around trust requires prework. Many community members across the four communities were not ready or willing to jump into a conversation about trust with public health, health care, and local government representatives. The mistrust ran

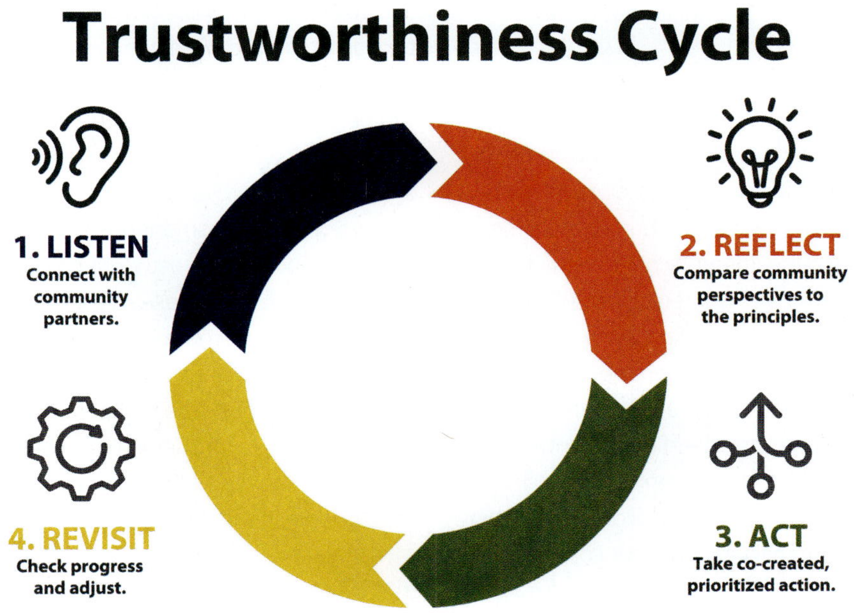

FIGURE 1— The Trustworthiness Cycle

too deep. As a first step, community members expressed a desire to be heard—for their public health and health care partners to simply listen to their experiences, histories, and perspectives. One community member from Omaha stated that this step is critical because "to know where you're going [becoming trustworthy], you must know where you have been." In response, two pilot sites independently developed "speak freely" sessions to provide community members a safe space to share lived experiences without fear or rebuttal. Those session guides are now a core component of the refreshed Toolkit.

The takeaway is that before developing interventions, public health policy, or tools—even before developing focus areas for interventions and policy—public health departments, health care systems and other organizations should bake in time for authentic listening to all communities they serve. Listening cannot be done on the fly, and it must not be perfunctory. Rather, it is a crucial, intentional, foundational, standalone first step for all our work.

REFLECT

Like many public health– and community health–focused efforts, our pilot program had limited resources and time, and our community partners had various competing interests. The Center's initial attempts to keep the program on time and on track were not well received. Teams felt rushed and that the Center team, despite our efforts and intention, had not done enough to demonstrate trustworthiness or to allow relationships to form between the four communities. It was a crucial reminder that trustworthiness must be demonstrated across levels—not just "on the ground" between organizations and community members but also between partners in the coalitions leading that on-the-ground work. After reflecting as a Center and then reflecting together with the four communities, we apologized and made significant changes to our timeline, expectations, and how we conducted our monthly meetings.

The takeaway is that we cannot shy away from tough conversations. Public health departments and other organizations should develop the capacity to pause, take accountability for past and present actions, and meaningfully adjust in real time. Mistakes will happen, but when there is a lack of accountability and adjustment, they become catalysts that hasten the degradation of trust.

ACT

Before convening the four communities, the Center had built a survey tool to assess community members' perceptions of local organizations' trustworthiness. Everyone across all four communities hated it. It was too long, and community members from all four pilot communities were generally wary of surveys given how extractive they can be. So, after reflection with our pilot partners, we decided to scrap the existing tool and to act collaboratively to develop 10 assessment questions, one per Principle of Trustworthiness. We then embedded those questions into three different data-collection strategies (survey, interview, listening session/talking circle) so that communities could decide for themselves which method to deploy. All three variations are available in the refreshed Toolkit.

The takeaway is that demonstrating trustworthiness hinges on acting in ways that show you have not only heard your community and multisector partners, but you have also meaningfully changed course or evolved because of that wisdom (even if those changes deviate from public health's or health care's "best laid plans").

REVISIT

The pilot program was the Center's attempt to revisit its work. We could have rested on the laurels received after the success of the 2021 version of the Toolkit, but the spirit of trustworthiness pushed us to dive deeper and hold ourselves and our work to account. Trustworthiness is fragile and requires constant refinement, adjustment, and more listening.

After the yearlong pilot, we still do not know if the Toolkit works. The Center abandoned that priority as it became clear that our community partners emphasized developing trustworthy processes, assessment tools, and relationships. We listened to them. We reflected together about the Center's mistakes and the Toolkit's shortcomings. We acted collectively to co-create a refreshed Toolkit more likely to be effective, one more likely to "work." And we continue to revisit our accomplishments and strategize ways to build on them. We are walking the talk.

The takeaway is that "revisiting" means everything is up for grabs, including, in our case, the initial objectives of the pilot program. It is impossible for public health departments or health care organizations to "meet communities where they are" if they are stuck in their own goals, priorities, and expectations.

CONCLUSION

We learned that establishing and building trust happens one relationship at a time, one community at a time, and that these encounters set the stage for how community residents perceive our institutions. At a time when trust is a main topic of public health and health care discourse and when trends related to the public's perception of our organizations' trustworthiness all point downward, the need for action-focused tools is more important than ever. These tools, however, will fail if we continue to create them from the top down, if we continue to rely on our theory and frameworks instead of on our community partners' lived experience, and if we focus exclusively on evidence generation and generalizability, to the exclusion of what works in specific places and spaces with unique contexts and histories.

Of course, we still hope to build evidence—local evidence—to support the Toolkit's effectiveness. Yet, despite a lack of evidence, one overarching takeaway has emerged: when it comes to demonstrating trustworthiness, the process is as important as the product. AJPH

CORRESPONDENCE

Correspondence should be sent to Jennifer K. Bretsch, MS, The Association of American Medical Colleges, 655 K St NW, Suite 100, Washington, DC 20001 (e-mail: jbretsch@aamc.org). Reprints can be ordered at https://www.ajph.org by clicking the "Reprints" link.

PUBLICATION INFORMATION

Full Citation: Alberti PM, Bretsch JK, Oto-Kent D, King KM. To demonstrate trustworthiness, public health must listen, reflect, act, and revisit. *Am J Public Health*. 2026;116(1):86–89.

Acceptance Date: October 14, 2025.

DOI: https://doi.org/10.2105/AJPH.2025.308329

ORCID iDs:

Philip M. Alberti https://orcid.org/0000-0002-3381-4882

Jennifer K. Bretsch https://orcid.org/0009-0000-9586-3199

CONTRIBUTORS

P. M. Alberti made substantial contributions to the conceptualization and design of the work and the acquisition, analysis, and interpretation of data for the work, and drafted and revised the work. J. K. Bretsch made substantial contributions to the design of the work and the acquisition, analysis, and interpretation of data for the work, and revised the work. D. Oto-Kent and K. M. King made substantial contributions to the acquisition, analysis, and interpretation of data for the work, and revised the work. All authors gave final approval of the version to be published.

ACKNOWLEDGMENTS

We extend our deepest gratitude to the communities in California, Georgia, Illinois, and Nebraska whose knowledge, lived experiences, and ongoing engagement have shaped and grounded this work. Their insight and resilience are central to advancing health equity. We also acknowledge the dedication and collaboration of our core team members, whose expertise, time, and commitment made this editorial possible. This work reflects a shared effort, and we are grateful to all who contributed to its vision and development.

CONFLICTS OF INTEREST

The authors report no conflicts of interest.

REFERENCES

1. Mackey K, Ayers CK, Kondo KK, et al. Racial and ethnic disparities in COVID-19–related infections, hospitalizations, and deaths: a systematic review. *Ann Intern Med.* 2021;174(3):362–373. https://doi.org/10.7326/M20-6306
2. Su D, Alshehri K, Ern J, et al. Racism experience among American adults during COVID-19: a mixed-methods study. *Health Equity.* 2022;6(1):554–563. https://doi.org/10.1089/heq.2022.0070
3. Shi L, Zhang D, Martin E, et al. Racial discrimination, mental health, and behavioral health during the COVID-19 pandemic: a national survey in the United States. *J Gen Intern Med.* 2022;37(10):2496–2504. https://doi.org/10.1007/s11606-022-07540-2
4. Mendez I, Alvarado CS, Alberti PM. Trust trends: US adults' gradually declining trust in institutions, 2021–2024. AAMC Center for Health Justice. February 18, 2025. Available at: https://www.aamchealthjustice.org/news/polling/trust-trends. Accessed September 3, 2025.
5. Akoy B, Harwell H, Kovaliukaite A, Eckel A. Measuring trust: a reinvestigation. *South Econ J.* 2018;84(4):992–1000. https://doi.org/10.1002/soej.12259
6. Richmond J, Anderson A, Cunningham-Erves J, et al. Conceptualizing and measuring trust, mistrust, and distrust: implications for advancing health equity and building trustworthiness. *Annu Rev Public Health.* 2024;45(1):465–484. https://doi.org/10.1146/annurev-publhealth-061022-044737
7. Hancock PA, Kessler TT, Kaplan AD, et al. How and why humans trust: a meta-analysis and elaborated model. *Front Psychol.* 2023;14:1081086. https://doi.org/10.3389/fpsyg.2023.1081086
8. AAMC Center for Health Justice. The Principles of Trustworthiness Toolkit. July 22, 2025. Available at: https://www.aamchealthjustice.org/our-work/trustworthiness/trustworthiness-toolkit. Accessed September 3, 2025.
9. Chinekezi O, Andress L, Agonafer EP, et al. From the national to the local: issues of trust and a model for community-academic engagement. *Front Public Health.* 2023;11:1068425. https://doi.org/10.3389/fpubh.2023.1068425
10. AAMC Center for Health Justice. AAMC CHARGE. Available at: https://www.aamchealthjustice.org/get-involved/aamc-charge. Accessed October 10, 2025.
11. Agency for Toxic Substances and Disease Registry. *Principles of Community Engagement.* 3rd ed. January 13, 2025. Available at: https://www.aamchealthjustice.org/media/8061/download?attachment. Accessed August 20, 2025.
12. AAMC Center for Health Justice. Principles of Trustworthiness Toolkit Project. Available at: https://www.aamchealthjustice.org/key-topics/trustworthiness/project. Accessed October 10, 2025.
13. AAMC Center for Health Justice. The Multisector Partner Group. Available at: https://www.aamchealthjustice.org/about-us/multisector-partner-group. Accessed October 10, 2025.

Fostering Collaboration and Trust to Address COVID-19–Related Disparities and Misinformation in South Central Texas

Tharani Ravi, MD, Jasmine Rodriguez, MPH, Robert L. Ferrer, MD, MPH, Alvin Estacio, MS, Ariel Gomez, MPH, Paula Winkler, MEd, and Erika L. Thompson, PhD, MPH, CPH

See also Trust in Public Health, pp. 31–94.

The Community Engagement Alliance (CEAL) Against COVID-19 is a national initiative to address disparities and misinformation surrounding COVID-19. The South Central Texas CEAL implemented community-based interventions to engage vulnerable populations, counter misinformation, and address the health impacts of COVID-19. Through community engagement, community-driven data gathering, and health information dissemination through trusted partners, this initiative fostered trust and collaboration among diverse community organizations, shared resources, and developed culturally tailored health messaging. This community-engaged program's success highlights its sustainability.
(*Am J Public Health*. 2026;116(1):90–94. https://doi.org/10.2105/AJPH.2025.308277)

AJPH January 2026, Vol. 116, No. 1

The South Central Texas Community Engagement Alliance (CEAL) initiative aimed to mitigate COVID-19's disproportionate impact on vulnerable populations by addressing health disparities and misinformation while fostering trust and collaboration among community organizations, in alignment with the national CEAL initiative.[1–3]

INTERVENTION AND IMPLEMENTATION

The objectives of the South Central Texas CEAL initiative were

1. Build sustainable partnerships with diverse, trusted community organizations.
2. Disseminate accurate, culturally tailored health information to vulnerable populations through trusted community leaders.
3. Collect community-driven data to identify health priorities and inform public health interventions.

Research Team

The South Central Texas CEAL is led by the Department of Family and Community Medicine at UT Health San Antonio together with the South Central Area Health Education Center.

Community Partnerships

The South Central Texas CEAL team focused on forming partnerships with organizations that were well-established within their communities and represented the area's diversity. The South Central Area Health Education Center played a pivotal role in identifying partners, drawing on its extensive knowledge of the region's community landscape. Initial partners included the local health authority, Ella Austin and WestCare (serving the predominantly Black Eastside), Alamo Colleges District (a network of community colleges that includes community health worker [CHW] training programs), and YWCA and Catholic churches (predominantly serving the Hispanic Westside of San Antonio). The team partnered with the local Translational Advisory Board, a group with experience in bridging community and academic research efforts. In year three, partners representing three surrounding rural counties, refugee, and immigrant communities were added.

Partners were selected on the basis of their strong, trusted presence in the community, which was essential for effectively sharing health information.[4] By choosing organizations that reflected the diversity of San Antonio and surrounding rural areas, the CEAL team aimed to ensure an equitable response to COVID-19.

Methods of Partner Engagement

Each year began with a breakfast meeting where partners and the research team gathered to cocreate a shared agenda for the year. The core engagement strategy centered on weekly 30-minute virtual meetings held on Monday mornings, bringing together representatives from partner organizations and the research team. Topics for discussion during the weekly meetings were determined by the partners and reflected the pressing concerns of their communities. Early in the pandemic, topics focused on emerging COVID-19 information and addressing misinformation as it arose in the communities. By 2021 and 2022, discussion topics included long COVID and mental health, which had become emerging concerns. In 2024, the focus shifted to chronic disease management and social determinants of health. These meetings facilitated regular, collaborative exchange of information and ideas among partners. They also connected clinical experts and community leaders to address key health issues, fostering collaboration to develop health messaging tailored to each community. Between meetings, communication continued via e-mail, with regular updates on outreach events and new developments, ensuring partners remained informed throughout the week.

Culturally Tailored Messaging

Health messaging topics were collaboratively identified by partners according to their communities' needs. Messaging was codeveloped through continuous, bidirectional communication and feedback, ensuring cultural relevancy and appropriate adaptations for specific populations.[5–8] Partners distributed this health information within their communities as trusted sources for information.[9,10] Many partner organizations distributed these materials through their CHWs, who had a strong presence in the community. Materials such as flyers, radio spots, and social media content were translated into Spanish and other languages (as requested) to reach refugee communities. This approach ensured that health information effectively resonated with the target audiences.

Community-Driven Information Gathering

The annual "Common Survey" was developed by the National Institutes of Health for all CEAL sites. The survey was designed to engage vulnerable communities and explore their attitudes and perceptions related to COVID-19, as well as assess the prevalence of chronic disease, social determinants of health, vaccine uptake, sources of health information, and trust.[11] South Central Texas CEAL partners contributed to these surveys by adding questions derived from local concerns. They distributed the surveys to their communities, using the results to inform outreach activities and apply for grants to address health disparities.

PLACE, TIME, AND PERSONS

This CEAL initiative began in October 2020 and continues today in urban Bexar County and surrounding rural counties. The South Central Texas CEAL team collaborated with community partners representing predominantly Hispanic low-income neighborhoods, immigrants, Black communities, refugees, and rural populations. About 80% of the partner organizations incorporated CHWs directly into their outreach efforts, relying on their trusted relationships to gather insights from the community and share culturally relevant health information.

PURPOSE

Hispanic populations in South Texas were disproportionately affected by COVID-19, making up 83% of cases in Bexar County despite representing 61% of the population. National data showed higher risks of hospitalization and death for Hispanics compared with non-Hispanic Whites.[1] These disparities were driven by structural inequities, including socioeconomic conditions, occupational exposure, and health care access barriers, compounded by misinformation and long-standing mistrust in health care systems.[1] In alignment with the national CEAL, South Central Texas CEAL aimed to foster sustainable academic–community partnerships to build trust, counter misinformation, and collaboratively address emerging health priorities, beginning with COVID-19.

EVALUATION AND ADVERSE EFFECTS

At the conclusion of each year, the team conducted reflection sessions to

AJPH January 2026, Vol. 116, No. 1

foster open discussions on the partnership's achievements, challenges, and areas for improvement. Partners completed anonymous surveys, providing candid feedback to inform future planning and activities. In addition, partner organizations submitted weekly reports detailing community outreach efforts (in-person and virtual events) and distribution of health messaging materials related to the collective impact. Minutes from the weekly virtual partner meetings were reviewed to document instances of resource sharing and collaboration.

Impact

Resource sharing. The weekly meetings served as a platform for partners to share information about upcoming community events and as an opportunity to share resources. There were instances where resource sharing otherwise would likely not have occurred. As an example, when one of our urban partners required additional COVID-19 vaccines for a health fair, our rural partner redirected her organization's surplus vaccines to that urban partner. Similarly, fresh produce left over from a summer camp event held by one of our partners was redirected to our Center for Refugee Services, which was in urgent need of food for their pantry. These examples show how the partnership addressed community needs and fostered trust that led to resource sharing and support.

Community messaging dissemination. The South Central Texas CEAL partnership facilitated mutual sharing of ideas for health message dissemination through various outlets including e-mail, health fairs, magazine ads, and radio. In the second year, the CEAL team began quantifying the number of events held by CEAL partner organizations. Collectively, in years two to three of CEAL, the South Central Texas CEAL partner organizations conducted 386 in-person community health events and 99 virtual events, and sent 116 759 messages related to vaccinations; CHW training and coordination; events supporting daily needs such as food aid, housing, utilities, and transportation; and other health-related events. Any messaging created through CEAL collaboration was sent through partner e-mail networks and distributed at community events (Table 1).

Capacity building. In response to CEAL partner organizations' pressing need to address COVID-19's impact on mental health, the team organized three Mental Health First Aid training sessions in 2024 with 65 people trained. In addition, expert-led discussions during the weekly meetings provided partners with valuable insights into emerging health concerns (e.g., measles), fostering continuous learning and collaboration.

Community's trust. Feedback from the CEAL partners' anonymous surveys and reflection sessions highlighted that their communities felt they received consistent, accurate health messaging from multiple trusted sources. This consistency contributes to building and strengthening their trust in health care systems (Box 1).

Adverse Effects

No adverse effects or unintended consequences were reported.

SUSTAINABILITY

The South Central Texas CEAL partnership demonstrated remarkable sustainability and adaptability. It grew from 10 urban partner groups in the first year

TABLE 1— Health Events and E-Mail Outreach Conducted by South Central Texas CEAL Community Partners: March 2022–March 2024

	In-Person Events	Virtual Events	E-Mail Distributions
Total no. of events	386	99	128
Community education on COVID-19–related topics	117	18	42
Vaccination event	164	1	2
Event supporting daily needs (e.g., food aid, housing, utilities, transportation)	56	7	3
Event for community health worker training or coordination	8	73	3
Other health and community well-being event	41	0	78
Total no. of people reached[a]	32 622	1 772	116 759

Note. CEAL = Community Engagement Alliance.
[a]Number of people could not be de-duplicated (i.e., the same person may have gone to multiple events).

BOX 1— Partner Feedback on the Impact of South Central Texas CEAL (From Anonymous Partner Surveys and Reflection Sessions)

Collaboration	Community Education or Health Messaging	Capacity Building	Trust
"From the beginning we meet weekly to discuss CEAL progress with our partners and leads. As a team we plan upcoming initiatives and collaboration opportunities." 'We can better serve our community by not working in silos and continue to brainstorm, collaborate as one team." 'We have built so many strong partnerships through our work with the CEAL and that is the primary thing we take back to our organization." 'Opportunity to network is priceless."	"We post CEAL informational offering[s] on our social media and offer them to the community at events, and we also provide pointers to our CHWs on how to build consistent messaging." "Good information from reliable sources to pass on to the people in our community center."	"The work we do in the community is information dissemination and capacity building, which is also what is done for our organization so that our staff can be credible messengers." "CEAL helped with putting out health messages. It made my community part of the team. . . . Even our priest was helping giving out [health] messages."	"We are already doing the most important part of this: creating consistent messaging and forming a united front to fight health disparities. It makes all the difference in the world that when a person goes to Ella Austin, Center for Refugee Services, or UTHSCSA, they will get the same message, which builds trust and, hence, engagement."

Note. CEAL = Community Engagement Alliance; CHW = community health worker; UTHSCSA = University of Texas Health Science Center at San Antonio.

to 17 partners by the third year, expanding to include rural organizations and those serving immigrant and refugee populations. Weekly meetings continued uninterrupted, underscoring the strength of the engagement model and its capacity to address evolving community needs. The partnership collaborated on a range of grant applications focused on health topics identified by the group, ensuring sustainability through ongoing funding and resources. This sustainability highlights the potential of this community-engaged strategy to create lasting impact in addressing public health challenges.

PUBLIC HEALTH SIGNIFICANCE

The South Central Texas CEAL initiative has had significant implications for public health. This collaborative partnership showed how even brief but consistent virtual meetings can build lasting and meaningful relationships among diverse community organizations. Impact was greatest when guided by the principles of meaningful engagement and inclusion of trusted leaders and individuals deeply in touch with community needs, such as CHWs. Such enduring collaborations created a unified voice that facilitated the delivery of consistent and accurate health information, thus strengthening the public's trust in the health care system. They also built community resilience by fostering trust, cooperation, and shared problem-solving among organizations. The collaborative sharing of resources and mutually reinforcing activities amplified their collective impact on community health. The initiative not only addressed the immediate COVID-19 challenges but also strengthened community resilience and established a foundation for addressing future public health challenges. The model's adaptability demonstrated its potential for broader application in diverse public health contexts. AJPH

ABOUT THE AUTHORS

Tharani Ravi and Jasmine Rodriguez are with the Department of Family and Community Medicine at University of Texas Health Science Center at San Antonio. Robert Ferrer was with the Department of Family and Community Medicine at University of Texas Health Science Center at San Antonio at the time of this study. Alvin Estacio is with the Department of Epidemiology, Human Genetics, and Environmental Sciences at University of Texas Health Science Center at Houston. Ariel Gomez and Paula Winkler are with South Central Area Health Education Center in San Antonio, TX. Erika L. Thompson is with the Department of Quantitative and Qualitative Health Sciences at University of Texas School of Public Health San Antonio.

CORRESPONDENCE

Correspondence should be sent to Tharani Ravi, 7703 Floyd Curl Drive, MC 7843, San Antonio, TX 78229 (e-mail: ravit@uthscsa.edu). Reprints can be ordered at https://www.ajph.org by clicking the "Reprints" link.

PUBLICATION INFORMATION

Full Citation: Ravi T, Rodriguez J, Ferrer RL, et al. Fostering collaboration and trust to address COVID-19–related disparities and misinformation in South Central Texas. *Am J Public Health*. 2026; 116(1):90–94.

Acceptance Date: August 16, 2025.

DOI: https://doi.org/10.2105/AJPH.2025.308277

ORCID iDs:

Tharani Ravi https://orcid.org/0009-0001-8995-784X

Jasmine Rodriguez https://orcid.org/0000-0002-9443-1658

Alvin Estacio https://orcid.org/0000-0002-1596-7025

Erika L. Thompson https://orcid.org/0000-0002-7115-0001

CONTRIBUTORS

T. Ravi made substantial contributions to the conceptualization and design of the work, analysis and interpretation of data, and article writing. J. Rodriguez made substantial contributions to the conceptualization and design of the work, analysis and interpretation of data, and revising the article critically. R. Ferrer and P. Winkler made substantial contributions to the conceptualization and design of the work. A. Estacio made substantial contributions to data analysis and interpretation of data. A. Gomez made substantial contributions to the conceptualization and design of the work and acquisition of the data. E. L. Thompson made substantial contributions to the conceptualization and design of the work and revision of the article. All authors provided final approval of the version to be published.

ACKNOWLEDGMENTS

This work was supported by the Texas Community Engagement Alliance (CEAL) Consortium, funded by the National Institutes of Health (1OT2HL156812).

We are deeply grateful to our South Central Texas CEAL community partners for their sustained collaboration and unwavering commitment to serving their diverse communities. These partners include Atascosa Health Center; Atascosa Inter-Agency Council Inc; Bexar, Frio, Karnes, and Atascosa Translational Advisory Boards; Center for Refugee Services; Domesticas Unidas; Ella Austin Community Center; Frio Regional Hospital; Health Confianza; Northwest Vista College – Community Health Worker Program; San Martin de Porres Catholic Church; South Central Texas Area Health Education Center; WestCare Texas; and the YWCA San Antonio. We also would like to acknowledge Junda Woo, MD, MPH, Lisa Kilpela, PhD, and Bob Clark, MD, for their mentorship.

CONFLICTS OF INTEREST

The authors report no conflicts of interest.

HUMAN PARTICIPANT PROTECTION

This study was approved by UT Health San Antonio's institutional review board. All surveys conducted by South Central Texas CEAL, including evaluation of partner activities, were also approved by UT Health San Antonio's institutional review board.

REFERENCES

1. Hosek MG, Sharma A, Nunn M, et al. Disproportionate burden of COVID-19 infection among Hispanic patients during the first COVID-19 surge in South Texas. *Health Equity.* 2022;6(1):546–553. https://doi.org/10.1089/heq.2021.0185
2. Mensah GA, Johnson LE, Zhang X, et al. Community Engagement Alliance (CEAL): a National Institutes of Health program to advance health equity. *Am J Public Health.* 2024;114(S1):S12–S17. https://doi.org/10.2105/AJPH.2023.307476
3. Webb Hooper M, Nápoles AM, Pérez-Stable EJ. COVID-19 and racial/ethnic disparities. *JAMA.* 2020;323(24):2466–2467. https://doi.org/10.1001/jama.2020.8598
4. George S, Duran N, Norris K. A systematic review of barriers and facilitators to minority research participation among African Americans, Latinos, Asian Americans, and Pacific Islanders. *Am J Public Health.* 2014;104(2):e16–e31. https://doi.org/10.2105/AJPH.2013.301706
5. Casillas A, Flores-Uribe E, Abhat A, et al. The language of COVID-19: health systems must now prioritize responsive in-language and culturally-tailored messaging. *Int J Disaster Risk Reduct.* 2022;77:103077. https://doi.org/10.1016/j.ijdrr.2022.103077
6. Velasquez D, Uppal N, Perez N. Equitable access to health information for non-English speakers amidst the novel coronavirus pandemic. *Health Affairs Forefront.* April 2, 2020. Available at: https://www.healthaffairs.org/content/forefront/equitable-access-health-information-non-english-speakers-amidst-novel-coronavirus. Accessed September 12, 2025.
7. Mack DH, Douglas M, Holiday R, et al. An equitable communication and dissemination model for linking culturally diverse communities to COVID-19 services. *Am J Public Health.* 2024;114(suppl 9):S718–S722. https://doi.org/10.2105/AJPH.2024.307813
8. Ryan RE, Silke C, Parkhill A, et al. Communication to promote and support physical distancing for COVID-19 prevention and control. *Cochrane Database Syst Rev.* 2023;10(10):CD015144. https://doi.org/10.1002/14651858.CD015144
9. Bekele F, Yu K, Archbold S, Mann E, Dawson-Hahn E, Aziz O. The Community Health Response Team: a culturally and linguistically tailored community response to COVID-19 addressing barriers to testing and vaccinations for refugee, immigrant and migrant communities in Atlanta, Georgia. *Front Public Health.* 2024;12:1362705. https://doi.org/10.3389/fpubh.2024.1362705
10. Nan X, Iles IA, Yang B, Ma Z. Public health messaging during the COVID-19 pandemic and beyond: lessons from communication science. *Health Commun.* 2022;37(1):1–19. https://doi.org/10.1080/10410236.2021.1994910
11. Walker RJ, Eisenhauer E, Thompson EL, et al. COVID-19 information, trust, and risk perception across diverse communities in the United States: initial findings from a multistate Community Engagement Alliance (CEAL). *Am J Public Health.* 2024;114(suppl 1):S112–S123. https://doi.org/10.2105/AJPH.2023.307504

The Association Between Vacant Lot Redevelopment and Violent/Firearm Violent Crime: A Difference-in-Difference Analysis From 2007 to 2023

Nicole Asa, MPH, Hiwot Y. Zewdie, PhD, MS, Ali Rowhani-Rahbar, MD, PhD, MPH, Bradley H. Wagenaar, PhD, MPH, and Stephen J. Mooney, PhD, MS

See also MacDonald, p. 18.

Objectives. To investigate the association between vacant lot redevelopment and violent crime and firearm violent crime.

Methods. We used a quasi-experimental study with a difference-in-difference (DID) design. The study population was 254 vacant lots located in Philadelphia, Pennsylvania. The exposure was redevelopment, defined as repurposing the vacant lot into a permanent structure (e.g., housing) between 2007 and 2023. The outcome was violent crime subtypes and firearm violent crime subtypes reported to the police. Our primary analysis used a staggered DID estimator.

Results. We found a negative association between redevelopment and aggravated assault (DID = −56.55 crimes per square mile per year; 95% confidence interval [CI] = −97.86, −15.24), firearm aggravated assault (DID = −35.11 crimes per square mile per year; 95% CI = −55.41, −14.82), and overall firearm violent crime (DID = −27.26 crimes per square mile per year; 95% CI = −52.97, −1.54). We did not find significant associations for the other outcomes tested.

Conclusions. Our results support the hypothesis that vacant lot redevelopment may prevent or displace violent crime.

Public Health Implications. Built environment investments may prevent or displace violence. (*Am J Public Health*. 2026;116(1):95–102. https://doi.org/10.2105/AJPH.2025.308269)

AJPH January 2026, Vol. 116, No. 1

Violence is a significant public health problem. The four most common violent crime categories are murder, rape, robbery, and aggravated assault.[1] In 2023, there were 1.2 million violent crimes reported in the United States.[1] Investment in the built environment by directly treating aspects of disinvested environments may prevent violence.[2,3]

Lot vacancy is a treatable aspect of disinvestment.[4] Many communities that experience high rates of gun violence also have a high volume of vacant lots and unmaintained land.[5] Vacant lots are hypothesized to contribute to nearby violence through 2 complementary mechanisms: (1) vacant lots indicate some level of abandonment, leading to the perception that there are fewer eyes on the street and thus a safer place to engage in potentially violent activities, and (2) an unmaintained vacant lot is an open and relatively deserted space where drugs or weapons can be stored.[2,3,6,7] Vacant land restoration has therefore emerged as a potential strategy for violence prevention.

Most of the vacant land restoration strategies for crime prevention focus on vacant lot greening. Greening vacant lots by removing trash, mowing and landscaping, and adding community cues to care such as gardens, have been shown to reduce overall and violent crime and improve perceptions of neighborhood safety.[6,8–13] For example, a study in Philadelphia, Pennsylvania, found that the odds of homicide were significantly lower in neighborhoods with maintained and greened vacant lots relative to those that did not have maintained and greened lots.[11] Similarly, another study in Philadelphia using a randomized controlled trial design found that all crimes, gun assaults, and burglaries were significantly reduced after a vacant lot greening intervention.[14]

Investment in housing and neighborhoods has been shown to reduce neighborhood violence.[15–18] For example, a study found that in Philadelphia, a housing repair intervention was associated with a 21.9% reduction in total crime.[15] It follows that redeveloping vacant lots into permanent structures such as housing may also reduce violence. However, perhaps because redevelopment is much more expensive on a per-lot basis than greening or repair, it has been less often studied as a violence prevention technique. Nonetheless, examining the effect of vacant lot redevelopment and violent crime and firearm violent crime could provide insight into potential mechanisms through which intervening on the built environment could help reduce crime in certain places.

We quantified the association between vacant lot redevelopment and violent crime and firearm violent crime reported to the police in Philadelphia from 2007 through 2023 using an analytic approach that accounted for staggered timing of vacant lot development. We hypothesized that there would be a reduction in violent crime and firearm violent crime as redevelopment removes the influence of abandonment and decreases the amount of open or deserted places.

METHODS

We conducted a quasi-experimental staggered difference-in-difference (DID) study to assess the relationship of vacant lot redevelopment with violent crime and firearm violent crime in Philadelphia from 2007 through 2023.

Study Population

We used the OpenDataPhilly Building Demolitions data set to identify vacant land parcels.[19] We aimed to combine contiguous lots within the data set, as they are likely perceived as a single land parcel. To construct contiguous vacant lots, we used the lot coordinates to cluster the addresses based on 1 point of contact within 26.2 feet and verified a random subsample (n = 10) using Google Street View (Google, Mountain View, CA) to double check our parameters were accurate. This process identified 2117 unique vacant lots. We randomly selected 300 vacant lots and subsequently excluded vacant lots (n = 46) that (1) only had 0 or 1 Street View images such that we were unable to assess when the lot was redeveloped or (2) had sufficiently blurry images that we were unable to locate the lot or determine its status. Our final study population consisted of 254 vacant lots in the City of Philadelphia. In our study population, demolitions occurred between 2007 and 2013. Lots entered the study population when the demolition was complete.

Exposure

Our exposure was vacant lot redevelopment. Two researchers (NA and HYZ) visually audited each vacant lot in the study sample using available Street View imagery for all available time points to determine whether anything had been constructed on the lot of interest, with the goal of identifying the first image showing redevelopment. We double-coded 62 randomly selected vacant lots. We identified no coding differences in type of redevelopment or year of redevelopment. We identified 6 discrepancies related to visual concerns, where raters were not able to accurately view the lot because of blurry images or removal of images on Street View. We removed these 6 lots from our study population.

From these images, we identified 3 forms of redevelopment: housing or business structures, impermeable fences, and other permanent structures (which included parking lots, sheds, and garages). We excluded permeable fences (e.g., split rail fences typically installed as part of the Philadelphia Horticultural Society's Land Care program[14]) as a form of redevelopment as they do not restrict access to the lot. We then created 2 exposure definitions of redevelopment for subsequent analyses. Our primary redevelopment definition tested the hypothesis that investment prevents or displaces violence. For this analysis, we defined redevelopment as new construction of housing or business structures, considering this to both visually indicate investment into the area and restrict public access to the no-longer-vacant lot. The secondary redevelopment definition tested the hypothesis that simply physically restricting access to the vacant lot (i.e., preventing drugs or weapons from being stored there) prevents or displaces violence. For this analysis, we defined redevelopment as fences (chain linked, wooden) and permanent structures (garages, sheds, or parking lots) in addition to housing or business structures, considering these to remove access to the lot, albeit with more variable signaling of investment. For both redevelopment definitions, we considered the lot to be redeveloped in the first year a Street View image showed redevelopment.

Outcome

Our outcome was violent crime and firearm violent crime reported to the police. We obtained georeferenced crime data from the Philadelphia Police Department from 2007 through 2023. Using police codes, we divided violent crime into the following four subtypes in line with the Uniform Crime Reporting Program: homicide, aggravated assault, robbery, and rape. We then separated firearm violent crime from 3 of the 4 subtypes to get a set of firearm violent crime subtypes: firearm homicide, firearm aggravated assault, and firearm robbery. There were no instances of firearm-related rape in our data set. Finally, we included an overall violent crime outcome, the sum of the 4 violent crime subtypes, and an overall firearm violent crime outcome, the sum of the 3 firearm violent crime subtypes.

We used kernel density estimation to generate a smoothed surface from georeferenced violent crime data for each crime type–year combination. For each surface, we used a quartic (biweight) kernel and specified a bandwidth of 500 feet to reflect the hypothesized spatial influence of vacant lot redevelopment on nearby violent crime and to reflect the average size of a Philadelphia block.[20–22] We estimated surfaces at a 100-foot resolution and applied an edge correction to correct for edge cases.[23] The resulting surfaces estimate the density of events per square mile for a given year for each violent crime subtype and firearm violent crime subtype. The density surfaces for each crime type were spatially linked to each vacant lot. We generated kernel density surfaces in RStudio version 4.2.2 using the "spatstat" package (Posit, Boston, MA).[24]

Statistical Analysis

We described Philadelphia census tract baseline characteristics using the 2010 American Community Survey data. Then, we estimated the association between redevelopment and violent crime and firearm violent crime densities using a DID design with a staggered estimator to account for redevelopment over different years. We estimated the average treatment effect after redevelopment using a binary variable with 1 for lots after redevelopment and 0 for lots before redevelopment or a lot that was never redeveloped. All regressions used ordinary least squares and included lot and year fixed effects. We implemented the heterogeneity-robust Gardner 2-stage estimator using the did2s package in RStudio.[25,26] We chose this approach as the Gardner 2-stage estimator uses all pretreatment data as a baseline, whereas other common estimator types use only the last pretreatment period as a baseline.[26,27] We felt incorporation of all pretreatment data was important given substantial year-over-year variation in violent crime and firearm violent crime. For ease of interpretation, we estimated relative change in addition to the absolute change in density.

A key identifying assumption for DID estimation is the parallel trends assumption—that the violence near lots in which redevelopment occurred would have continued along their same trajectories in the absence of redevelopment. Although the true parallel trends assumption is untestable, consistent with DID best practices, we can assess the parallel trends assumption by examining preintervention trends using event study analyses.[27,28] The event study evaluates the pretreatment dynamics between the treatment and control group by including an additional term that indicates the leads and lags of the treatment variable.[28] If violent crime and firearm violent crime rates for redeveloped and nonredeveloped lots were trending similarly before redevelopment, we expect estimated coefficients for event times before redevelopment to be small and statistically insignificant.

We conducted spillover analyses to measure immediate spatial displacement of crime to areas near the vacant lots included in this study. To do this, we used a "donut versus donut hole" buffer zone approach.[14] First, we captured occurrence of crime as counts per year within a 152.4-meter bandwidth (~500 feet) of vacant lots and then captured occurrence of crime as counts per year within 152.4 meters to 304.8 meters bandwidth (~500 to 1000 feet) of vacant lots. We then used the same approach described for the primary analysis and estimated the association between redevelopment and police-reported violent crime and firearm violent crime outcomes using a DID design with a staggered estimator, ordinary least squares regression, and year and lot fixed effects (Table A, available as a supplement to the online version of this article at https://ajph.org).

We conducted all analyses in RStudio version 4.2.2. We conducted data analysis from March 2024 through December 2024. We determined statistical significance at the level of $P < .05$.

RESULTS

When we used the primary redevelopment definition (housing or business structures), 41 (16.1%) of lots were redeveloped. Lots that were redeveloped were clustered around Philadelphia's Center City District (Figure 1). For the

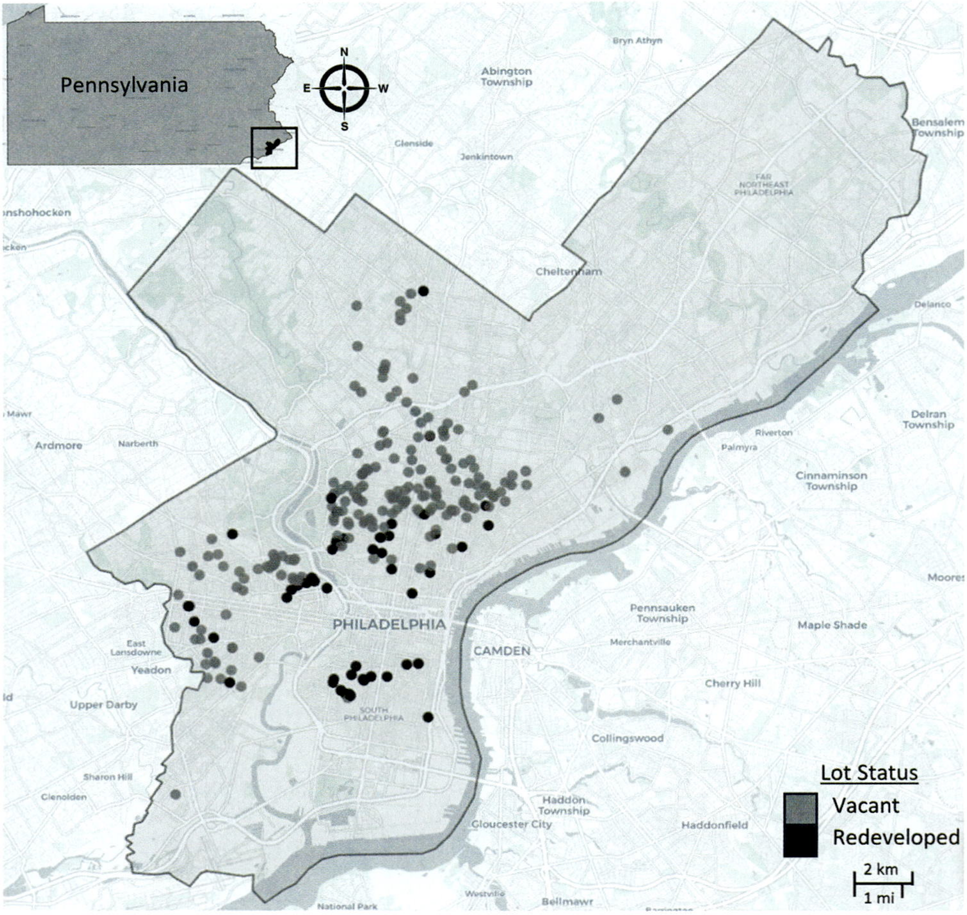

FIGURE 1— Spatial Distribution of Redeveloped Lots and Vacant Lots in Philadelphia, PA: 2007–2023

secondary redevelopment definition (housing or business structures, permanent structures, fences), 143 (59.3%) lots were redeveloped over the study period. Lots that were redeveloped were more likely to be areas with a higher average percentage of White respondents (20.5% vs 9.9%), higher average median income per year ($24 981 vs $21 156), and lower poverty percentage (38.6% vs 41.1%) compared with areas without vacant lot redevelopment (Table 1).

Redevelopment and Violent Crime

For the primary redevelopment definition using housing or business structures, we found a statistically significant negative association between redevelopment and aggravated assault, firearm aggravated assault, and overall firearm violent crime, consistent with our hypothesis that redevelopment may prevent or displace violent crime and firearm violent crime (Table 2). When we compared the difference between postredevelopment and predevelopment years among lots that were redeveloped with the difference during that time in lots that were not redeveloped, the average aggravated assault rate was 56.6 crimes per square mile per year lower (95% confidence interval [CI] = −97.9, −15.2) representing a roughly 30.1% decrease in aggravated assaults (95% CI = −29.0%, −31.2%). Similarly, the average firearm aggravated assault rate was 35.1 crimes per square miles per year lower (95% CI = −55.4, −14.8), or about a 30.8% decrease (95% CI = −29.0%, −32.6%), and the average overall firearm violent crime rate was 27.3 crimes per square mile per year lower (95% CI = −53.0, −1.5) or a 14.7% decrease (95% CI = −13.1%, −16.3%; Table 2). There were no significant associations between the primary redevelopment definition and other violent crime and firearm violent crime outcomes.

For the secondary redevelopment definition (housing or business structures, permanent structures, and fences),

TABLE 1— Census Tract Characteristics for Lots: Philadelphia, PA, 2010

Characteristic[a]	Lot Status[b]	
	Vacant Lots	Redeveloped Lots
White, mean %	9.9	20.5
Poverty, mean %	41.1	38.6
Median yearly income, mean $	21 156	24 981

[a]Characteristics pulled from the 2010 American Community Survey.
[b]Each lot was attributed to the corresponding census tract, and the characteristics are averaged across census tract stratified by lot status. Vacant lots remained vacant throughout the entire study period, whereas redeveloped lots were redeveloped at some point during the study period.

TABLE 2— Difference-in-Difference (DID) Estimates of Violent Crime and Firearm Violent Crime per Square Mile per Year Comparing Redeveloped and Vacant Lots: Philadelphia, PA, 2007–2023

Outcome	DID Estimate[a] (95% CI)
Primary redevelopment definition: housing or business structures[b]	
Overall violent crime	−37.57 (−92.86, 17.73)
Aggravated assault	−56.55 (−97.86, −15.24)
Homicide	2.62 (−4.47, 9.71)
Rape	−0.05 (−6.71, 6.60)
Robbery	16.41 (−9.42, 42.25)
Overall firearm violent crime	−27.26 (−52.97, −1.54)
Firearm aggravated assault	−35.11 (−55.41, −14.82)
Firearm homicide	−3.30 (−7.11, 0.52)
Firearm robbery	11.15 (−4.59, 26.90)
Secondary redevelopment definition: housing or business structures, permanent structures, fences[b]	
Overall violent crime	−8.48 (−52.00, 35.03)
Aggravated assault	−5.11 (−37.90, 27.69)
Homicide	−6.59 (−16.32, 3.15)
Rape	−5.75 (−13.42, 1.92)
Robbery	8.96 (−13.69, 31.61)
Overall firearm violent crime	11.42 (−16.98, 39.82)
Firearm aggravated assault	8.05 (−13.24, 29.34)
Firearm homicide	−6.99 (−13.95, −0.02)
Firearm robbery	10.36 (−3.46, 24.18)

[a]DID regressions used Gardner's 2-stage estimator, used ordinary least squares regression, and included year and lot fixed effects with standard errors clustered at the lot level. The unit of the DID estimates is crimes per square mile per year.
[b]The primary redevelopment definition includes housing or business structures only. The secondary redevelopment definition includes housing or business structures, along with permanent structures and fences.

we found a statistically significant negative association between redevelopment and firearm homicide. The average firearm homicide rate was 7.0 crimes per square mile per year lower comparing postredevelopment and preredevelopment years among lots that were redeveloped contrasting with the change during that time in lots that were not redeveloped (95% CI = −14.0, −0.02) or a decrease of 29.8% (95% CI = −26.7%, −32.7%; Table 2). No other changes in violence were associated with our secondary redevelopment definition beyond what might be expected by chance.

Spillover analyses of the police-reported violent crime and firearm violent crime outcomes showed no indication of spatial displacement. In none of the outcomes did we see that there was a significant reduction in the 152.4-meter buffer surrounding vacant lots that was coupled with significant increases in the ring surrounding the vacant lots (Table A).

Event Study Findings

Event study specifications, which were used to evaluate the parallel trends assumption, are presented for the primary redevelopment definition in Figures A1 and A2 (available as a supplement to the online version of this article at https://ajph.org). Figures A1 and A2 show differences in the rates of violent crime and firearm violent crime before redevelopment, comparing vacant lot clusters that were redeveloped and those that remained vacant. The event study detected minor and variable differences in violent crime and firearm violent crime rates 4 years before redevelopment, though this estimate is small. However, the event study did not detect differences in violent crime and firearm violent crime in the other years before in lots that were redeveloped compared with lots that were not.

DISCUSSION

To our knowledge, this is the first study assessing the association between vacant lot redevelopment and violent crime and firearm violent crime. We found an association between vacant lot redevelopment and lower rates of aggravated assault, firearm aggravated assault, and overall firearm violent crime. However, our results did not hold when we included permanent structures and fences into the redevelopment definition (secondary redevelopment definition). This suggests that redevelopment of vacant lots into housing or business structures might hold a greater impact on aggravated assaults than more modest investments. More broadly, our results support the hypothesis that interventions that invest in neighborhoods (such as housing structures) may prevent or displace (that is, violent crime moving from one area to another) violent crime.

Our results are consistent with those from other studies exploring similar neighborhood violence-prevention mechanisms. One potential mechanism in which redevelopment may prevent or displace violence is through clear ownership of the lot. Replacing unsupervised lots with housing may force unwanted activities to relocate or be reduced,[29] suggesting more neighbors in place may increase collective efficacy, or the perception of mutual trust and willingness to help each other.[30,31] One study created a collective efficacy measure from neighborhoods in Chicago, Illinois, that reflected a combination of factors related to cohesion, social trust, shared experiences, and the willingness of neighborhood residents to act in support of these values, and found that areas with higher collective efficacy measures had lower rates of violence.[30]

Another mechanism through which redevelopment may prevent or displace violence is through removing signs of abandonment. Findings from studies targeting this mechanism are mixed.[15,16,18,32] One study assessed abandoned housing and vacant land remediation through home repairs, full gut rehabilitation, and new builds in relation to all and violent crime in Columbus, Ohio, using synthetic control methods[18] and found no significant effects on assaults or robberies across an 11-year time period.[18] Another study assessing the 2011 Doors and Windows Ordinance in Philadelphia, which required property owners of abandoned buildings to install working doors and windows in all structural openings, found implementation of the ordinance was associated with a decrease in all assaults (−2% change) and firearm assaults (−4% change) over a 2-year time period.[32]

Our secondary redevelopment definition, which focused on restricted access to the lot (i.e., by construction of housing, permanent structures, and fences rather than only housing), resulted in weaker findings than the primary redevelopment definition. We identified an association consistent with prevention of firearm homicides, which we were concerned may have arisen by chance as we had not specifically hypothesized an impact on homicide alone. It is possible that the differences between the primary and secondary redevelopment definitions represent housing or business redevelopment having a more consistent impact on violent crime compared with fences or permanent structures. One study assessing residents' perceptions of the quality and benefits of green space from 2 neighborhoods in the Netherlands found that green areas that were accessible and usable mattered more than the mere amount of green space.[33] By analogy, the quality and utility of vacant lot redevelopment may impact violence differentially, which may explain the patterns we identified across redevelopment types.

Lastly, our study found no evidence of spatial spillover or displacement. This is in line with previous research that shows that given the methods we have available to capture displacement, displacement is often inconsequential.[34,35] Although we did not expect displacement to be present, our displacement analysis likely faces significant methodological problems in measuring displacement or diffusion.[34] Understanding and improving the methods used to quantify and assess spatial displacement is an important area for future research.

Limitations

First, our quasi-experimental design is subject to substantial assumptions that affect any causal interpretation. In particular, we observed that many of the redeveloped lots were in and around the Center City District of Philadelphia, whereas undeveloped lots were spread about the city. It is thus possible that redevelopment is occurring in a location in which violence was already dropping. While our parallel trends test did not indicate lack of parallelism and our staggered DID models account for time trends, an exchangeability violation could still lead to a biased estimate of the causal effect.

Second, we could not control for neighborhood block-level time-varying factors that could have changed over the study period differentially by lot—for example, if small-scale gentrification encourages redevelopment and displaces violent crime, residual confounding would still be present in our findings.

Third, as the range in which redevelopment might affect violence is not well defined, our analytic approach could not account for possible spatial spillover or displacement or relocation of violence to other areas. Although we did include a spillover analysis to assess displacement, these methods may not accurately capture displacement or diffusion.

Fourth, owing to lack of support for Poisson or negative binomial model specification in staggered DID software packages, we modeled violence density as a continuous variable—that is, our estimators assumed a Gaussian (normal) distribution, despite the fact that violence densities are constrained to be nonnegative. This likely did not affect our results for assaults, which are relatively common, but may have impacted our rarer outcomes, such as firearm homicides. For this reason, we have less confidence in our finding of the broader redevelopment definition preventing or displacing firearm homicide than we do in the narrower definition preventing or displacing assaults.

Fifth, our analysis only included violence reported to the police, and unreported violence may be common in areas with high vacancies. If redevelopment causes more violence to be reported, it would cause a bias toward the null.

Finally, although our event study was consistent with the hypothesis that violence near vacant lots before redevelopment was independent of whether a lot was developed, we cannot fully disentangle redevelopment processes from gentrification processes that affect neighborhood poverty, a root cause of violence.

Public Health Implications

Our work supports calls for sustainable interventions to prevent violence by modifying the built environment. The relationship between neighborhood physical environments and violent crime is of critical interest to public health and local governments seeking to address root causes of violence. These results may be useful to policymakers considering vacant land redevelopment as a component of neighborhood violence prevention. AJPH

ABOUT THE AUTHORS

Nicole Asa and Ali Rowhani-Rahbar are with the Department of Epidemiology, School of Public Health, University of Washington, and the Firearm Injury and Policy Research Program, School of Medicine, University of Washington, Seattle. Hiwot Y. Zewdie was with the Department of Epidemiology, School of Public Health, University of Washington, Seattle, at the time of this study. Bradley H. Wagenaar is with the Department of Epidemiology and the Department of Global Health, School of Public Health, University of Washington, Seattle. Stephen J. Mooney is with the Department of Epidemiology, School of Public Health, University of Washington, Seattle.

CORRESPONDENCE

Correspondence should be sent to Nicole Asa, 3980 15th Ave NE, Seattle, WA 98122 (e-mail: nasa3@uw.edu). Reprints can be ordered at https://www.ajph.org by clicking the "Reprints" link.

PUBLICATION INFORMATION

Full Citation: Asa N, Zewdie HY, Rowhani-Rahbar A, Wagenaar BH, Mooney SJ. The association between vacant lot redevelopment and violent/firearm violent crime: a difference-in-difference analysis from 2007 to 2023. *Am J Public Health*. 2026;116(1):95–102.

Acceptance Date: August 8, 2025.

DOI: https://doi.org/10.2105/AJPH.2025.308269

ORCID iDs:

Nicole Asa https://orcid.org/0000-0002-3334-1704

Hiwot Y. Zewdie https://orcid.org/0000-0003-1642-1574

Ali Rowhani-Rahbar https://orcid.org/0000-0002-2705-4485

Bradley H. Wagenaar https://orcid.org/0000-0002-3351-7175

CONTRIBUTORS

All authors contributed equally to the work including substantial contributions to the concept and design, analysis and interpretation of data, drafting the work and revising it critically, and final approval of the version to be published.

ACKNOWLEDGMENTS

This work was supported by Arnold Ventures.

We thank Michael Urciuoli at the Philadelphia Police Department for facilitating access to the crime data.

CONFLICTS OF INTEREST

The authors declare no conflicts of interest.

HUMAN PARTICIPANT PROTECTION

This study did not require institutional review board approval as it did not involve human participants.

REFERENCES

1. Statista. Violent crime statistics in the US. December 16, 2024. Available at: https://www.statista.com/topics/1750/violent-crime-in-the-us. Accessed January 15, 2025.
2. Cozens P, Love T. A review and current status of crime prevention through environmental design (CPTED). *J Plan Lit.* 2015;30(4):393–412. https://doi.org/10.1177/0885412215595440
3. Bogar S, Beyer KM. Green space, violence, and crime: a systematic review. *Trauma Violence Abuse.* 2016;17(2):160–171. https://doi.org/10.1177/1524838015576412
4. Newman GD, Bowman AOM, Jung Lee R, Kim B. A current inventory of vacant urban land in America. *J Urban Des (Abingdon).* 2016;21(3):302–319. https://doi.org/10.1080/13574809.2016.1167589
5. Branas CC, Rubin D, Guo W. Vacant properties and violence in neighborhoods. *ISRN Public Health.* 2013;2012:246142. https://doi.org/10.5402/2012/246142
6. Garvin E, Branas C, Keddem S, Sellman J, Cannuscio C. More than just an eyesore: local insights and solutions on vacant land and urban health. *J Urban Health.* 2013;90(3):412–426. https://doi.org/10.1007/S11524-012-9782-7
7. Lanfear CC, Matsueda RL, Beach LR. Broken windows, informal social control, and crime: assessing causality in empirical studies. *Annu Rev Criminol.* 2020;3:97–120. https://doi.org/10.1146/ANNUREV-CRIMINOL-011419-041541
8. Macdonald J, Nguyen V, Jensen ST, Branas CC. Reducing crime by remediating vacant lots: the moderating effect of nearby land uses. *J Exp Criminol.* 2022;18(3):639–664. https://doi.org/10.1007/S11292-020-09452-9
9. Branas CC, Cheney RA, MacDonald JM, Tam VW, Jackson TD, Ten HTR. A difference-in-differences analysis of health, safety, and greening vacant urban space. *Am J Epidemiol.* 2011;174(11):1296–1306. https://doi.org/10.1093/AJE/KWR273
10. Branas CC, Kondo MC, Murphy SM, South EC, Polsky D, MacDonald JM. Urban blight remediation

as a cost-beneficial solution to firearm violence. *Am J Public Health.* 2016;106(12):2158–2164. https://doi.org/10.2105/AJPH.2016.303434

11. Culyba AJ, Jacoby SF, Richmond TS, Fein JA, Hohl BC, Branas CC. Modifiable neighborhood features associated with adolescent homicide. *JAMA Pediatr.* 2016;170(5):473–480. https://doi.org/10.1001/JAMAPEDIATRICS.2015.4697
12. Sivak CJ, Pearson AL, Hurlburt P. Effects of vacant lots on human health: a systematic review of the evidence. *Landsc Urban Plan.* 2021;208:104020. https://doi.org/10.1016/J.LANDURBPLAN.2020.104020
13. Kondo MC, Morrison C, Jacoby SF, et al. Blight abatement of vacant land and crime in New Orleans. *Public Health Rep.* 2018;133(6):650–657. https://doi.org/10.1177/0033354918798811
14. Branas CC, South E, Kondo MC, et al. Citywide cluster randomized trial to restore blighted vacant land and its effects on violence, crime, and fear. *Proc Natl Acad Sci U S A.* 2018;115(12):2946–2951. https://doi.org/10.1073/PNAS.1718503115
15. South EC, Macdonald J, Reina V. Association between structural housing repairs for low-income homeowners and neighborhood crime. *JAMA Netw Open.* 2021;4(7):e2117067. https://doi.org/10.1001/JAMANETWORKOPEN.2021.17067
16. MacDonald JM, Knorre A, Mitre-Becerril D, Chalfin A. Place-based approaches to reducing violent crime hot spots: a review of the evidence on public health approaches. *Aggress Violent Behav.* 2024;78:101984. https://doi.org/10.1016/J.AVB.2024.101984
17. Freedman M, Owens EG. Low-income housing development and crime. *J Urban Econ.* 2011;70(2-3):115–131. https://doi.org/10.1016/J.JUE.2011.04.001
18. Kondo M, Esposti MD, Jay J, et al. Changes in crime surrounding an urban home renovation and rebuild programme. *Urban Studies.* 2022;59(5):1011–1030. https://doi.org/10.1177/0042098021995141
19. OpenDataPhilly. Building demolitions. 2017. Available at: https://opendataphilly.org/datasets/building-demolitions. Accessed January 26, 2025.
20. Hipp JR. *The Spatial Scale of Crime: How Physical and Social Distance Drive the Spatial Location of Crime.* New York, NY: Taylor and Francis; 2022. https://doi.org/10.4324/9781003262879
21. Braga AA, Turchan B, Papachristos AV, Hureau DM. Hot spots policing of small geographic areas effects on crime. *Campbell Syst Rev.* 2019;15(3):e1046. https://doi.org/10.1002/CL2.1046
22. Hart T, Zandbergen P. Kernel density estimation and hotspot mapping: examining the influence of interpolation method, grid cell size, and bandwidth on crime forecasting. *Policing.* 2014;37(2):305–323. https://doi.org/10.1108/PIJPSM-04-2013-0039
23. Diggle P. A kernel method for smoothing point process data. *J R Stat Soc Ser C Appl Stat.* 1985;34(2):138–147. https://doi.org/10.2307/2347366
24. Baddeley A, Rubak E, Turner R. *Spatial Point Patterns: Methodology and Applications With R.* New York, NY: Chapman and Hall/CRC; 2015. https://doi.org/10.1201/B19708
25. Butts K. Two-stage difference-in-differences following Gardner. 2021. Available at: https://github.com/kylebutts/did2s_stata. Accessed March 1, 2023.
26. Gardner J, Butts K, Wang T. Two-stage differences in differences. Preprint. Posted online July 13, 2022. arXiv 2207.05943. https://doi.org/10.48550/arXiv.2207.05943
27. Wang G, Hamad R, White JS. Advances in difference-in-differences methods for policy evaluation research. *Epidemiology.* 2024;35(5):628–637. https://doi.org/10.1097/EDE.0000000000001755
28. Miller DL. An introductory guide to event study models. *J Econ Perspect.* 2023;37(2):203–230. https://doi.org/10.1257/jep.37.2.203
29. Shepley M, Sachs N, Sadatsafavi H, Fournier C, Peditto K. The impact of green space on violent crime in urban environments: an evidence synthesis. *Int J Environ Res Public Health.* 2019;16(24):5119. https://doi.org/10.3390/IJERPH16245119
30. Maxwell CD, Garner JH, Skogan WG. Collective efficacy and violence in Chicago neighborhoods: a reproduction. *J Contemp Crim Justice.* 2018;34(3):245–265. https://doi.org/10.1177/1043986218769988
31. Cohen DA, Inagami S, Finch B. The built environment and collective efficacy. *Health Place.* 2008;14(2):198–208. https://doi.org/10.1016/J.HEALTHPLACE.2007.06.001
32. Kondo MC, Keene D, Hohl BC, MacDonald JM, Branas CC. A difference-in-differences study of the effects of a new abandoned building remediation strategy on safety. *PLoS One.* 2015;10(7):e0129582. https://doi.org/10.1371/JOURNAL.PONE.0129582
33. Zhang Y, Van den Berg AE, Van Dijk T, Weitkamp G. Quality over quantity: contribution of urban green space to neighborhood satisfaction. *Int J Environ Res Public Health.* 2017;14(5):535. https://doi.org/10.3390/IJERPH14050535
34. Weisburd D, Wyckoff LA, Ready J, Eck JE, Hinkle JC, Gajewski F. Does crime just move around the corner? A controlled study of spatial displacement and diffusion of crime control benefits. *Criminology.* 2006;44(3):549–592. https://doi.org/10.1111/J.1745-9125.2006.00057.x
35. Telep CW, Weisburd D, Gill CE, Vitter Z, Teichman D. Displacement of crime and diffusion of crime control benefits in large-scale geographic areas: a systematic review. *J Exp Criminol.* 2014;10(4):515–548. https://doi.org/10.1007/S11292-014-9208-5

Congenital Syphilis: From Near-Elimination to Crisis

Chad J. Abresch, PhD, Irene A. Stafford, MD, MS, MPH, Regan M. Johnson, MPH, Kayode Olabanji, Ashleigh M. Sutphen, MPH, Helen E. Cejtin, MD, MPH, and Ashley Hoover, MPH

See also Stafylis and Klausner, p. 21.

This analytic essay examines the transformation of congenital syphilis (CS) in the United States from near-elimination to crisis. Drawing from the January 2025 Congenital Syphilis Summit in Atlanta, Georgia—convening public health leaders, Tribal health departments, the National Coalition of STD Directors, and Centers for Disease Control and Prevention experts—we contrast prevention systems during near-elimination (1998–2005) with the current crisis (2018–2025).

Evidence revealed how dismantling public health infrastructure produced dramatically different outcomes, with CS cases increasing 937% over the past decade and racial/ethnic disparities worsening. American Indian/Alaska Native communities face rates up to 100 times higher than White populations in some regions, illustrating the multiplicative effects of system failures on vulnerable communities.

We identify 5 critical system failures: cyclical boom-and-bust funding, workforce deterioration, fragmented surveillance, disconnected health care systems, and health equity failures. We present policy proposals for rebuilding prevention infrastructure through a deliberate phased approach transitioning from crisis response to sustained maintenance, ensuring prevention systems receive continuous support rather than episodic investments that have characterized past approaches. (*Am J Public Health*. 2026;116(1):103–112. https://doi.org/10.2105/AJPH.2025.308266)

AJPH January 2026, Vol. 116, No. 1

This essay examines the dramatic transformation of congenital syphilis (CS) in the United States—from a disease nearly eliminated in the early 2000s, with fewer than 4 cases per 100 000 people,[1] to a resurging public health crisis today. Congenital syphilis is a severe, preventable infection that occurs when *Treponema pallidum*, the bacterium that causes syphilis, is transmitted from an infected pregnant person to their fetus during pregnancy, most often via the placenta, or less commonly during delivery. Untreated CS can result in stillbirth, infant death, or lifelong complications. In 2005, there were 334 cases of CS reported nationwide.[2] By 2022, reported cases had risen to 3761 cases.[3] An analysis of the systemic changes between these eras illuminates how dismantling prevention infrastructure has produced starkly different outcomes and worsened health inequities.

In January 2025, public health leaders gathered in Atlanta, Georgia, to confront this escalating crisis. The summit (hereafter, CS 2025 Summit), convened by CityMatCH (a national maternal and child health organization—citymatch.org) and the Centers for Disease Control and Prevention (CDC), highlighted how CS has reemerged as a critical threat. Data from 2022 revealed that cases had increased by 937% in the past decade,[2–5] with preliminary data suggesting continued increases across 2023 and 2024.[6] This resurgence occurred despite widespread understanding of effective prevention strategies and definitive treatment with penicillin, which prevents 98% of cases when properly administered.[7]

The contrast between eras also reveals how the systematic dismantling of public health infrastructure disproportionately affects communities with preexisting vulnerabilities. Racial and ethnic disparities in CS rates have widened dramatically, with the highest burden falling on communities already experiencing limited health care access and socioeconomic challenges.[4] These disparities are pronounced in American Indian/Alaska Native (AI/AN), Black, and Hispanic/Latinx populations, reflecting how system failures disproportionately impact marginalized communities, where the erosion of public health infrastructure compounds existing barriers.

Syphilis biology creates unique prevention challenges that current fragmented systems struggle to address. As the disease progresses, treatment becomes increasingly complex, with penicillin remaining the only effective intervention during pregnancy. This becomes particularly problematic given nationwide penicillin shortages[5] and the challenges faced by allergic patients who require desensitization procedures. Timing is also critical. Treatment must begin more than 30 days before delivery to prevent CS and hospitalization for treatment. Further complicating matters, the infection is often asymptomatic, allowing for undetected reinfection during pregnancy. Transmission risk to the fetus is also variable, ranging from nearly 100% in early stages to 10% in later stages. These biological realities create a narrow prevention window requiring both rapid response and continuous monitoring—our current fragmented systems consistently fail to deliver this essential integration.[8,9]

The following sections contrast the coordinated public health infrastructure, sustained funding, and integrated health care delivery systems of the early 2000s with current systemic failures. This analysis identifies essential components for rebuilding effective prevention systems. Understanding both historical success factors and current system failures is crucial for developing sustainable solutions that can once again bring CS under control while addressing the fundamental inequities driving its resurgence.

THE NECESSITY OF CONTINUOUS SYSTEM MAINTENANCE

While nominal federal sexually transmitted infection (STI) funding remained steady at $157 to $160 million annually from 2003 to 2019, this represents a 40% inflation-adjusted decline. This decline occurred even as primary and secondary syphilis rates more than tripled—from approximately 12 per 100 000 in 2003 to 38 per 100 000 in 2019—and the US population increased by approximately 50 million people.[1,4,10] This funding collapse triggered cascading system failures: closure or limitation of testing centers, loss of experienced public health workforce, weakened surveillance systems, and diminished capacity for partner services.[5] In many jurisdictions, local health departments simultaneously faced budget cuts that forced reductions in clinical services, including screening and treatment of STIs, at precisely the time when such services were most needed.[10]

The impact extends beyond direct service provision. By early 2010, more than half of local health departments in the United States were experiencing reductions in their core STI funding.[1,10] Without adequate staffing, even basic prevention activities become difficult to maintain. Many reported having to close or severely limit hours and staff, decreasing opportunities for testing and treatment.[5] The occurrence of repeated public health crises, the most recent and notable being the COVID-19 pandemic, further depleted already thinned capacity by shifting focus and resources.

This system deterioration occurred despite no change in the fundamental science of CS prevention—the same diagnostic tests and penicillin treatment that made elimination achievable remain highly effective. During the CS 2025 Summit, presentations sharing the experiences of Tribal health departments emphasized that treatment resources like penicillin frequently remained ineffective because of inadequate funding for staffing, testing, and patient follow-up.[11]

This pattern reveals a fundamental truth about public health systems: prevention systems require continuous active maintenance rather than passive existence. The mere presence of effective interventions proves insufficient without sustained infrastructure and a workforce to deploy them.

MULTIPLICATIVE EFFECTS OF SYSTEM FAILURE

While CS rates have increased across all populations, AI/AN communities have emerged as a sentinel population that reveals the full scope of compounded system failures. This reality is acutely illustrated in South Dakota, where CS affects 1 in 42 AI/AN births compared with just 1 in 3988 White births—a nearly 100-fold disparity.[3,12] For reference, Black and Hispanic/Latinx populations face disparities of 3 to 3.5 times higher than White populations nationally.[3,5,12]

The extreme disparities in AI/AN communities reflect the interaction of multiple system failures. For example, health care facility closures across rural America, including in areas where AI/AN communities reside, have created expansive regions where patients must drive more than 100 miles to access basic prenatal services, including syphilis testing and treatment.[13] This distance barrier compounds with historical and contemporary trauma experienced by AI/AN communities, resulting in ongoing mistrust of medical systems. When syphilis care is sought, follow-up is required to ensure treatment was successful and reinfection did not occur. This requires communication and coordination across providers and facilities;

however, fragmented data systems impede coordination. Further barriers are created through punitive policies for substance use in pregnancy (e.g., criminal prosecution for substance use during pregnancy, mandatory reporting to child protective services, incarceration for drug-related offenses). Such policies undermine effective CS prevention.[14] Together, these system failures create nearly insurmountable obstacles to syphilis care and CS prevention among AI/AN communities, explaining the unfathomable nearly 100-fold disparities seen in South Dakota.

Data sovereignty emerged as another critical barrier for AI/AN communities at the CS 2025 Summit. In South Dakota, federal and state authorities' refusal to share surveillance data with the regional Tribal Health Board and Tribal Epidemiology Center has undermined their ability to protect Indigenous community health.[15] During the first year of the COVID-19 pandemic, this lack of data sovereignty came to a head. The dearth of syphilis surveillance, combined with a shift in attention to pandemic response, resulted in an 8-fold statewide spike in syphilis case counts.[14,15] Despite the spike in active CS caseloads, attention remained fixed on severe acute respiratory syndrome coronavirus 2 (SARS-CoV-2), allowing syphilis transmission to accelerate unchecked.

These examples illuminate a darker reality of public health systems: system failures compound multiplicatively rather than additively. Each breakdown in the system amplifies the impact of others, creating cascade effects that disproportionately affect vulnerable populations, whether through geographic barriers, criminalization of substance use, data sovereignty restrictions, or other structural inequities.

THE PARADOX OF PREVENTION

Perhaps most perplexing is how the very success of CS prevention efforts in the early 2000s may have contributed to their undoing. When cases dropped to historic lows, suggesting elimination was possible, attention and investments shifted elsewhere—most notably toward rising syphilis rates among gay, bisexual, and other men who have sex with men.[16] The CDC's syphilis elimination efforts officially ended in December 2013, reflecting a broader pattern of reduced prioritization following apparent success.[3]

This pattern exemplifies what public health researchers refer to as Brown's Law—the tendency for prevention programs to be scaled back just as they become most effective, leading to subsequent increases in transmission rates.[17] As cases decrease, the urgency of maintaining prevention infrastructure becomes less apparent. Funding gets redirected to more visible crises, experienced staff move to other priorities, and surveillance systems atrophy—creating conditions for disease resurgence.

The current crisis demonstrates how quickly these cycles can reverse decades of progress. In 2022, the United States reported 3755 CS cases (102.5 per 100 000 live births), compared with only 529 cases (13.4 per 100 000 live births) in 2000.[1] This dramatic reversal returned US rates to levels not seen since the early 1990s.[4,18]

Here lies a central paradox of public health: the very visibility of system success can ultimately undermine its maintenance. Successful prevention becomes invisible, making it difficult to sustain support for the systems that created success.

DUAL CHALLENGE OF HORIZONTAL AND VERTICAL TRANSMISSION

The CS crisis suggests that addressing diseases with both horizontal and vertical transmission requires prevention systems that can bridge separate domains of public health. While sexually transmitted syphilis prevention and CS prevention are inextricably linked—without cases in adults, there would be no vertical transmission—they demand distinct yet coordinated prevention approaches. Traditional STI control systems evolved primarily to address horizontal transmission through testing, treatment, and partner services for nonpregnant adults. These systems were not designed to address the unique urgency, timeline constraints, and clinical complexities of preventing vertical transmission.[19–21]

The early 2000s demonstrated that effective coordination between these distinct prevention systems is achievable. During that period, well-integrated prevention systems successfully drove CS cases to near-elimination levels. Currently, 88% to 90% of CS cases represent preventable missed opportunities, with approximately 50% involving inadequate maternal treatment despite timely syphilis diagnosis.[22] When prevention systems operate in isolation as they do today, their separate domains create gaps at critical transition points. Pregnant patients seeking emergency care, for example, frequently encounter structural disconnects—STI clinics without established prenatal care referral protocols, prenatal providers lacking expertise in syphilis treatment, and test results that fail to transfer between health care systems.[23]

These realities were validated by data presented at the CS 2025 Summit from

AJPH January 2026, Vol. 116, No. 1

the Illinois Perinatal Syphilis Warmline, which provides clinical consultation for syphilis treatment in pregnancy and the newborn period. More than 40% of consultation requests received by the Warmline involve coordination challenges between obstetric and infectious disease services, demonstrating how providers from each specialty area commonly lack crucial information from the other.[24]

The University of Texas Health Science Center's Preg-OUT program was also presented during the summit. Approximately 40% of CS cases reported nationwide are among children born to people with little or no prenatal care who nonetheless utilize emergency departments during their pregnancies.[22] The Preg-OUT program implements opt-out syphilis screening for pregnant patients in emergency departments with rapid point-of-care testing and immediate treatment. During evaluation, the program demonstrated dramatic impact, increasing syphilis testing among pregnant emergency department patients from 2% (6 of 302) to 56.4% (114 of 202 approached) and identifying 4 positive cases, indicating a 3.5% prevalence rate.[25] By deliberately creating systems that work across traditional boundaries, Preg-OUT demonstrates that effective prevention requires intentional integration rather than parallel operation of separate efforts. The most successful interventions address transitions between systems—providing navigation support at handoff points, implementing shared data systems, and coordinating funding streams.[23,25,26]

The broader lesson for public health system design is clear: vertical transmission highlights the inherent complexity of building effective prevention systems across traditionally siloed domains. Disease will spread through any available pathway, and prevention systems must be equally adaptable to effectively interrupt all transmission routes.

PROPOSALS FOR REBUILDING CONGENITAL SYPHILIS PREVENTION

Box 1 summarizes the stark contrasts between the near-elimination era systems and current crisis systems. The dramatic resurgence of CS highlights the need for innovative approaches to rebuilding prevention infrastructure that can withstand political and economic fluctuations. Analyzing successful models from both historical CS prevention and other disease elimination efforts reveals several essential components for sustainable system reconstruction. Box 2 summarizes the 5 critical system failures identified in this analysis alongside corresponding policy proposals for rebuilding effective CS prevention infrastructure.

SUSTAINABLE FUNDING MODELS

The cyclic nature of CS prevention funding—expanding during crises and contracting during periods of success—creates inherently unstable systems. The 40% inflation-adjusted reduction in federal STI funding since 2000 and subsequent dismantling of prevention infrastructure directly illustrate why moving from grant-based to infrastructure-based funding is a needed paradigm shift. Infrastructure-based funding refers to sustained financial support directed at maintaining core public health functions and systems rather than specific time-limited initiatives.

While short-term categorical grants remain politically expedient during crises, they create structural instability in prevention systems. The near elimination of CS in the early 2000s demonstrates that sustained investment in core prevention activities can drive case rates to historic lows. However, without mechanisms to maintain an appropriate level of investment during periods of success, prevention systems become vulnerable to funding cuts that ultimately lead to disease resurgence.

Two alternative funding policies merit consideration. First, bundling vertical transmission prevention across multiple conditions offers a promising approach. By packaging similar prevention efforts addressing vertically transmittable diseases like HIV, syphilis, and hepatitis B, public health systems could create economies of scale and more resilient funding structures. This syndemic approach, highlighted by CDC representatives at the CS 2025 Summit,[6] better reflects the interconnected nature of these conditions and could help maintain essential prevention infrastructure through fluctuations in individual disease rates.

Second, existing maternal and child health funding through Title V of the Social Security Act offers an instructive model that could be expanded to include vertical transmission prevention with appropriate funding increases. Unlike the cyclical grant-based STI funding that expands and contracts with disease prevalence, Title V provides stable infrastructure support through ongoing block grants to all states and territories. Enhanced maternal and child health block grants that specifically include CS prevention funding would address the funding instability that undermines prevention efforts. Furthermore, this organizational structure would leverage the unique expertise of maternal and child health professionals

BOX 1— Comparison of Congenital Syphilis (CS) Prevention Systems Between Near-Elimination and Crisis Eras

System Component	Near-Elimination Era (1998–2005)	Current Crisis Era (2018–2025)
Funding and resources	• Strong federal support for STI prevention (~$167 million in 2003, inflation-adjusted) • Dedicated CS elimination funding • Sustained, reliable funding streams	• 40% reduction in federal STI funding since 2000 (~$105 million in 2019, inflation-adjusted) • Grant-based, time-limited funding • Competing priorities within public health
Workforce and infrastructure	• Specialized DIS workforce • Dedicated STI clinics • Comprehensive partner services	• Shrinking public health workforce • Clinic closures, limited hours • Reduced partner services capacity
Surveillance and data systems	• Active case-finding strategies • Coordinated, real-time reporting systems • Rapid response to detected cases	• Fragmented, outdated data systems • Delays in case identification • Limited coordination across jurisdictions, particularly with Tribal public health agencies
Health care integration	• Strong connection between STI and prenatal care • Coordinated screening protocols • Clear referral pathways	• STI and maternal health systems operate in silos • Gaps at system intersections • Discontinuity in care across specialties
Testing and treatment access	• Extensive network of STI clinics and testing sites • Reliable penicillin supply • Multiple accessible treatment locations	• Clinic closures and reduced testing capacity because of reduced STI funding • Penicillin shortages • Geographic disparities in access
Health equity approach	• Early recognition of disparities • Universal protocols with limited cultural adaptation	• Worsening racial/ethnic disparities (3–12 times higher) • Insufficient response to structural barriers • Minimal community engagement
Primary outcomes	• Cases declined to historic lows • Fewer than 4 cases per 100 000 population • Elimination appeared achievable	• 937% increase in cases over the decade • Return to 1950s case levels • 100-fold disparities in most affected communities

Note. DIS = disease intervention specialist; STI = sexually transmitted infection. Table based on analysis of published literature, Centers for Disease Control and Prevention surveillance reports, and presentations from the 2025 Congenital Syphilis Summit.

and bring valuable perspectives on prenatal care systems, care coordination across the perinatal period, and 2-generation approaches to public health programming (i.e., interventions that address the health and social needs of parents and children in a coordinated and simultaneous manner).

Prevention consistently costs substantially less than treatment of established cases. With 3882 CS cases in 2023[4] requiring extensive medical intervention and follow-up, the current crisis represents both a public health failure and significant economic waste.[27] Given current federal fiscal constraints, rebuilding prevention infrastructure will require creative solutions that emphasize cross-program coordination and administrative efficiency. Prevention infrastructure will require continuous maintenance, not the episodic investment patterns that have characterized past approaches.

WORKFORCE DEVELOPMENT

The near-elimination of CS in the early 2000s relied on a robust public health workforce that has since deteriorated significantly.[10] As documented in the presentations at the CS 2025 Summit, workforce deficiencies directly contribute to prevention failures across multiple domains. Rebuilding this workforce will require systematic strengthening through 3 distinct but complementary strategies.

First, disease intervention specialists (DISs) provide the foundation for CS prevention through case investigation, partner services, and outbreak response activities for adult syphilis. These positions require specialized technical knowledge combined with relationship-building skills that develop over years of practice. Given the established pattern of implementation failures driving the current crisis, maintaining a subsistence level of experienced DIS personnel is critical. Regions that eliminate these positions cannot rapidly reconstitute effective case investigation and partner notification services when emergency funding becomes available, as these functions rely on institutional knowledge and community relationships that require significant time to develop. AI/AN communities already receive some direct funding through CDC's Tribal Epidemiology Centers and infrastructure cooperative agreements. However, recruitment and deployment of DISs still rely primarily on state-managed resources. Direct funding of

BOX 2— System Failures and Policy Proposals for Congenital Syphilis (CS) Prevention

System Failure	Observed Impact	Policy Proposal
Discontinuous funding	• 40% reduction in STI prevention funding since 2000 • Clinic closures • Staff reductions	• Shift from grant-based to infrastructure-based funding models • Bundle vertical transmission prevention across conditions (HIV, syphilis, hepatitis B) • Consider a block grant funding model • Fully incorporate the MCH workforce into CS prevention
Workforce deterioration	• Loss of experienced DIS personnel • Knowledge gaps between specialties • Limited community outreach	• Maintain minimum subsistence-level experienced DIS personnel • Establish specific funding streams for DIS in Tribal communities • Establish cross-specialty consultation networks • Integrate community health workers into prevention systems
Fragmented surveillance	• Delayed case identification • Lack of coordination across jurisdictions • Reactive rather than proactive response	• Develop early warning indicators for system performance (beyond case counts) • Implement case review methodologies like FIMR/HIV • Create real-time data exchange between clinical, public health, and Tribal health systems
Siloed health care systems	• Gaps at intersections of STI and maternal health systems • Disconnected care pathways • Missed opportunities for intervention	• Embed clinical decision support systems in EHRs • Establish telehealth consultation networks • Implement standardized care pathways spanning the prevention cascade • Screen at nontraditional sites (EDs, corrections, substance use treatment)
Health equity failures	• 12:1 racial disparities nationally • 100:1 disparities in AI/AN communities in some regions • Disproportionate impact of system failures	• Develop culturally responsive prevention approaches • Address structural barriers to care • Engage affected communities in prevention system design • Implement trauma-informed care approaches

Note. AI/AN = American Indian and Alaska Native; DIS = disease intervention specialist; ED = emergency department; EHR = electronic health record; FIMR = Fetal and Infant Mortality Review; MCH = maternal and child health; STI = sexually transmitted infection.

DIS positions to Tribal health departments would address this gap—ensuring culturally responsive, locally controlled implementation of partner services and case investigation in communities facing the highest burden.

Second, cross-specialty consultation services represent a promising model for addressing knowledge gaps between maternal care and infectious disease domains. As demonstrated by the Illinois Perinatal Syphilis Warmline experience, specialized consultative resources can efficiently bridge workforce knowledge gaps without requiring all providers to develop expertise across multiple specialties.[24] This approach recognizes the distinct but complementary knowledge bases in obstetrics, pediatrics, and infectious disease, allowing each specialty to maintain focus while accessing needed expertise through structured consultation pathways. Implementing similar consultation networks nationally could significantly improve clinical decision-making for CS prevention with minimal additional staffing requirements.

Third, community health workers (CHWs) have emerged as a critical yet frequently overlooked component of successful CS prevention systems. As the striking South Dakota example demonstrated, CHWs are not merely service extenders but essential cultural bridges that have a direct impact on prevention outcomes. Their unique ability to navigate fragmented health care systems while building trust in communities with historical reasons for health care system distrust underscores the need for sustainable CHW funding streams.[28,29] Prevention systems should integrate CHWs as core team members with dedicated funding lines rather than as supplemental staff dependent on grant cycles. This approach would help maintain these critical connections between clinical systems and communities even during funding fluctuations.

A comprehensive workforce development strategy must integrate these interconnected dimensions to rebuild effective CS prevention capacity. Strategic investment in this multifaceted workforce represents an essential foundation capable of once again approaching—and sustaining—elimination.

SURVEILLANCE SYSTEM MODERNIZATION

Effective CS prevention requires cross-jurisdictional surveillance systems that identify cases in real time and account for syphilis's unique challenges—tracking both initial treatment and monitoring throughout pregnancy to address reinfection risks. The current fragmented reporting infrastructure across and within jurisdictions—including between state, local, Tribal, and territorial systems, as well as between state health departments and large municipal jurisdictions—prevents effective response and can delay patient care while entities determine data ownership. At the CS 2025 Summit, presenters emphasized how this fragmentation provides only lagging indicators, hindering timely case identification and treatment. Surveillance system redesign should prioritize approaches that detect deteriorating system performance before incidence increases. Several promising models address these surveillance challenges.

First, early warning indicators that monitor prevention system performance rather than just case counts could provide more timely signals of infrastructure deterioration. These might include treatment completion time frames, partner services follow-up rates, and the proportion of syphilis cases identified through routine screening versus symptomatic presentation. By continuously monitoring process metrics in addition to outcome measures, communities could identify system weaknesses before they manifest as increased transmission.

Second, case review methodologies originally developed for investigating adverse events have been successfully adapted to examine gaps in perinatal infection prevention systems. The Fetal and Infant Mortality Review–HIV Prevention Methodology (FIMR-HIV) offers a structured approach that has proven effective for identifying and addressing system-level barriers to care.[30] This methodology uses a combination of medical record abstraction, maternal interviews, and multidisciplinary case reviews to generate recommendations for system improvement. Similar approaches have been applied to CS, often borrowing FIMR-HIV committees to pivot into CS investigation as perinatal HIV cases diminish nationally.

Third, real-time data exchange mechanisms between clinical systems and state, local, and Tribal public health agencies could significantly improve prevention efforts. Current reporting systems often involve substantial delays between testing, result notification, treatment, and case reporting. Electronic laboratory reporting has improved timeliness but does not typically include treatment information. Integrated systems that track the entire prevention cascade—from testing through treatment completion—could identify and address gaps as they emerge rather than months later through retrospective surveillance.

While enhanced surveillance alone cannot solve the CS crisis, modernizing these systems represents an essential foundation for effective and timely intervention. Implementation of these improvements would require a sustained level of investment, but alternative funding approaches presented here could more readily enable needed expenditures.

HEALTH CARE SYSTEM INTEGRATION

The disconnect between STI prevention and prenatal care systems represents a fundamental structural vulnerability in CS prevention. Effective prevention requires deliberately designed integration rather than parallel operation of separate systems. Drawing on successful models presented at the CS 2025 Summit and broader evidence of effective integrated care approaches, several promising policy directions merit consideration.

First, clinical decision support systems embedded in electronic health record systems can significantly improve adherence to screening and treatment protocols. The University of Texas Health Science Center's Best Practice Alert system, presented during the CS 2025 summit, demonstrated the power of this approach. This system prompted providers about required syphilis testing during pregnancy, increasing appropriate third trimester and delivery testing from 3% to 89% and reducing CS cases from 22 of 8697 deliveries (0.25%) to 5 of 5367 (0.09%) in participating facilities.[23,31] This dramatic improvement occurred without additional staff or significant infrastructure costs, suggesting a scalable approach that could be implemented across health care systems with electronic health records.

Second, telehealth and virtual consultation networks offer scalable infrastructure for bridging expertise gaps between maternal care and infectious disease domains without requiring physical colocation of specialists or comprehensive cross-training. The Illinois Perinatal Syphilis Warmline demonstrates this approach's effectiveness.[24] National expansion through hub-and-spoke models centered on academic medical centers or regional expertise centers would extend specialized knowledge to rural, underresourced, and historically marginalized communities where access to in-person specialists remains limited. Integrating these virtual networks into standard care protocols could significantly reduce treatment delays, improve clinical decision-making, and address the geographic maldistribution of specialists that currently undermines CS prevention efforts.

Third, nontraditional screening sites represent an essential component of comprehensive prevention given the gaps in traditional prenatal care access. The Maternal and Congenital Syphilis Prevention (OPTINS) Program implemented in Houston emergency departments demonstrated how integration can capture crucial missed opportunities. By implementing universal opt-out syphilis screening for pregnant patients regardless of chief complaint, this program identified previously undiagnosed infections in 3.8% of pregnant patients and significantly increased treatment completion through dedicated linkage coordination.[32] Similar approaches in nonpregnant people engaging in emergency department services have been demonstrated successful in identifying asymptomatic syphilis cases.[32] These approaches in nontraditional venues could identify and treat cases missed by conventional prenatal screening approaches, particularly for those avoiding care because of fear of criminalization for substance use during pregnancy.[28]

Implementing these health care system integration strategies requires policy changes at multiple levels. Federal agencies should establish integration requirements for grant recipients, incentivize electronic health record adoption of syphilis-specific decision support, and fund model demonstration projects. State health departments must mandate standardized screening and referral protocols, establish consultation networks, and develop care coordination systems that bridge traditional and nontraditional care settings. Finally, professional organizations need to develop standardized guidelines for integrated

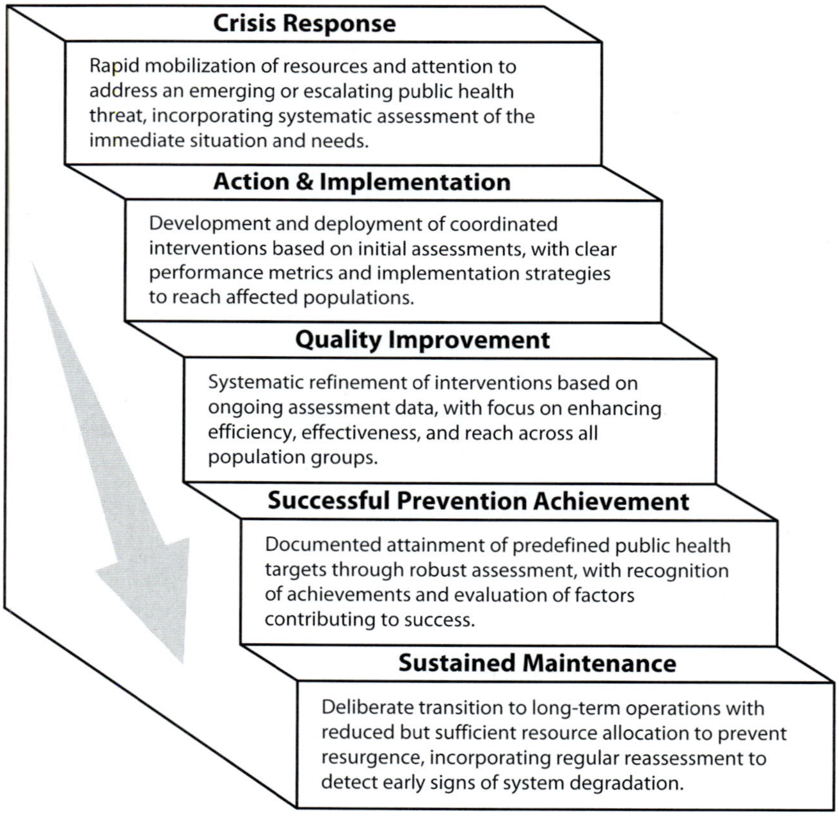

FIGURE 1— Stepped Prevention System Model

Note. Transitioning from crisis response to sustained maintenance with intentional design at each phase and decreased expenditure and prevention intensity throughout.

care across obstetric and infectious disease specialties.

REIMAGINING PREVENTION SYSTEMS

The cyclical pattern documented throughout this analysis—where prevention systems are built during crises, only to be dismantled when successful—demands a fundamental reimagining of how we approach public health infrastructure. Rather than accepting this destructive boom-and-bust cycle as inevitable, we must design prevention systems with sustained maintenance in mind from the outset.

This requires conceptualizing prevention not as a single sustained effort but as a series of distinct steps—from crisis response through action and implementation, quality improvement, successful prevention achievement, and, finally, sustained maintenance. Figure 1 presents this proposed Stepped Prevention System Model. The figure depicts how each step requires different activities, metrics, and appropriate funding levels. By explicitly planning for this full sequence from the outset, we can create more resilient systems that do not collapse at the first sign of success.

This reimagined approach requires not just technical solutions but a cultural shift in how we conceptualize prevention success. Instead of celebrating the end of programs when cases decline, we should celebrate the transition to sustainable maintenance—acknowledging that ongoing vigilance, albeit at a reduced level, represents the true victory in public health. While uncommon, this approach is not completely unprecedented. The Global Polio Eradication Initiative[33] offers lessons through its postcertification strategies that address virus reintroduction risks by maintaining surveillance, preserving laboratory capacity, and planning for outbreak response. This approach recognizes elimination as a transition to a different phase of vigilance rather than an endpoint. If we are to truly protect future generations from CS, we must commit to building systems that sustain prevention not just during crises but through the long, quiet work of maintenance that follows success. AJPH

ABOUT THE AUTHORS

Chad J. Abresch, Regan M. Johnson, Kayode Olabanji, and Ashleigh M. Sutphen are with the Department of Health Promotion, College of Public Health, University of Nebraska Medical Center, Omaha. Irene A. Stafford is with the Department of Obstetrics, Gynecology, and Reproductive Sciences, Division of Maternal–Fetal Medicine, McGovern Medical School at UTHealth, Houston. Helen E. Cejtin is with the Department of Obstetrics and Gynecology, Feinberg School of Medicine, Northwestern University, Chicago, IL. Ashley Hoover is with The Raven Collective, Multnomah County, Grayslake, IL.

CORRESPONDENCE

Correspondence should be sent to Chad J. Abresch, PhD, 984365 Nebraska Medical Center, Omaha, NE 68198-4365 (e-mail: cabresch@unmc.edu). Reprints can be ordered at https://ajph.org by clicking the "Reprints" link.

PUBLICATION INFORMATION

Full Citation: Abresch CJ, Stafford IA, Johnson RM, et al. Congenital syphilis: from near-elimination to crisis. *Am J Public Health*. 2026;116(1):103–112.

Acceptance Date: August 8, 2025.

DOI: https://doi.org/10.2105/AJPH.2025.308266

ORCID iDs:

Chad J. Abresch https://orcid.org/0000-0001-7210-0279

Kayode Olabanji https://orcid.org/0000-0002-9430-1773

Ashleigh M. Sutphen https://orcid.org/0009-0002-7957-1422

Ashley Hoover https://orcid.org/0009-0009-5449-509X

CONTRIBUTORS

C. J. Abresch served as lead author, contributed to the conceptualization and design of the work, convened the 2025 Congenital Syphilis Summit, contributed to data acquisition and interpretation, and led the drafting of the article. I. A. Stafford, H. E. Cejtin, and A. Hoover participated in the 2025 Congenital Syphilis Summit providing valuable information used in the article and contributed substantively to the development and editing of the article. R. M. Johnson convened the 2025 Congenital Syphilis Summit, contributed to data acquisition, and contributed substantively to the development and editing of the article. K. Olabanji assisted with the drafting of the article and led revisions of the article following peer review. A. M. Sutphen convened the 2025 Congenital Syphilis Summit and contributed substantively to the development and editing of the article. All authors provided final approval of the version to be published and agree to be accountable for all aspects of the work in ensuring that questions related to the accuracy or integrity of any part of the work are appropriately investigated and resolved.

ACKNOWLEDGMENTS

This work was supported by the Centers for Disease Control and Prevention's (CDC's) National Center for HIV, Viral Hepatitis, STDs, and TB Prevention. We are grateful to our CDC project officers for their ongoing guidance and support throughout this work.

We extend our sincere appreciation to all participants of the 2025 Congenital Syphilis Summit, particularly community members with lived experience of HIV and syphilis who shared their insights and expertise. Their perspectives were invaluable in helping us understand prevention system failures and identify pathways toward more effective and equitable approaches.

CONFLICTS OF INTEREST

The authors declare no conflicts of interest.

HUMAN PARTICIPANT PROTECTION

This analytic essay was developed from a national summit and did not involve human participant research requiring institutional review board approval.

REFERENCES

1. Clement ME, Hicks CB. Syphilis on the rise: what went wrong? *JAMA*. 2016;315(21):2281–2283. https://doi.org/10.1001/jama.2016.7073
2. Centers for Disease Control and Prevention. Congenital syphilis—United States, 2003–2008. *MMWR Morb Mortal Wkly Rep*. 2010;59(14):413–417.
3. Centers for Disease Control and Prevention. *Sexually Transmitted Infections Surveillance 2022*. March 12, 2025. Available at: https://www.cdc.gov/sti-statistics/media/pdfs/2024/11/2022-STI-Surveillance-Report-PDF.pdf. Accessed March 11, 2025.
4. Centers for Disease Control and Prevention. National overview of STIs in 2023. March 12, 2025. Available at: https://www.cdc.gov/sti-statistics/annual/summary.html. Accessed March 11, 2025.
5. Mohtasham D. Syphilis cases surge in the US, CDC says. National Public Radio. January 31, 2024. Available at: https://www.npr.org/2024/01/31/1228195107/syphilis-cases-soar-in-us-cdc-says. Accessed March 11, 2025.

6. McDonald R, Miele K. The current state of syphilis and congenital syphilis. Oral presentation at: CityMatCH Congenital Syphilis Meeting; January 14, 2025; Atlanta, GA.
7. Alexander J, Sheffield J, Sanchez P, Mayfield J, Wendel G. Efficacy of treatment for syphilis in pregnancy. *Obstet Gynecol.* 1999;93(1):5–8. https://doi.org/10.1016/s0029-7844(98)00338-x
8. Sheffield JS, Sánchez PJ, Morris G, et al. Congenital syphilis after maternal treatment for syphilis during pregnancy. *Am J Obstet Gynecol.* 2002;186(3):569–573. https://doi.org/10.1067/mob.2002.121541
9. Rac MWF, Bryant SN, McIntire DD, et al. Progression of ultrasound findings of fetal syphilis after maternal treatment. *Am J Obstet Gynecol.* 2014;211(4):426.e1–426.e6. https://doi.org/10.1016/j.ajog.2014.05.049
10. National Academies of Sciences, Engineering, and Medicine; Health and Medicine Division; Board on Population Health and Public Health Practice; Committee on Prevention and Control of Sexually Transmitted Infections in the United States, Crowley JS, Geller AB, Vermund SH, eds. STI economics, public-sector financing, and program policy. In: *Sexually Transmitted Infections: Adopting a Sexual Health Paradigm.* Washington, DC: National Academies Press; 2021.
11. Hoover A, Leston J. Considerations for addressing congenital syphilis in Indigenous communities. Oral presentation at: CityMatCH Congenital Syphilis Meeting; January 14, 2025; Atlanta, GA.
12. Centers for Disease Control and Prevention. Syphilis surveillance supplemental slides, 2018–2022. January 2024. Available at: https://www.cdc.gov/std/statistics/syphilis-supplement/default.htm. Accessed February 3, 2025.
13. Fontenot J, Brigance C, Lucas R, Stoneburner A. Navigating geographical disparities: access to obstetric hospitals in maternity care deserts and across the United States. *BMC Pregnancy Childbirth.* 2024;24(1):350. https://doi.org/10.1186/s12884-024-06535-7
14. Simon R, Giroux J, Chor J. Effects of substance use disorder criminalization on American Indian pregnant individuals. *AMA J Ethics.* 2020;22(10):E862–E867. https://doi.org/10.1001/amajethics.2020.862
15. Landman K. How a fight over data made South Dakota's bad syphilis outbreak worse. Vox. December 19, 2023. Available at: https://www.vox.com/24006120/south-dakota-syphilis-congenital-indigenous-tribal-native-american-meghan-oconnell-health-board. Accessed May 10, 2025.
16. Solomon MM, Mayer KH. Evolution of the syphilis epidemic among men who have sex with men. *Sex Health.* 2015;12(2):96–102. https://doi.org/10.1071/SH14173
17. Chesson HW, Pinkerton SD, Holtgrave DR. Distribution of prevention resources and impact on sexual health in the USA. In: Aral SO, Fenton KA, Lipshutz JA, eds. *The New Public Health and STD/HIV Prevention.* New York, NY: Springer; 2013:129–149. https://doi.org/10.1007/978-1-4614-4526-5_7
18. Centers for Disease Control and Prevention. *Sexually Transmitted Disease Surveillance, 2000.* Atlanta, GA: US Department of Health and Human Services; September 2001.
19. Mutabazi JC, Zarowsky C, Trottier H. The impact of programs for prevention of mother-to-child transmission of HIV on health care services and systems in sub-Saharan Africa—a review. *Public Health Rev.* 2017;38(1):28. https://doi.org/10.1186/s40985-017-0072-5
20. Fuertes-Bucheli JF, Buenaventura-Alegría DP, Rivas-Mina AM, Pacheco-López R. Congenital syphilis prevention challenges, Pacific Coast of Colombia, 2018–2022. *Emerg Infect Dis.* 2024;30(5):890–899. https://doi.org/10.3201/eid3005.231273
21. Centers for Disease Control. Guidelines for the prevention and control of congenital syphilis. *MMWR.* 1988;37(suppl 1). Available at: https://www.cdc.gov/mmwr/preview/mmwrhtml/00026330.htm. Accessed September 18, 2025.
22. McDonald R, O'Callaghan K, Torrone E, et al. Vital signs: Missed opportunities for preventing congenital syphilis—United States, 2022. *MMWR Morb Mortal Wkly Rep.* 2023;72(46):1269–1274. https://doi.org/10.15585/mmwr.mm7246e1
23. Stafford I. Programmatic strategies to reduce maternal & congenital syphilis. Oral presentation at: CityMatCH Congenital Syphilis Meeting; January 14, 2025; Atlanta, GA.
24. Cejtin H. Illinois Perinatal Syphilis Warmline. Oral presentation at: CityMatCH Congenital Syphilis Meeting; January 14, 2025; Atlanta, GA.
25. Stafford IA, Bakunas C, Haydamous J, et al. Implementation of an opt-out and rapid point-of-care syphilis testing program for pregnant patients presenting to the emergency department. *Sex Transm Dis.* 2025;52(6):352–355. https://doi.org/10.1097/OLQ.0000000000002131
26. Wall KM, Workowski K, Young M, Stafford IA. Point-of-care testing to combat congenital syphilis—the time is now. *JAMA.* 2025;333(13):1115. https://doi.org/10.1001/jama.2025.0171
27. Chen HY, Klausner JD, Stafford IA. Congenital syphilis in live births: adverse outcomes, hospital length of stay, and costs. *Obstet Gynecol.* 2024;144(2):207–214. https://doi.org/10.1097/AOG.0000000000005642
28. Seiler N, Horton K, Organick-Lee P, et al. Use of community health workers to help end the epidemic of sexually transmitted infections. *Public Health Rep.* 2024;139(3):271–276. https://doi.org/10.1177/00333549231199481
29. Hammack AY, Bickham JN, Gilliard I, 3rd, Robinson WT. A community health worker approach for ending the HIV epidemic. *Am J Prev Med.* 2021;61(suppl 1):S26–S31. https://doi.org/10.1016/j.amepre.2021.06.008
30. Warren MD, Pilkey D, Joshi DS, Collier A. Fetal, infant, and child death review: a public health approach to reducing mortality and morbidity. *Pediatrics.* 2024;154(suppl 3):e2024067043B. https://doi.org/10.1542/peds.2024-067043B
31. Chen HY, Stafford IA. Lack of prenatal care in pregnancies complicated by syphilis: trend, risk factors and outcomes. *Sex Transm Infect.* 2025;101(6):386–394. https://doi.org/10.1136/sextrans-2024-056453
32. Stanford KA, Hazra A, Friedman E, et al. Opt-out, routine emergency department syphilis screening as a novel intervention in at-risk populations. *Sex Transm Dis.* 2021;48(5):347–352. https://doi.org/10.1097/OLQ.0000000000001311
33. Lopez Cavestany R, Eisenhawer M, Diop OM, Verma H, Quddus A, Mach O. The last mile in polio eradication: program challenges and perseverance. *Pathogens.* 2024;13(4):323. https://doi.org/10.3390/pathogens13040323

Opioid Overdose Mortality Among Patients Receiving a Peer-Delivered, Emergency Department–Based Nonfatal Opioid Overdose Intervention in New York City, 2017–2022

Kelsey L. Kepler, MPH, Alice E. Welch, DrPH, MPH, RPh, Ellenie Tuazon, MPH, Dominique Chambless, MPH, Joseph Kennedy, MPH, and Angela Jeffers, MA

See also Henry and Moulin, p. 24.

Objectives. To measure risk of fatal opioid overdose within 1 year of engagement with Relay's nonfatal overdose response initiative and characterize differences in demographics, substance use, and overdose risk factors by service engagement.

Methods. We assessed the mortality status of 5006 patients who presented to Relay's partnered emergency departments (EDs) in New York City for a suspected nonfatal opioid overdose (2017–2022) and accepted peer-delivered overdose prevention services in the ED, grouped by agreement to and subsequent receipt of post-ED follow-up.

Results. Compared with those declining follow-up, the risk of fatal overdose was not significantly higher among those consenting (adjusted hazard ratio [AHR] = 1.24; 95% confidence interval [CI] = 0.94, 1.65). Among those accepting follow-up, risk was lower for those who were reached (AHR = 0.64; 95% CI = 0.48, 0.84) compared with those who were not.

Conclusions. Peer-delivered ED interventions such as Relay may be effective in reducing fatal overdose risk for individuals with fewer risk factors, and post-ED services are essential for those at higher risk. Approaches should be tailored to more effectively deliver post-ED services to this group. (*Am J Public Health*. 2026;116(1):113–123. https://doi.org/10.2105/AJPH.2025.308270)

AJPH January 2026, Vol. 116, No. 1

In 2023, drug overdose deaths reached historic levels in New York City, largely driven by fentanyl, which was present in 80% of 3046 overdose deaths.[1] Overdose mortality disproportionately affects Black and Latino/a New Yorkers, reflecting the health inequities caused by structural racism and inequitable access to quality health care, treatment, and services.[2–4]

Experiencing a nonfatal overdose increases the risk of future fatal overdose,[5] and emergency departments (EDs) are an opportune setting to deliver an overdose risk reduction intervention. Numerous ED-based interventions have been implemented to deliver opioid overdose risk reduction services, which can include naloxone distribution and overdose prevention education, medication for opioid use disorder (MOUD) initiation, and referrals to substance use disorder treatment and behavioral counseling.[6] The inclusion of peers with lived experience of substance use in the delivery of overdose risk reduction services is an essential component of the current response to the overdose crisis.[7]

In response to rising rates of fatal overdose, the New York City Health Department's Bureau of Alcohol and Drug Use launched Relay, a peer-delivered ED intervention, in June 2017.[8] Relay is currently operating 24 hours a day, 7 days a week, in

14 nonpublic EDs across New York City. Collaborating EDs are selected to target the areas with the highest rates of overdose in New York City. Relay dispatches trained peer wellness advocates, who possess a peer or substance use–related certification or at least 2 years of commensurate peer experience, to engage patients arriving at collaborating EDs after a suspected nonfatal opioid overdose. Using a harm reduction approach, wellness advocates offer peer support, personalized overdose risk reduction education, naloxone and overdose rescue training, and referrals to other service providers to all patients engaged in the ED. Patients who accept Relay services in the ED and feel they need additional support may also consent to receive 90 days of follow-up, during which a wellness advocate will provide ongoing support, education, and assistance accessing resources. The frequency and method (i.e., in person, telephone call, or text message) of follow-up varies based on the needs and preferences of each participant, but in-person contact is encouraged when possible.

Previous research assessing participant outcomes of peer-delivered ED interventions for overdose risk reduction has primarily focused on subsequent nonfatal overdoses, health care utilization, and connection to substance use disorder treatment.[9–12] To date, there has been little published research examining fatal opioid overdose following a peer-delivered ED intervention. We measured opioid overdose mortality risk within 1 year of engagement with Relay's nonfatal overdose response initiative and characterized differences in demographics, substance use, and overdose risk factors based on level of service engagement.

METHODS

For this analysis, we included patients aged 18 years or older who (1) arrived at any of Relay's partnered EDs in New York City for an unintentional opioid overdose between program launch in June 2017 through December 2022, and (2) were eligible for and accepted Relay services in the ED. We did not consider patients who were in police custody or were physically or cognitively incapable of providing consent at the time of the ED encounter eligible for Relay, and we excluded them from this analysis. We did not match patients who did not provide their name or did not reside in New York City at the time of their initial ED encounter to mortality records, and we excluded them from this analysis.

Measures

We grouped patients by whether they consented to follow-up and, among those who consented, whether they received at least 1 contact (i.e., in-person meeting, telephone call, or text message exchange) after the initial ED encounter. We used the date of the patient's initial ED encounter as the index event. When selecting the index ED encounter date for patients with multiple eligible ED encounters, we prioritized encounters with the highest level of Relay engagement. If a patient had multiple encounters in the same category, we selected the earliest encounter.

The primary outcome was unintentional fatal opioid overdose within 1 year of the initial ED encounter. We matched eligible patients to all-cause mortality data that the New York City Health Department's Bureau of Vital Statistics maintains and reports. We matched patient records to death certificates that the Bureau of Vital Statistics maintains based on exact and near matches of identifying data, including first and last name, date of birth, and address.

Two members of the study team (K. L. K. and A. E. W.) reviewed all potential matches by comparing records from both data sources. We identified unintentional opioid overdose deaths from the New York City Health Department's Bureau of Alcohol and Drug Use's overdose surveillance,[1] which combines death certificates with the New York City Office of Chief Medical Examiner postmortem investigations. We reviewed death certificate multiple cause codes (from the *International Classification of Diseases, 10th Revision*; Geneva, Switzerland: World Health Organization; 1992) for accidental poisonings (X40–X44) and for substance use or abuse (F11–F16, F18–F19, excluding chronic use or dependence), with New York City Office of Chief Medical Examiner records and toxicology for opioid involvement. We categorized patients as not deceased, deceased from a fatal opioid overdose, or deceased from other causes.

Covariates included demographic characteristics, circumstances of the initial overdose event, current MOUD and syringe service program (SSP) engagement, and history of previous overdose. During the initial encounter, wellness advocates collected self-reported demographic characteristics from all patients, including gender identity, race/ethnicity, age, and housing status. We considered patients unstably housed if they reported experiencing homelessness or living in a shelter, transitional housing, single-room occupancy, hotel, or drug treatment facility. We considered them living with others if they reported that they were couch surfing or staying with family or friends and stably housed if they reported living in their own home or apartment or in a nursing home or assisted living facility. Additionally, wellness advocates collected data on the circumstances of the overdose event for all patients.

Patients were asked to self-report which substance or substances they intended to take before their overdose; the route or routes of administration; whether they are currently prescribed MOUD, including methadone or buprenorphine; and whether they were currently engaged with an SSP for harm reduction services. Lifetime history of overdose was based primarily on patients' self-report but also included any Relay encounters before the encounter selected as the initial event. Wellness advocates entered data on patient demographics, circumstances of overdose, and details of all encounters in the ED as well as follow-up contacts into Maven Public Health Solutions version 6.11.1 (Conduent Public Health Solutions, Florham Park, NJ), Relay's patient management system.

Statistical Analysis

We used logistic regression to calculate bivariate odds ratios (ORs) and 95% confidence intervals (CIs) for the odds of the patient consenting to Relay follow-up and, among those who did consent, the odds of being reached for follow-up. We used the Cox proportional hazards model to calculate hazard ratios of fatal opioid overdose for each covariate, adjusted for gender identity, race/ethnicity, and age group. We included only covariates with less than 10% missing data in the model. We censored individuals who died of other causes at their date of death.

We conducted all statistical analyses with SAS 9.4 (SAS Institute, Cary, NC).

RESULTS

From program launch in June 2017 through December 2022, Relay was called to respond to 10 239 suspected nonfatal opioid overdoses among 7917 unique patients at its collaborating EDs (Figure 1). Of those, 6738 patients were engaged in the ED and 5702 were determined to be eligible for Relay services, of whom 5292 accepted services. There was no notable difference in demographic characteristics between patients who declined services and those who accepted services (data not shown). For this analysis, we excluded individuals whose initial nonfatal overdose was intentional (n = 57) or whose records had no names or a non–New York City addresses to be matched to New York City mortality records (n = 229).

In our analysis, we included 5006 unique New York City residents who

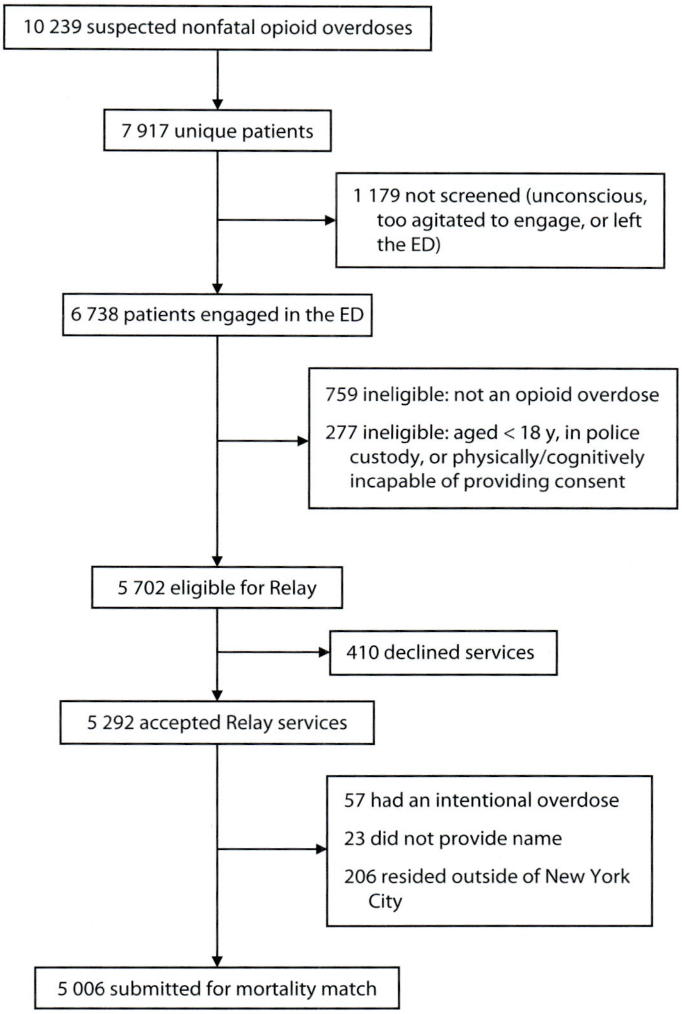

FIGURE 1— Flow Diagram of Eligibility for Relay Services and Mortality Matching: New York City (NYC), June 1, 2017–December 31, 2022

Note. ED = emergency department. Relay is a peer-delivered ED intervention launched by the NYC Health Department's Bureau of Alcohol and Drug Use in June 2017.

received Relay services in the ED after surviving an unintentional opioid overdose. Of the 3477 patients (69.5%) who agreed to follow-up, 2055 (59.1%) were successfully reached at least once. Within 1 year of their initial overdose encounter, 269 (5.4%) patients died of an unintentional opioid overdose and 121 (2.4%) died from other causes.

Table 1 describes mortality, patient demographics, and select substance use and risk factor information among patients at their initial overdose. The largest proportions of patients identified as men (76.5%) and Latino/a (43.0%), and about half (52.6%) were aged 45 years or older. Nearly one third (31.7%) of patients were unstably housed. Most patients (83.4%) reported having intentionally taken an opioid before the initial overdose, with 68.3% reporting they had taken heroin. Fewer patients (18.5%) reported taking cocaine or crack, and of these, half (51.1%) did not report intentionally taking any opioid. The majority (63.4%) of patients reported having snorted their drugs, and 18.0% reported injection drug use. Most patients receiving Relay services were not engaged in substance use or harm reduction services at the time of their initial encounter: 18.6% were prescribed MOUD and 5.4% were engaged with an SSP for harm reduction services. Table A (available as a supplement to the online version of this article at http://www.ajph.org) further describes the number and proportion of patients by each covariate.

Relay Engagement

The odds of consenting to Relay follow-up were greater among patients who were in the older (45–54, 55–64, and 65 years and older) age groups (ORs = 1.44, 1.61, and 1.73, respectively) as well as among those who were

TABLE 1— Demographic, Substance Use, and Overdose Risk Factor Characteristics of Eligible Patients Receiving Relay Services: New York City (NYC), June 1, 2017–December 31, 2022

Characteristic	Total, No. (%)
Overall	5006
1-year mortality status	
Deceased from opioid overdose	269 (5.4)
Deceased from other cause	121 (2.4)
Not deceased	4616 (92.2)
Consented to Relay follow-up	
Yes	3477 (69.5)
No	1529 (30.5)
Received Relay follow-up	
Yes	2055 (59.1)
No	1422 (40.9)
NA	1529
Gender identity	
Man	3754 (76.5)
Woman	1150 (23.5)
Unknown	102
Race/Ethnicity	
White	1294 (26.8)
Black/African-American	1230 (25.4)
Latino/a	2080 (43.0)
Another race or races[a]	229 (4.7)
Unknown	172
Age, y	
18–24	282 (5.7)
25–34	1073 (21.6)
35–44	1006 (20.2)
45–54	1043 (21.0)
55–64	1146 (23.0)
≥ 65	426 (8.6)
Unknown	30
Housing status[b]	
Stable (Ref)	1864 (43.0)
Living with others	1096 (25.3)
Unstable	1373 (31.7)
Unknown	673
Self-reported substances intentionally taken before overdose[c]	
Any opioid	3751 (83.4)
Heroin	3075 (68.3)
Cocaine or crack	831 (18.5)
Cocaine or crack with no opioid	425 (9.5)
Opioid analgesics	521 (11.6)
Fentanyl	160 (3.6)
Unknown	506

Continued

TABLE 1— Continued

Characteristic	Total, No. (%)
Self-reported routes of administration before overdose[d]	
Injected	733 (18.0)
Snorted	2581 (63.4)
Smoked	397 (9.8)
Ingested orally	963 (23.7)
Unknown/not asked	935
Self-reported lifetime history of overdose	
Yes	1570 (41.4)
No	2219 (58.6)
Unknown	1217
Currently prescribed medication for opioid use disorder (self-reported)	
Yes	771 (18.6)
No	3374 (81.4)
Unknown	861
Current syringe service provider participant (self-reported)	
Yes	215 (5.4)
No	3752 (94.6)
Unknown	1039

Note. NA = not available because patient did not consent. Relay is a peer-delivered emergency department intervention launched by the NYC Health Department's Bureau of Alcohol and Drug Use in June 2017.
[a]Includes Asian, Middle Eastern, American Indian or Alaska Native, Native Hawaiian or Pacific Islander, and multiracial groups.
[b]Stable: living in their own home or apartment, or in a nursing home or assisted living facility; living with others: couch surfing or staying with family or friends; unstable: experiencing homelessness (sheltered or unsheltered), or living in transitional housing, single-room occupancy, hotel, or drug treatment facility.
[c]Patients may report ≥ 1 substance, so percentages may add up to > 100%. Combinations of substances are not exhaustive because participants may have taken other substances in addition to the substances listed.
[d]Patients may report ≥ 1 route of administration, so percentages may add up to > 100%. Route of administration is only collected for heroin, cocaine or crack, opioid analgesics, methadone, and benzodiazepines.

unstably housed (OR = 1.31; 95% CI = 1.12, 1.54) or living with others (OR = 1.22; 95% CI = 1.03, 1.45). We also observed higher odds for patients who reported taking any opioid (OR = 2.16; 95% CI = 1.83, 2.54), specifically heroin (OR = 2.01; 95% CI = 1.75, 2.31) or fentanyl (OR = 1.49; 95% CI = 1.01, 2.21), before their initial overdose; who reported snorting their drugs before their initial overdose (OR = 1.21; 95% CI = 1.05, 1.40); who had ever overdosed before (OR = 1.78; 95% CI = 1.53, 2.08); or who were currently prescribed MOUD (OR = 1.35; 95% CI = 1.11, 1.64).

The odds of consenting were lower among those who reported taking opioid analgesics (OR = 0.75; 95% CI = 0.91, 0.91) or cocaine or crack without any intentional opioid use (OR = 0.56; 95% CI = 0.45, 0.69) before their initial overdose. Among patients who consented to follow-up, those who reported taking cocaine or crack without any intentional opioid use before their initial overdose were more likely to be successfully reached at least once (OR = 1.33; 95% CI = 1.02, 1.74).

Those less likely to be reached included patients who identified as Black (OR = 0.81; 95% CI = 0.67, 0.98); were unstably housed (OR = 0.48; 95% CI = 0.41, 0.57) or living with others (OR = 0.82; 95% CI = 0.68, 0.98); reported taking any opioid (OR = 0.81; 95% CI = 0.66, 1.00), specifically heroin (OR = 0.72; 95% CI = 0.61, 0.85) before their initial overdose; reported injecting (OR = 0.72; 95% CI = 0.60, 0.87) or smoking (OR = 0.66; 95% CI = 0.52, 0.84) their drugs before their initial overdose; had previously overdosed (OR = 0.81; 95% CI = 0.70, 0.94); or were currently engaged with an SSP (OR = 0.67; 95% CI = 0.49, 0.92; Table 2).

Opioid Overdose Mortality

Table 3 presents adjusted hazard ratios (AHRs) of opioid overdose death within 1 year of initial nonfatal overdose by consent to and receipt of Relay follow-up, patient demographics, and select substance use and risk factor covariates. There was no significant difference in the risk of fatal opioid overdose within 1 year of initial Relay encounter between patients who consented to Relay follow-up and those who did not, adjusted for age, race/ethnicity, and gender (AHR = 1.24; 95% CI = 0.94, 1.65). Among patients who agreed to Relay follow-up, those who were successfully reached at least once were at 46% lower risk of a fatal overdose within 1 year of their initial Relay encounter compared with those who were not reached, adjusted for age, race/ethnicity, and gender (AHR = 0.64; 95% CI = 0.48, 0.84).

There were no significant differences in the risk of fatal opioid overdose by gender, race/ethnicity, or housing status. Individuals aged 45 to 54, 55 to 64, and 65 years and older had significantly higher risks of a fatal overdose

TABLE 2— Associations Between Demographic, Substance Use, and Overdose Risk Factor Characteristics and Consent to or Receipt of Relay Follow-Up: New York City (NYC), June 1, 2017–December 31, 2022

Characteristic	Consented to Follow-Up, OR (95% CI)	Received Follow-Up, OR (95% CI)
Women	1.10 (0.95, 1.27)	1.28 (1.09, 1.50)
Race/Ethnicity		
White (Ref)	1	1
Black/African-American	1.14 (0.96, 1.35)	0.81 (0.67, 0.98)
Latino/a	1.07 (0.92, 1.25)	0.89 (0.75, 1.05)
Another race or races[a]	0.67 (0.50, 0.89)	0.99 (0.69, 1.43)
Age, y		
18–24	1.33 (1.00, 1.77)	1.18 (0.85, 1.64)
25–34	1.16 (0.97, 1.39)	0.99 (0.80, 1.23)
35–44 (Ref)	1	1
45–54	1.44 (1.19, 1.73)	0.95 (0.76, 1.17)
55–64	1.61 (1.34, 1.94)	1.07 (0.87, 1.32)
≥65	1.73 (1.34, 2.24)	1.14 (0.86, 1.49)
Housing status[b]		
Stable (Ref)	1	1
Living with others	1.22 (1.03, 1.45)	0.82 (0.68, 0.98)
Unstable	1.31 (1.12, 1.54)	0.48 (0.41, 0.57)
Self-reported substances intentionally taken before overdose[c]		
Any opioid	2.16 (1.83, 2.54)	0.81 (0.66, 1.00)
Heroin	2.01 (1.75, 2.31)	0.72 (0.61, 0.85)
Cocaine or crack with no opioid	0.56 (0.45, 0.69)	1.33 (1.02, 1.74)
Opioid analgesics	0.75 (0.61, 0.91)	1.53 (1.21, 1.94)
Fentanyl	1.49 (1.01, 2.21)	0.74 (0.52, 1.06)
Self-reported routes of administration before overdose[d]		
Injected	1.20 (0.99, 1.46)	0.72 (0.60, 0.87)
Snorted	1.21 (1.05, 1.40)	1.08 (0.93, 1.25)
Smoked	1.21 (0.94, 1.55)	0.66 (0.52, 0.84)
Ingested orally	0.94 (0.79, 1.10)	1.50 (1.26, 1.79)
Self-reported lifetime history of overdose	1.78 (1.53, 2.08)	0.81 (0.70, 0.94)
Currently prescribed MOUD (self-reported)	1.35 (1.11, 1.64)	1.14 (0.95, 1.36)
Current SSP participant (self-reported)	1.14 (0.81, 1.58)	0.67 (0.49, 0.92)

Note. CI = confidence interval; MOUD = medication for opioid use disorder; OR = odds ratio; SSP = syringe service program. We used binary logistic regression to calculate ORs among all 5006 eligible patients for odds of consenting to follow-up and among the 3477 patients who consented to follow-up for odds of receiving follow-up. Relay is a peer-delivered emergency department intervention launched by the NYC Health Department's Bureau of Alcohol and Drug Use in June 2017.

[a]Includes Asian, Middle Eastern, American Indian or Alaska Native, Native Hawaiian or Pacific Islander, and multiracial groups.

[b]Stable: living in their own home or apartment, or in a nursing home or assisted living facility; living with others: couch surfing or staying with family or friends; unstable: experiencing homelessness (sheltered or unsheltered), or living in transitional housing, single-room occupancy, hotel, or drug treatment facility.

[c]Patients may report ≥1 substance. Combinations of substances are not exhaustive because participants may have taken other substances in addition to the substances listed.

[d]Patients may report ≥1 route of administration. We collected the route of administration only for heroin, cocaine or crack, opioid analgesics, methadone, and benzodiazepines.

TABLE 3— Associations Between Demographic, Substance Use, and Overdose Risk Factor Characteristics and Fatal Opioid Overdose: New York City (NYC), June 1, 2017–December 31, 2022

Characteristic	AHR (95% CI)
Consented to Relay follow-up	1.24 (0.94, 1.65)
Received Relay follow-up[a]	0.64 (0.48, 0.84)
Woman	0.89 (0.66, 1.20)
Race/Ethnicity	
White (Ref)	1
Black/African-American	0.96 (0.69, 1.35)
Latino/a	0.84 (0.62, 1.13)
Another race or races[b]	0.76 (0.38, 1.52)
Age, y	
18–24	1.05 (0.55, 2.01)
25–34	0.88 (0.57, 1.37)
35–44 (Ref)	1
45–54	1.59 (1.08, 2.35)
55–64	1.63 (1.11, 2.39)
≥ 65	1.92 (1.20, 3.06)
Housing status[c]	
Stable (Ref)	1
Living with others	0.96 (0.68, 1.35)
Unstable	0.98 (0.73, 1.32)
Self-reported substances intentionally taken before overdose[d]	
Any opioid	1.66 (1.09, 2.51)
Heroin	1.50 (1.11, 2.03)
Cocaine or crack with no opioid	0.56 (0.32, 0.99)
Opioid analgesics	0.81 (0.52, 1.26)
Fentanyl	1.07 (0.55, 2.08)
Self-reported routes of administration before overdose[e]	
Injected	1.20 (0.85, 1.69)
Snorted	1.06 (0.80, 1.41)
Smoked	1.00 (0.64, 1.56)
Ingested orally	0.81 (0.58, 1.13)
Self-reported lifetime history of overdose	1.53 (1.16, 2.02)
Currently prescribed MOUD (self-reported)	0.58 (0.38, 0.86)
Current SSP participant (self-reported)	1.65 (1.00, 2.71)

Note. AHR = adjusted hazard ratio; CI = confidence interval; MOUD = medication for opioid use disorder; SSP = syringe service program. We used the Cox proportional hazards model to calculate risk of fatal opioid overdose, adjusted for gender identity, race/ethnicity, and age group. Relay is a peer-delivered emergency department intervention launched by the NYC Health Department's Bureau of Alcohol and Drug Use in June 2017.

[a]We calculated the AHR for receiving Relay follow-up among the 3477 patients who consented to follow-up.

[b]Includes Asian, Middle Eastern, American Indian or Alaska Native, Native Hawaiian or Pacific Islander, and multiracial groups.

[c]Stable: living in their own home or apartment, or in a nursing home or assisted living facility; living with others: couch surfing or staying with family or friends; unstable: experiencing homelessness (sheltered or unsheltered), or living in transitional housing, single-room occupancy, hotel, or drug treatment facility.

[d]Patients may report ≥ 1 substance. Combinations of substances are not exhaustive because participants may have taken other substances in addition to the substances listed.

[e]Patients may report ≥ 1 route of administration. We collected the route of administration only for heroin, cocaine or crack, opioid analgesics, methadone, and benzodiazepines.

when compared with those aged 35 to 44 years (AHRs = 1.59, 1.63, and 1.92, respectively).

Individuals who reported having intentionally taken any opioid had a significantly greater risk of experiencing a fatal opioid overdose than did those who did not (AHR = 1.66; 95% CI = 1.09, 2.51), as did those who reported using heroin specifically (AHR = 1.50; 95% CI = 1.11, 2.03). Patients who reported taking cocaine or crack but did not report any intentional opioid use were at lower risk of opioid overdose death than were other patients (AHR = 0.56; 95% CI = 0.32, 0.99). Individuals who had previously experienced a nonfatal opioid overdose before the overdose leading to their Relay engagement had a 53% higher risk of opioid overdose death than did those who had not (AHR = 1.53; 95% CI = 1.16, 2.02). Individuals currently prescribed MOUD at the time of their initial overdose were at lower risk of experiencing a fatal opioid overdose (AHR = 0.58; 95% CI = 0.38, 0.86), whereas those who reported receiving harm reduction services at an SSP were at higher risk (AHR = 1.65; 95% CI = 1.00, 2.71). The number and proportion of overdose decedents by each characteristic are presented in Table B (available as a supplement to the online version of this article at http://www.ajph.org).

DISCUSSION

Peer-delivered overdose response initiatives have shown promising outcomes in terms of connections to substance use treatment and harm reduction services, but few studies have examined their impacts on postintervention overdose mortality.[8,11–14] The cohort of individuals accepting Relay services after surviving an opioid overdose were mostly opioid overdose decedents in New York City: the largest proportions were men, Latino/a, and middle aged or older.[1] Individuals experiencing homelessness were disproportionately represented among the Relay patient population, reflecting the high burden of drug-related death among homeless individuals in New York City.[15] Although Relay operates in areas with the highest rates of overdose in New York City, we found that the majority of individuals receiving Relay services were not engaged in other substance use treatment or services at the time of their overdose, despite 41% having overdosed before. Our findings underscore the importance of expanding access to life-saving harm reduction services and tailoring targeted interventions to meet the needs of communities most affected by opioid use.

Overdose Risk by Relay Engagement

Among patients who consented to Relay follow-up services, those successfully reached for follow-up experienced lower rates of fatal overdose within 1 year of Relay engagement than did those who were not, demonstrating the benefit of postoverdose follow-up services for people who use opioids. Several factors associated with high overdose risk—lack of stable housing,[16] intentional opioid use, and lifetime history of overdose[5]—were positively associated with requesting follow-up but negatively associated with receiving it. This suggests that those at highest overdose risk are likely to accept services following peer engagement but face barriers to retention.

Despite intensive outreach efforts, we were unable to reach a large proportion of patients. Individuals targeted by interventions such as Relay are not inherently hard to reach but rather are "hardly reached" by inadequate approaches to address barriers to engagement. To inform the future of Relay and similar interventions, we must address these barriers, including stigmatization of substance use, infrastructure, incarceration history, and lack of social support.[17] For example, among patients experiencing homelessness or poverty, challenges to providing follow-up include competing priorities and a lack of reliable contact information (e.g., a telephone, address, or consistent hangout location).[18] Additionally, the COVID-19 pandemic presented significant barriers to in-person engagement and follow-up.

Patients who self-selected to receive only ED services did not have a significantly greater risk of fatal overdose than those who consented to follow-up. These patients were more likely to be younger and stably housed and less likely to have intentionally used an opioid, injected their drugs, or previously overdosed than were their counterparts. For individuals with fewer overdose-related risk factors, additional follow-up may not be needed to reduce the risk of fatal overdose after an ED-based intervention such as Relay.

Additional Overdose Risk Factors

The risk of fatal opioid overdose was significantly lower among those who self-reported using cocaine without intentional opioid use, which was half of all individuals reporting cocaine use and was most prevalent in the group that declined follow-up. In light of the increased presence of fentanyl in the unregulated drug supply,[19] it is critical that individuals who do not intentionally use opioids receive tailored overdose prevention education and naloxone. Our findings suggest that providing these services after a nonfatal opioid overdose, even without additional follow-up, may be effective in preventing future fatal opioid overdoses.

Conversely, our findings also suggest that for individuals who do intentionally use opioids or have experienced multiple nonfatal overdoses, an ED intervention alone may not be sufficient. For example, individuals who use opioids and are experiencing homelessness face numerous barriers to engagement and retention in substance use and social services programs.[20–21] Consequently, follow-up approaches need to be tailored to reach populations who are underserved by existing models of substance use and overdose prevention services.

The majority of patients seen by Relay were not connected to substance use services, specifically receiving harm reduction services at an SSP (5%) or taking MOUD (19%). It is likely that the higher risk of overdose death among SSP participants—of whom the largest proportion consented to but did not receive follow-up—reflects underlying differences in housing status and substance use patterns. Many SSP participants fall into the highest risk population of people who use opioids: those who are unhoused or unstably housed, use drugs frequently, or engage in polysubstance use.[22] Our finding that those who were taking MOUD at the time of their initial overdose were less likely to have a fatal opioid overdose supports the evidence base for MOUD as a protective factor against overdose and highlights the importance of connecting patients to MOUD postoverdose.[23]

Limitations

This study has several limitations. First, all individuals included in this analysis received Relay services in the ED. Without a comparison group of individuals who did not receive any intervention, we were unable to fully assess the impact of Relay services in reducing overdose risk. A randomized controlled trial comparing Relay to site-directed care at 4 of Relay's partnered EDs has been conducted to assess the effectiveness of Relay overall[24]; results are forthcoming. In our current analysis, we were unable to determine whether, or quantify to what extent, the reduction in risk of fatal overdose among those reached for follow-up is attributable to the effect of follow-up itself or is because the patients at highest risk are also those hardly reached. Patients may not have been reached because they died during the follow-up period.

Furthermore, we did not assess the extent of Relay follow-up participants received: we grouped individuals receiving frequent, in-depth follow-ups with those who may have received only 1 brief contact. Future analyses should examine type and intensity of follow-up services. We were also able to match only to New York City vital statistics data, so it is possible that there were deaths outside New York City that were not included.

A final limitation is our reliance on self-reported data for housing status, substance use behaviors, and connections to substance use treatment and services. In addition to potentially introducing bias, this resulted in a high degree of missing data, which limited our ability to control for these factors in AHR calculations. However, peers collected the data, which may have reduced social desirability bias; people who use drugs have reported in qualitative interviews that they feel more comfortable opening up to peer workers.[25] Other studies measuring mortality following a nonfatal overdose have used only medical record data and have not included any patient history or substance use behavior information.[26–28]

Public Health Implications

Relay is a novel peer-delivered public health intervention that supports people who experience nonfatal overdose both while in the ED and afterward. Information gleaned from this analysis allows a better understanding of risk and protective factors for a fatal opioid overdose within 1 year of experiencing a nonfatal opioid overdose. The intensity of Relay services that patients received aligned with their vulnerability to a future fatal overdose and demonstrates how Relay was able or unable to support them. Recognizing that peer interventions for ED patients exist among structural barriers—including lack of affordable housing, inadequate access to MOUD and harm reduction services, criminalization of drug use, and a volatile unregulated drug supply—we have several recommendations for future programs.

Expanding the reach and accessibility of harm reduction (e.g., Overdose Prevention Centers, extensive naloxone distribution, point-of-care drug-checking at SSPs) and substance use disorder treatment services (e.g., low-threshold access to MOUD), particularly for those currently underserved and hardly reached by existing models of service, is critical for addressing some of the inequities we observed in overdose and overdose mortality.

Peer-delivered ED-based initiatives such as Relay can continue to fill these gaps by providing services and connections to care to individuals at risk for overdose who are not otherwise engaged in substance use services, particularly those whose immediate needs can be met in the ED, including those who do not intentionally use opioids. However, novel approaches are needed to follow up post-ED more effectively with hardly reached individuals, such as contingency management, providing participants with prepaid cell phones, hosting drop-in spaces, or conducting robust street outreach. AJPH

ABOUT THE AUTHORS

Kelsey L. Kepler, Alice E. Welch, Ellenie Tuazon, Dominique Chambless, and Angela Jeffers are with the Bureau of Alcohol and Drug Use, Division of Mental Hygiene, New York City Department of Health and Mental Hygiene, New York, NY. Joseph Kennedy is with the Bureau of Vital Statistics, Center for Population Health Data Science, New York City Department of Health and Mental Hygiene, New York, NY.

CORRESPONDENCE

Correspondence should be sent to Kelsey L. Kepler, 42-09 28th St, Long Island City, NY 11101 (e-mail: kkepler@health.nyc.gov). Reprints can be ordered at https://www.ajph.org by clicking the "Reprints" link.

PUBLICATION INFORMATION

Full Citation: Kepler KL, Welch AE, Tuazon E, Chambless D, Kennedy J, Jeffers A. Opioid overdose mortality among patients receiving a peer-delivered, emergency department–based nonfatal opioid overdose intervention in New York City, 2017–2022. *Am J Public Health*. 2026;116(1): 113–123.

Acceptance Date: August 12, 2025.

DOI: https://doi.org/10.2105/AJPH.2025.308270

ORCID iDs:

Kelsey L. Kepler https://orcid.org/0000-0003-0209-6686

Alice E. Welch https://orcid.org/0000-0002-9157-4987

Ellenie Tuazon https://orcid.org/0000-0002-8779-1604

CONTRIBUTORS

K. L. Kepler performed the data analyses. K. L. Kepler and A. E. Welch drafted the article. K. L. Kepler, A. E. Welch, D. Chambless, and A. Jeffers contributed to the design and implementation of the Relay initiative, including data collection and acquisition. E. Tuazon and J. Kennedy contributed to the acquisition of mortality data. All authors contributed to the study design, data interpretation, and revision of the final article.

ACKNOWLEDGMENTS

The authors would like to thank the Relay Wellness Advocates and Wellness Advocate Supervisors, as well as all of the individuals seen by Relay. We would also like to thank Rebecca Linn-Walton, Shivani Mantha, and Hannah Helmy for their thoughtful review and feedback.

CONFLICTS OF INTEREST

The authors have no conflicts of interest to disclose.

HUMAN PARTICIPANT PROTECTION

This study was reviewed and approved by the institutional review board of the New York City Department of Health and Mental Hygiene.

REFERENCES

1. Tuazon E, Sun T, Weitz A, et al. Unintentional drug poisoning (overdose) deaths in New York City in 2023. *Epi Data Brief.* 2024;142:1–9. Available at: https://www.nyc.gov/assets/doh/downloads/pdf/epi/databrief142.pdf. Accessed September 26, 2025.
2. Kunins HV. Structural racism and the opioid overdose epidemic: the need for antiracist public health practice. *J Public Health Manag Pract.* 2020;26(3):201–205. https://doi.org/10.1097/PHH.0000000000001168
3. Gramlich J. Recent surge in US drug overdose deaths has hit Black men the hardest. January 21, 2022. Available at: https://www.pewresearch.org/fact-tank/2022/01/19/recent-surge-in-u-s-drug-overdose-deaths-has-hit-black-men-the-hardest. Accessed June 26, 2025.
4. Cohen A, Vakharia SP, Netherland J, Frederique K. How the war on drugs impacts social determinants of health beyond the criminal legal system. *Ann Med.* 2022;54(1):2024–2038. https://doi.org/10.1080/07853890.2022.2100926
5. Caudarella A, Dong H, Milloy MJ, Kerr T, Wood E, Hayashi K. Non-fatal overdose as a risk factor for subsequent fatal overdose among people who inject drugs. *Drug Alcohol Depend.* 2016;162:51–55. https://doi.org/10.1016/j.drugalcdep.2016.02.024
6. Chen Y, Wang Y, Nielsen S, Kuhn L, Lam T. A systematic review of opioid overdose interventions delivered within emergency departments. *Drug Alcohol Depend.* 2020;213:108009. https://doi.org/10.1016/j.drugalcdep.2020.108009
7. Mercer F, Miler JA, Pauly B, et al. Peer support and overdose prevention responses: a systematic "state-of-the-art" review. *Int J Environ Res Public Health.* 2021;18(22):12073. https://doi.org/10.3390/ijerph182212073
8. Welch AE, Jeffers A, Allen B, Paone D, Kunins HV. Relay: a peer-delivered emergency department-based response to nonfatal opioid overdose. *Am J Public Health.* 2019;109(10):1392–1395. https://doi.org/10.2105/AJPH.2019.305202
9. Santos C, Ramdin C, Becceril J, Al Kik B, Jefri M, Nelson L. The impact of an emergency department peer navigator (EDPN) program in improving clinical outcomes and healthcare utilization in an urban setting. *Am J Emerg Med.* 2023;68:10–16. https://doi.org/10.1016/j.ajem.2023.02.031
10. Chambers LC, Li Y, Hallowell BD, et al. Effect of a peer-led emergency department behavioral intervention on non-fatal opioid overdose: 18-month outcome in the Navigator randomized controlled trial. *Addiction.* 2024;119(12):2116–2128. https://doi.org/10.1111/add.16581
11. Treitler P, Crystal S, Cantor J, et al. Emergency department peer support program and patient outcomes after opioid overdose. *JAMA Netw Open.* 2024;7(3):e243614. https://doi.org/10.1001/jamanetworkopen.2024.3614
12. Watson DP, Tillson M, Taylor L, et al. Results from the POINT pragmatic randomized trial: an emergency department-based peer support specialist intervention to increase opioid use disorder treatment linkage and reduce recurrent overdose. *Subst Use Addict J.* 2024;45(3):378–389. https://doi.org/10.1177/29767342231221054
13. Waye KM, Goyer J, Dettor D, et al. Implementing peer recovery services for overdose prevention in Rhode Island: an examination of two outreach-based approaches. *Addict Behav.* 2019;89:85–91. https://doi.org/10.1016/j.addbeh.2018.09.027
14. Avalone L, Lalane M, King C, Pfeiffer K, Linn-Walton R, Barron C. Integrating substance use peer support and screening brief intervention and referral to treatment services in the emergency department: a descriptive study of the ED leads program. *Addict Sci Clin Pract.* 2024;19(1):15. https://doi.org/10.1186/s13722-024-00445-x
15. Brand D. Drug overdoses continue to rise inside New York City homeless shelters. June 30, 2022. Available at: https://citylimits.org/drug-overdoses-continue-to-rise-inside-nyc-homeless-shelters. Accessed June 26, 2025.
16. Yamamoto A, Needleman J, Gelberg L, Kominski G, Shoptaw S, Tsugawa Y. Association between homelessness and opioid overdose and opioid-related hospital admissions/emergency department visits. *Soc Sci Med.* 2019;242:112585. https://doi.org/10.1016/j.socscimed.2019.112585
17. Sokol R, Fisher E, Hill J. Identifying those whom health promotion hardly reaches: a systematic review. *Eval Health Prof.* 2015;38(4):518–537. https://doi.org/10.1177/0163278715605883
18. Routhier G, Freeman R, Welch AE, et al. Understanding engagement with an emergency department-based peer navigator intervention for opioid overdose prevention for a subset of patients experiencing homelessness. *J Soc Distress Homeless.* 2025;1–11. https://doi.org/10.1080/10530789.2025.2473760
19. Wagner KD, Fiuty P, Page K, et al. Prevalence of fentanyl in methamphetamine and cocaine samples collected by community-based drug checking services. *Drug Alcohol Depend.* 2023;252:110985. https://doi.org/10.1016/j.drugalcdep.2023.110985
20. Fine DR, Lewis E, Weinstock K, Wright J, Gaeta JM, Baggett TP. Office-based addiction treatment retention and mortality among people experiencing homelessness. *JAMA Netw Open.* 2021;4(3): e210477. https://doi.org/10.1001/jamanetworkopen.2021.0477
21. Paradise RK, Desmarais J, O'Malley SE, et al. Perspectives and recommendations of opioid overdose survivors experiencing unsheltered homelessness on housing, overdose, and substance use treatment in Boston, MA. *Int J Drug Policy.* 2023;119:104127. https://doi.org/10.1016/j.drugpo.2023.104127

22. Erath TG, LaCroix R, O'Keefe E, Higgins ST, Rawson RA. Substance use patterns, sociodemographics, and health profiles of harm reduction service recipients in Burlington, Vermont. *Harm Reduct J*. 2024;21(1):76. https://doi.org/10.1186/s12954-024-00995-y
23. Substance Abuse and Mental Health Services Administration. *Medications for Opioid Use Disorder*. Treatment Improvement Protocol (TIP) Series 63 Publication No. PEP21-02-01-002. Rockville, MD; 2021. Available at: https://library.samhsa.gov/sites/default/files/pep21-02-01-002.pdf. Accessed September 26, 2025.
24. Doran KM, Welch AE, Jeffers A, et al. Study protocol for a multisite randomized controlled trial of a peer navigator intervention for emergency department patients with nonfatal opioid overdose. *Contemp Clin Trials*. 2023;126:107111. https://doi.org/10.1016/j.cct.2023.107111
25. Kennedy MC, Boyd J, Mayer S, Collins A, Kerr T, McNeil R. Peer worker involvement in low-threshold supervised consumption facilities in the context of an overdose epidemic in Vancouver, Canada. *Soc Sci Med*. 2019;225:60–68. https://doi.org/10.1016/j.socscimed.2019.02.014
26. Spencer MR, White DG, Jackson G. National Hospital Care Survey demonstration projects: mortality following nonfatal opioid overdose visits to the emergency department. *Natl Health Stat Report*. 2023;187:1–8.
27. Samples H, Nowels MA, Williams AR, Olfson M, Crystal S. Buprenorphine after nonfatal opioid overdose: reduced mortality risk in Medicare disability beneficiaries. *Am J Prev Med*. 2023;65(1):19–29. https://doi.org/10.1016/j.amepre.2023.01.037
28. Jones CM, Shoff C, Blanco C, Losby JL, Ling SM, Compton WM. Overdose, behavioral health services, and medications for opioid use disorder after a nonfatal overdose. *JAMA Intern Med*. 2024;184(8):954–962. https://doi.org/10.1001/jamainternmed.2024.1733

Political Polarization During Disease Outbreaks: A Meta-Analysis of Archival Survey Data From Polio to COVID-19

Caitlin L. McMurtry, PhD, SM, and Rachana Cheu, MPH

See also Nuzzo, p. 26.

Objectives. To assess how political polarization during COVID-19 compares with that in past disease outbreaks in the United States.

Methods. Using random-effects meta-analyses and mixed-effects meta-regressions, we searched the Roper Center for Public Opinion Research and estimated the association between polarization during COVID-19 and during non–COVID-19 disease outbreaks.

Results. The study included 170 polls spanning 13 outbreaks over nearly 70 years. Polarization during COVID-19 was 5 and 12 times greater than in past disease outbreaks in terms of concern about infection and vaccine hesitancy, respectively. After we controlled for survey-level characteristics, COVID-19 was associated with 20.23 (95% confidence interval [CI] = 12.30, 28.17) and 25.89 (95% CI = 6.63, 45.16) additional percentage points of polarization regarding concern about infection and vaccine hesitancy, respectively—far higher than historical trends would predict.

Conclusions. In terms of concern about infection and vaccine hesitancy, polarization during COVID-19 was substantially higher than in any other disease outbreak in modern American history for which we have relevant data.

Public Health Implications. High levels of polarization do not appear endemic to disease outbreaks, suggesting such division may be preventable in the future. (*Am J Public Health*. 2026;116(1):124–136. https://doi.org/10.2105/AJPH.2025.308226)

AJPH January 2026, Vol. 116, No. 1

Political polarization can inhibit effective responses to public health crises like infectious disease outbreaks. This is because ideological polarization is associated with legislative gridlock—the growing inability of legislative bodies like Congress or state legislatures to pass laws—since members of each party have less incentive to compromise as they move apart.[1,2] Legislative gridlock, in turn, is associated with lagging social and economic policies, which can hamper the government's ability to effectively respond to constituent needs in a crisis.[2,3] In situations like disease outbreaks, where conditions are changing rapidly, these policy lags are associated with waning risk protection, especially for the least powerful.[4] Affective polarization—the growing tendency of partisans to distrust and dislike members of the other party[5]—is also associated with legislative gridlock and declining trust in government,[6] which can jeopardize public health in several ways. First, preventive behaviors crucial to controlling the spread of diseases during outbreaks (e.g., masking, social distancing, vaccination) are strongly correlated with partisanship[7–11] and trust in government in the United States.[12] In fact, trust in government has been identified as a key determinant of COVID-19 vaccine uptake globally[13–15] and influenza vaccination in the United States.[16,17] Not only are vaccines integral to curbing the incidence of severe disease and death from infectious diseases, but increasing vaccination is inversely correlated with hospitalizations,[18] which may prevent excess morbidity and mortality from overwhelmed health systems.[19] Thus, increasing polarization and declining trust in government can threaten pandemic preparedness.

Political polarization is not new; research indicates it has been growing since the mid-1970s.[20] American politics scholars largely agree that political parties have become more polarized over time and, as voters improve their ability to choose parties that align with their ideological views, society has followed.[1,21–25] Despite this rise in party sorting, studies show that the views of the public remain largely moderate, even on controversial issues like abortion.[23,24,26–28] However, it is unclear how levels of polarization observed during COVID-19 compare with historical trends.

This study addresses the question: How did political polarization during the coronavirus pandemic compare with polarization during past disease outbreaks in the United States? Perhaps polarization is a natural consequence of public health emergencies and, in times of crisis, we should expect that partisans will retreat to their ideological corners. If levels of polarization during COVID-19 were akin to levels during contentious outbreaks like anthrax and HIV, polarization should be reversible with existing strategies. On the other hand, if polarization during the pandemic was substantially higher, past tactics may prove ineffective. Using a meta-analysis of 170 public opinion polls across 13 disease outbreaks over nearly 70 years, we show that although some partisan separation is routine, pandemic-era levels of polarization were far higher than in any other disease outbreak in modern US history for which we have relevant data. Additionally, high levels of polarization continue to linger, indicating that research on and new approaches to reducing societal divisions are urgently needed.

METHODS

To generate a list of disease outbreaks with associated polling data, we searched the Roper Center for Public Opinion Research's iPoll database, the largest polling archive in the world, for disease-related terms and general ones such as "flu," "virus," "fever," "disease," "illness," "outbreak," "epidemic," "infection," and "pandemic." To compare across outbreaks, we looked for questions with wording that remained stable over time and that were used by multiple organizations to measure attitudes during a given crisis. This produced 2 outcomes of interest: concern about infection and intention to receive a vaccine. We measured the first outcome by variations of the question, "How concerned are you that you or someone you know will get infected with [a given disease]?" We measured the second outcome using variations of the question, "Do you plan to get vaccinated for [a given disease] when a vaccine becomes available to you?" Full question wording is available in Appendixes D and E (available as a supplement to the online version of this article at http://www.ajph.org).

We then combined terms related to our outcomes with disease terms to search the database. For concern about infection, our outcome-related search terms included "worried" or "concerned"; for vaccine intention, we used the terms "vaccine," "vaccination," "vaccinate," "vaccinated," "shot," "inoculate," and "inoculation." These were paired with specific disease-related terms (e.g., "H5N1," "HIV"); general terms (e.g., "immune deficiency," "sarcoma"); and colloquial terms, including some commonly used pejorative phrases that reflected news coverage at the time (e.g., "bird flu," "Asian flu," "gay cancer"). For diseases associated with vaccines already in widespread use (e.g., diphtheria, chickenpox, influenza) we added search terms to focus on one's likelihood of vaccination during a given health threat (e.g., "likely," "plan," "would," and "probably"), rather than past receipt, to keep comparisons standard over time.

Inclusion Criteria

In the first screening phase, we used a database filter to return only polls with downloadable data sets. We copied these results into an Excel file. Polls were then screened for relevant question wording. Third, we reviewed full-text questions to determine whether they met inclusion criteria. A poll was considered eligible if it (1) asked about concern on a 4-point response scale or vaccine intention on a binary or 4-point scale, (2) included party affiliation, (3) did not use prejudicial terms, (4) asked about an outbreak within the first 5 years of its emergence or resurgence into the national discourse, and (5) sampled adults nationwide. Study searching occurred from April to July 2021, and an update was conducted from January to April 2024. One reviewer (C. L. M.) conducted the primary search, and both authors (C. L. M. and R. C.) conducted the update. Discrepancies were discussed and resolved. Because most major news organizations in the United States archive their data sets at the Roper Center regardless of their results, publication bias is unlikely to be a concern. Assessments of poll quality based on survey organization ratings are available in online Appendix H.

Polls that surveyed adults in certain states, of certain ages, or only registered voters were excluded for not being nationally representative. We also excluded polls that asked questions on dissimilar scales because differences in the underlying distribution of responses could be mistakenly interpreted as changes in opinion. We did not include polls that contained prejudicial terms such as "safe" or "effective" regarding vaccines and phrases such as "seriously ill" regarding concern. These qualifiers were considered meaningful departures in wording that could exaggerate differences between partisans if, for example, Democrats were more likely than Republicans to believe in the reported safety or effectiveness of a vaccine. Polls on HIV/AIDS conducted in the 1990s were also excluded to ensure that surveys asking about disease outbreaks captured attitudes while the threat remained relatively novel and thus comparable in timing to COVID-19. Additionally, we excluded polls that asked if one worried about infection yesterday and vaccine polls that asked about receipt, rather than intention.

Data Extraction

To preserve survey weights (present in $k = 160/170$) that ensure a poll's sample is nationally representative at the time of its fielding, each poll was analyzed individually (by C. L. M.). The proportions of self-identified Democrats and Democratic-leaners ("Democrats") and Republicans and Republican-leaners ("Republicans") who said they were "very concerned" about infection or who did not intend to get a vaccine when one became available to them were estimated for each poll using the *svy* package in Stata version 17.0 (StataCorp LP, College Station, TX). Some vaccine polls ($k = 52$) used a 4-point likeliness scale for responses, ranging from "very likely" to "not at all likely." To enable comparisons to questions on a binary yes–no scale ($k = 37$), this variable was dichotomized by aggregating responses into a "likely" group and an "unlikely" group.

Ten polls conducted before 1988 did not have survey weights but instead used area-based probability sampling techniques. To obtain standard errors for point estimates from these polls, we created survey weights of 1 to generate uncertainty estimates without affecting accuracy or precision. Additionally, 2 polls used a duplicate card system for survey weighting, which can artificially inflate the sample size and statistical power of a poll. To correct this, we multiplied each poll's duplicate card weight by the inverse mean of all the weights in the sample to create a new weight centered around the total weight mean. This preserved the original sample size and the relative magnitude of the weights.

Statistical Analyses

We conducted a random effects meta-analysis to analyze the mean difference between partisans. Specifically, our principal summary measure was the percentage-point difference between Democrats and Republicans (or, for vaccine hesitancy, Republicans and Democrats). Our subgroups allowed us to compare polarization during the pandemic and during noncoronavirus outbreaks. A random-effects model was selected a priori because whereas fixed-effects models assume 1 true effect size across all studies, random-effects models allow effect sizes to vary between studies and assume that included studies "represent a random sample of effect sizes that could have been observed."[29(p71)] Given the Roper Center's archiving practices, we assumed that this condition was satisfied. We used restricted maximum likelihood estimation to estimate between-study variability.[30]

Mixed-effects meta-regression explored sources of heterogeneity and assessed the relationship between COVID-19 and polarization for each outcome. Moderator variables adjusted for variation in question wording and response options, where applicable; survey administration mode (e.g., telephone, web); the presence of survey weights; months until the next election; the party of the president in power; and, where sample size allowed, so-called "house effects"—differences in sampling and weighting techniques unique to individual survey organizations.[31] Additionally, by fitting our meta-regression model to prepandemic data, we obtained a predicted level of polarization in December 2023 to evaluate whether COVID-19 fell along a trend of rising polarization over time. Because of sample size limitations, moderator variables in the predictive models adjusted for variation in question wording and response options, house effects (for concern about infection), the presence of survey weights (vaccine hesitancy), months until the next election, and party of the president in power. We evaluated moderator associations based on coefficients and 95% confidence intervals (95% CIs), and meta-regressions used the Knapp–Hartung adjustment to help account for uncertainty in the estimate of τ^2.[30] We examined residual heterogeneity by estimating τ^2 using restricted maximum likelihood estimation and I^2, and employing Cochran's Q test, where the null hypothesis was that all studies share a common effect.[29] We conducted all meta-analyses and meta-regressions in R version 4.1.3 (R Foundation for Statistical Computing, Vienna, Austria), using the *metafor* package (Viechtbauer, 2010).

RESULTS

The search yielded 6095 surveys for preliminary screening: 2474 pertaining to concern about infection and 3621 to vaccine hesitancy. After we removed those without downloadable data sets, 2950 surveys were screened for inclusion across both outcomes and 369 received full-text review. Ultimately, 170 unique surveys met inclusion criteria, of which 90 asked questions on concern about infection and 89 asked about vaccine hesitancy. These polls included a total sample size of 158 143 partisans, of which 87 412 identified as or leaned Democrat and 70 731 identified as or leaned Republican.

Study Characteristics

Table 1 summarizes the characteristics of the included polls. The online Appendices include our PRISMA flow diagram (Appendix A), search terms and results (B and C), and full question wording with sample size for each poll (D and E). Regarding concern about infection, 42% of polls examined COVID-19, whereas the rest covered 8 other outbreaks dating back to HIV/AIDS in 1985. Seventeen survey organizations polled on this outcome, the most common of which was Ipsos (23%). Just under half (43%) asked about one's level of concern about being infected by, becoming ill with, or getting sick from a given disease. About a quarter (28%) asked about catching, contracting, or getting a disease, and a similar proportion (22%) asked about being exposed to or affected by a given disease. Just 4 (4%) asked about being a victim of a given disease. Most (71%) were conducted via telephone, followed by web only (23%), telephone and web (4%), and face-to-face (1%). All polls used survey weights and 73% were fielded during a Republican presidential administration. On average, these polls were conducted 10 months before the next election, with about 452 self-identified Democrats (and leaners) and about 373 Republicans (and leaners).

Regarding vaccine hesitancy, 71% of polls examined COVID-19 whereas the rest covered 8 other outbreaks dating back to polio in 1954. Seventeen survey organizations conducted polls on this outcome, 51% of which were conducted by Ipsos. Half (51%) were conducted via web only, followed by telephone only (36%), face-to-face (11%), and a combination of telephone and web (2%). Most polls (58%) used a 4-point likeliness scale, whereas 42% used a binary yes–no response scale. Ten (11%) lacked survey weights, and 56% were conducted during a Democratic presidential administration. On average, vaccine hesitancy polls were conducted about 14 months before the next election, with about 558 self-identified Democrats (and leaners) and about 448 Republicans (and leaners).

Meta-Analysis

Pooled estimates of polarization regarding concern about infection during COVID-19 and non–COVID-19 disease outbreaks are displayed in Figure 1. Before the pandemic, the weighted average difference between Democrats and Republicans who said they were "very concerned" that they or someone they know would be infected with a given disease was about 5.04 percentage points ($k = 38$; 95% CI = 4.15, 5.93). During the pandemic, this rose to 24.66 percentage points ($k = 52$; 95% CI = 21.39, 27.93). Tests indicate high levels of heterogeneity (non–COVID-19: $Q = 73.35$, $P < .05$, $\tau^2 = 3.00$, $I^2 = 29.3\%$; COVID-19: $Q = 242.48$, $P < .001$, $\tau^2 = 85.94$, $I^2 = 86.2\%$), which is not unusual for public opinion over time. We can reject the null hypothesis that polarization regarding concern about infection is the same for COVID-19 and non–COVID-19 outbreaks ($Q_M = 9.07$; $P < .001$).

Figure 2 displays pooled estimates of polarization regarding vaccine hesitancy, during COVID-19 and non–COVID-19 disease outbreaks. Before the pandemic, the weighted average difference between Republicans and Democrats who said they were unlikely to or would not receive a vaccine for a given disease when one became available to them was about 1.90 percentage points ($k = 26$; 95% CI = −0.16, 3.97). During the pandemic, this rose to 23.85 percentage points ($k = 63$; 95% CI = 22.10, 25.59). Tests again indicate high levels of heterogeneity (non–COVID-19: $Q = 66.32$, $P < .01$, $\tau^2 = 16.81$, $I^2 = 66.5\%$; COVID-19: $Q = 311.59$, $P < .01$, $\tau^2 = 37.37$, $I^2 = 77.5\%$). We can reject the null hypothesis that polarization regarding vaccine hesitancy is the same for COVID-19 and non–COVID-19 outbreaks ($Q_M = 23.63$; $P < .001$).

Meta-Regression

Regarding concern about infection, COVID-19 was associated with significantly higher levels of polarization (20.23; 95% CI = 12.30, 28.17; $P < .001$) in our meta-regression models (Figure 3a). Regarding vaccine hesitancy, COVID-19

TABLE 1— Characteristics of Included Polls: United States, May 2, 1954–December 31, 2023

	Concern About Infection (n = 90), No. of Studies (%) or Mean (95% CI)	Vaccine Hesitancy (n = 89), No. of Studies (%) or Mean (95% CI)
Disease		
COVID-19	38 (42)	63 (71)
Zika	8 (9)	0
Ebola	5 (6)	1 (1)
H1N1 (2009)	4 (4)	7 (8)
H5N1	5 (6)	0
SARS	11 (12)	0
West Nile	1 (1)	0
Smallpox	0	5 (6)
Anthrax	9 (10)	1 (1)
HIV/AIDS	9 (10)	2 (2)
H1N1 (1976)	0	3 (3)
H2N2	0	2 (2)
Polio	0	5 (6)
Survey organization		
Associated Press	0	1 (1)
Beacon Research/Shaw & Co. Research	0	1 (1)
CBS News	1 (1)	1 (1)
CBS News/*New York Times*	1 (1)	1 (1)
Gallup	10 (11)	11 (12)
Harris Interactive	2 (2)	1 (1)
Hart-Teeter Research Companies	0	1 (1)
International Communications Research	7 (8)	2 (2)
Ipsos	21 (23)	45 (51)
Langer Research Associates	10 (11)	6 (7)
Los Angeles Times	3 (3)	0
Marist	0	9 (10)
National Opinion Research Center at the University of Chicago	4 (4)	2 (2)
Opinion Research Corporation	2 (2)	2 (2)
Peter D. Hart Research Associates	1 (1)	0
Princeton Survey Research Associates International	11 (12)	0
Public Religion Research Institute	1 (1)	0
SSRS (formerly Social Science Research Solutions)	9 (10)	1 (1)
Stony Brook University Center for Survey Research	1 (1)	1 (1)
The Roper Organization	0	2 (2)
TNS Intersearch	5 (6)	2 (2)
Yankelovich Clancy Shulman	1 (1)	0
Question wording: impact of disease		
Being exposed to/affected by	22 (24)	...
Catching/contracting/getting	25 (28)	...
Being infected by/becoming ill/getting sick	39 (43)	...
Being a victim of	4 (4)	...

Continued

TABLE 1— Continued

	Concern About Infection (n = 90), No. of Studies (%) or Mean (95% CI)	Vaccine Hesitancy (n = 89), No. of Studies (%) or Mean (95% CI)
Survey mode		
Web only	21 (23)	45 (51)
Web and telephone	4 (4)	2 (2)
Telephone only	64 (71)	32 (36)
Face-to-face	1 (1)	10 (11)
Response choice		
Binary choice (yes/no)	. . .	37 (42)
Four-point likeliness scale (very/somewhat/not too/not at all)	. . .	52 (58)
Presence of survey weights		
With weights	90 (100)	79 (89)
Without weights	0	10 (11)
Party of the president in power		
Democrat	24 (27)	50 (56)
Republican	66 (73)	39 (44)
Proximity to next election: months until Election Day	10 (−3, 23)	14 (1, 28)
Weighted sample size		
Democrats and leaners	452 (−165, 1070)	558 (−1084, 2200)
Republicans and leaners	373 (−32, 777)	448 (−713, 1609)

Note. CI = confidence interval. Full question wording, response options, and sample size figures are provided in Appendices D and E (available as a supplement to the online version of this article at http://www.ajph.org). Percentages may not add to 100 because of rounding.

(25.89; 95% CI = 6.63, 45.16; $P < .05$), the polling firm Stony Brook University Center for Survey Research (17.03; 95% CI = 1.93, 32.12; $P < .05$), and months until Election Day (0.25; 95% CI = 0.08, 0.41; $P < .01$) were significantly associated with higher levels of polarization (Figure 3b). Meanwhile, having a Republican president (−8.03; 95% CI = −10.64, −5.43; $P < .001$) was significantly associated with lower levels of polarization (Figure 3b).

To test whether polarization underwent a discrete jump during the pandemic, we predicted levels of polarization in December 2023 under a Democratic president using prepandemic data. Results indicate that the observed level of polarization regarding concern about infection during COVID-19 was 10.5 percentage points (1.09 times) greater than what would be predicted based on historical trends (9.64; 95% prediction interval [PI] = 3.44, 15.84). For vaccine hesitancy, results indicate that the observed level of polarization during COVID-19 was 24.3 percentage points (14.91 times) greater than what would be predicted based on historical trends (1.63; 95% PI = −11.30, 14.55).

Robustness Checks

We conducted 3 checks to test whether these findings were robust to alternate specifications. First, we replaced all polls (concern: $k = 2$; vaccine: $k = 8$) with a negative difference between partisans by using the absolute value. Second, we removed all polls that occurred before and during party realignment in the United States from 1954 to 1980 ($k = 10$)—a procedure that only affected vaccine hesitancy and removed all but 1 poll that did not employ survey weights (Associated Press and Media General, April 1987). Third, we tested alternative specifications of polarization. For concern about infection, we analyzed responses from the opposite end of the response scale—those who said they were "not at all concerned" about infection. One poll from the HIV/AIDS epidemic (Rolling Stone, September 1987) was dropped for this test because the lowest response category used different wording. For vaccine intention, analyses examined enthusiasm, measuring those who said they did intend to get a vaccine. Overall, these procedures had few substantive impacts on our findings; full results are available in online Appendices I through R.

AJPH January 2026, Vol. 116, No. 1

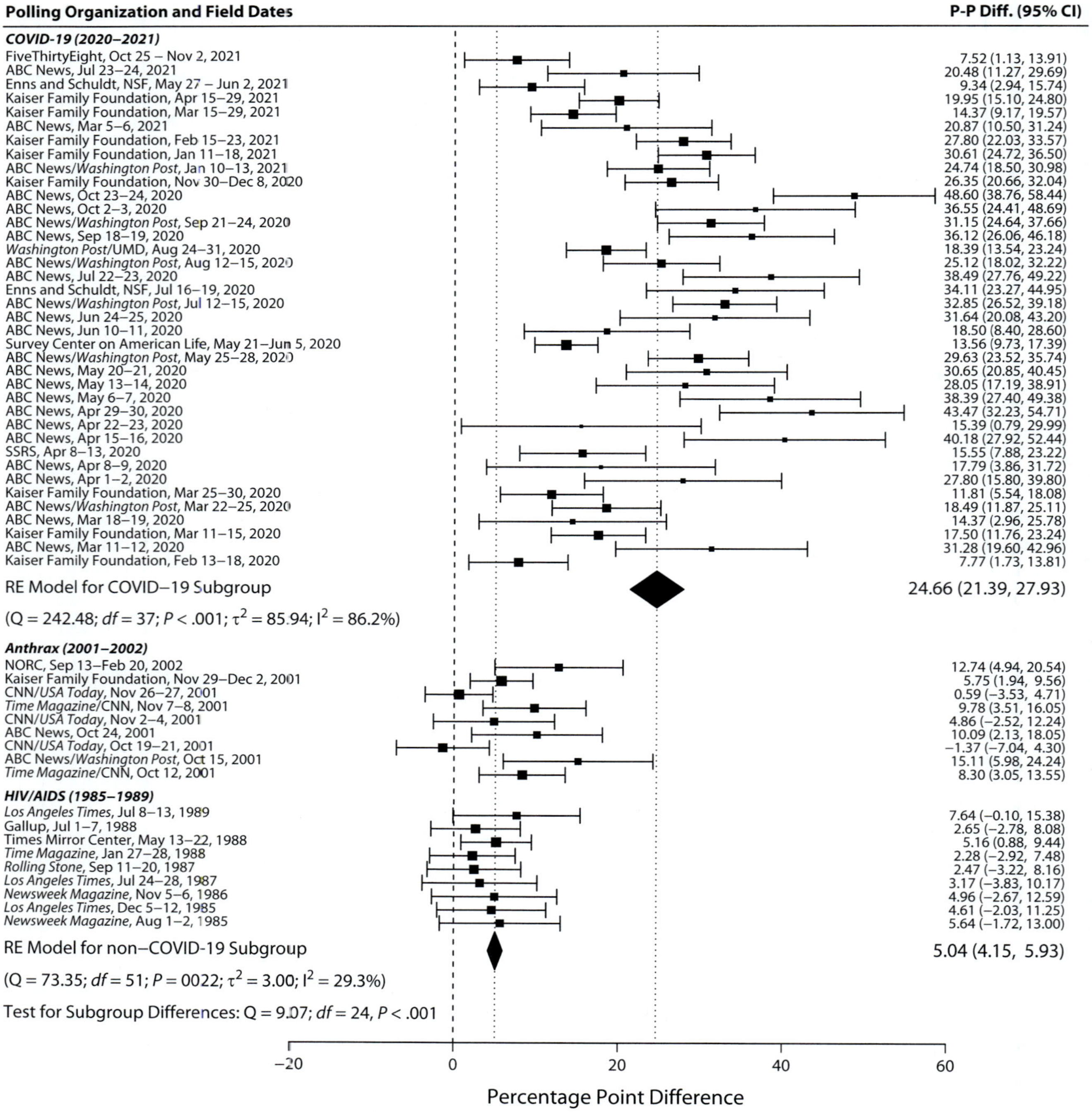

FIGURE 1— Percentage-Point Difference Between Democrats and Republicans Expressing High Concern About Infection, by Disease Subgroup: United States, August 1, 1985–December 31, 2023

Note. CI = confidence interval; NORC = National Opinion Research Center; NSF = National Science Foundation; P-P Diff = the percentage-point difference between Democrats and Republicans who said they were "very concerned" that they or someone they know would get a given disease; RE = random effects; SSRS = Social Science Research Solutions; UMD = University of Maryland. Weighted percentages reflect the use of survey weights to match known population parameters for the adult US population at the time of the survey. This figure was abbreviated for space. For the full figure, please see Appendix F (available as a supplement to the online version of this article at https://www.ajph.org).

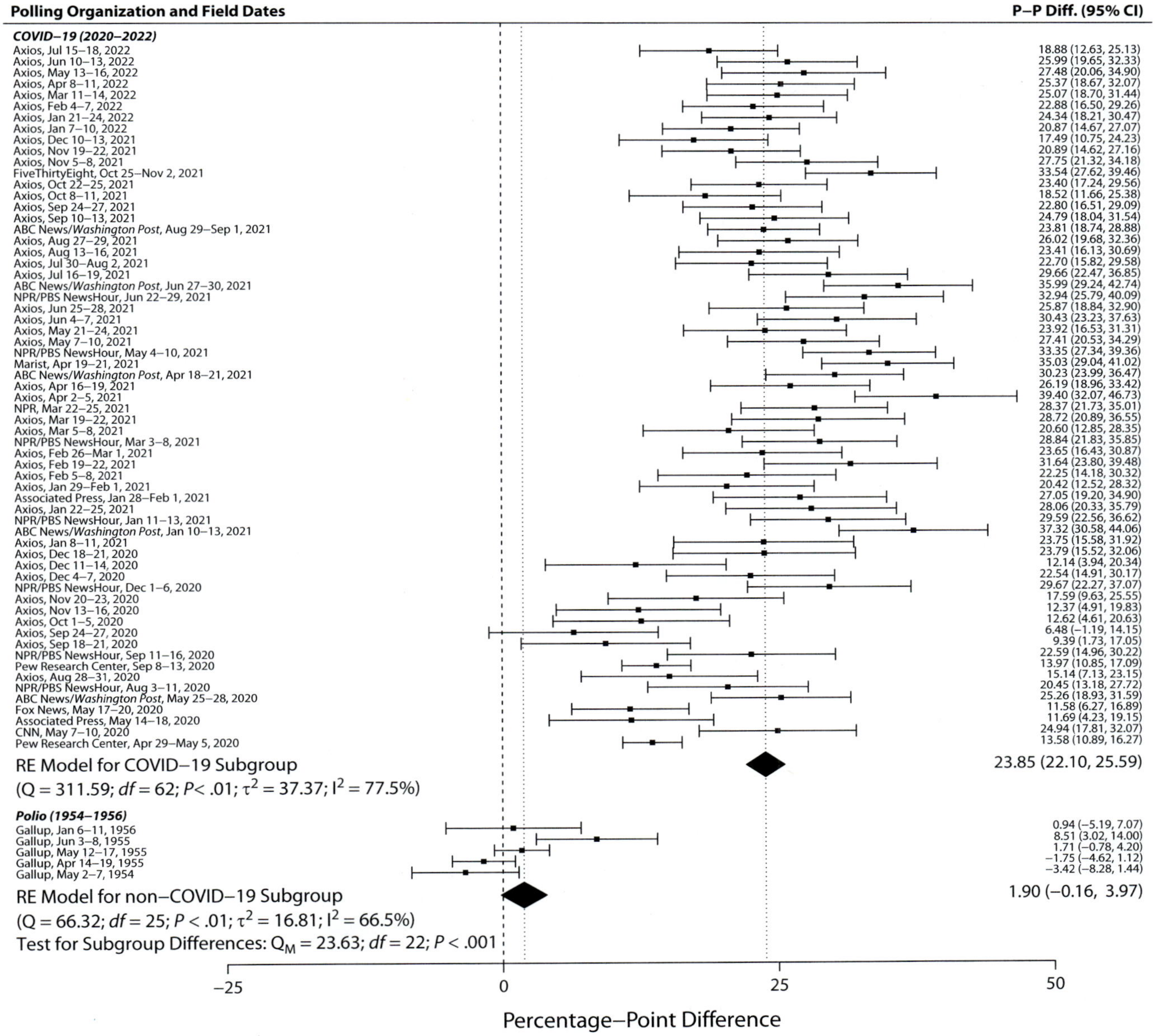

FIGURE 2— **Percentage-Point Difference Between Democrats and Republicans Expressing Vaccine Hesitancy, by Disease Subgroup: United States, May 2, 1954–December 31, 2023**

Note. CI = confidence interval; P-P Diff. = the percentage point difference between Republicans and Democrats who say they will not or are unlikely (somewhat unlikely or very unlikely) to receive a vaccine for a given disease when one becomes available to them; RE = random effects. Weighted percentages reflect the use of survey weights to match known population parameters for the adult US population at the time of the survey. Seven polls in this study conducted before 1960 did not employ survey weights; neither did 2 H1N1 polls conducted in late 1976, nor the HIV/AIDS poll conducted in April 1987. Three polls conducted between May 1, 1954 and May 31, 1955 asked about one's intention to get their child vaccinated with the polio vaccine. Full question wording and information about survey weights are available in the Appendices (available as a supplement to the online version of this article at http://www.ajph.org). This figure was abbreviated for space. For the full figure, please see Appendix G.

DISCUSSION

Our findings indicate that political polarization during COVID-19 was about 5 times greater than in any other disease outbreak for which we have public opinion data regarding concern about infection (non–COVID-19: 5.04; COVID-19: 24.66) and more than 12 times greater regarding vaccine hesitancy (non–COVID-19: 1.90; COVID-19: 23.85). Furthermore, it appears that high levels of polarization continue to linger, suggesting reversal may be difficult. Although COVID-19 was superlative in

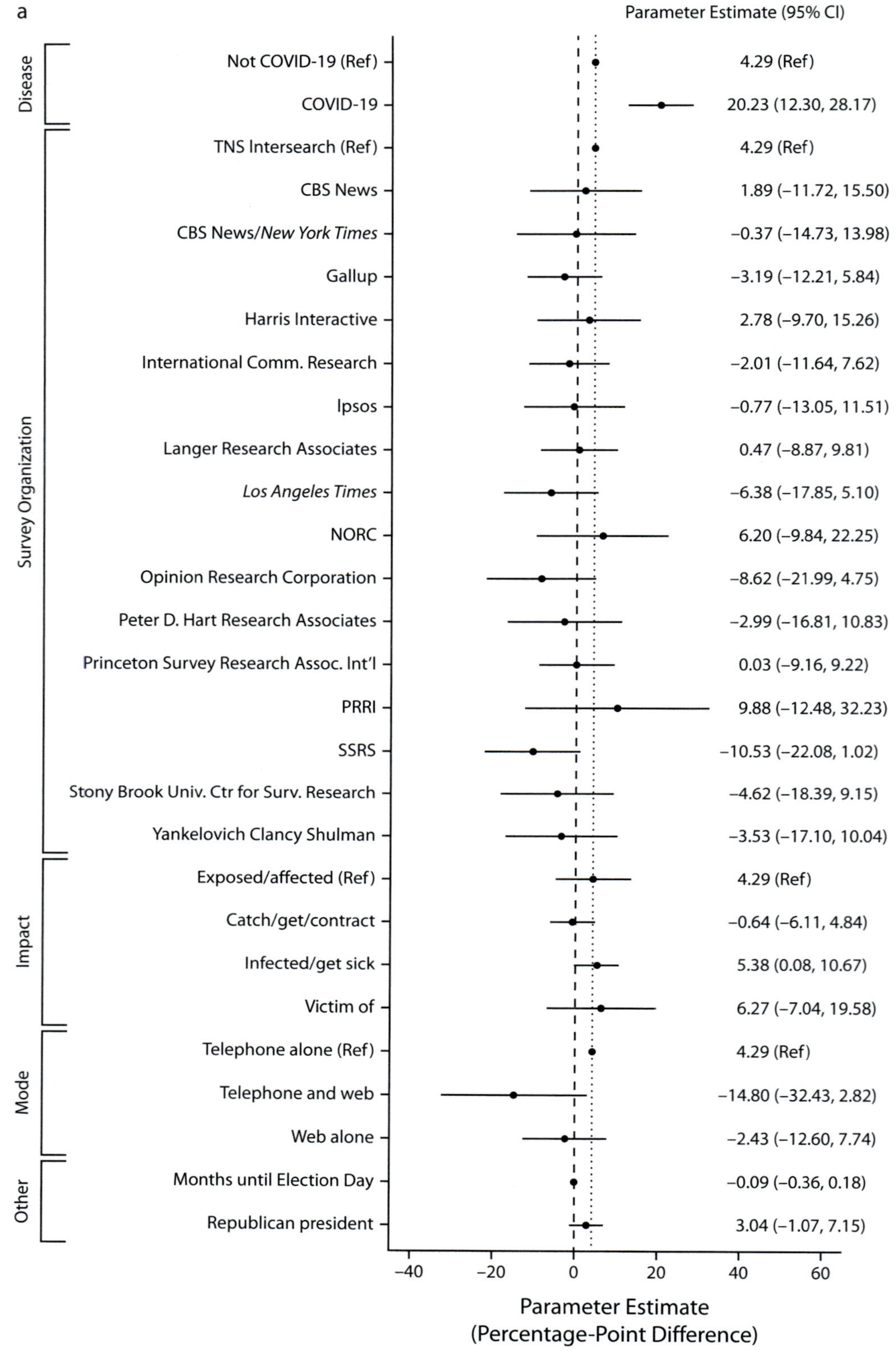

Model Summary: Q = 197.31; $P < .001$; $I^2 = 70.47\%$; $\tau^2 = 23.99$; $R^2 = 80.29\%$

FIGURE 3— Mixed-Effects Meta-Regression of the Association Between Study-Level Characteristics and Polarization for (a) Concern About Infection and (b) Vaccine Hesitancy: United States, May 2, 1954–December 31, 2023

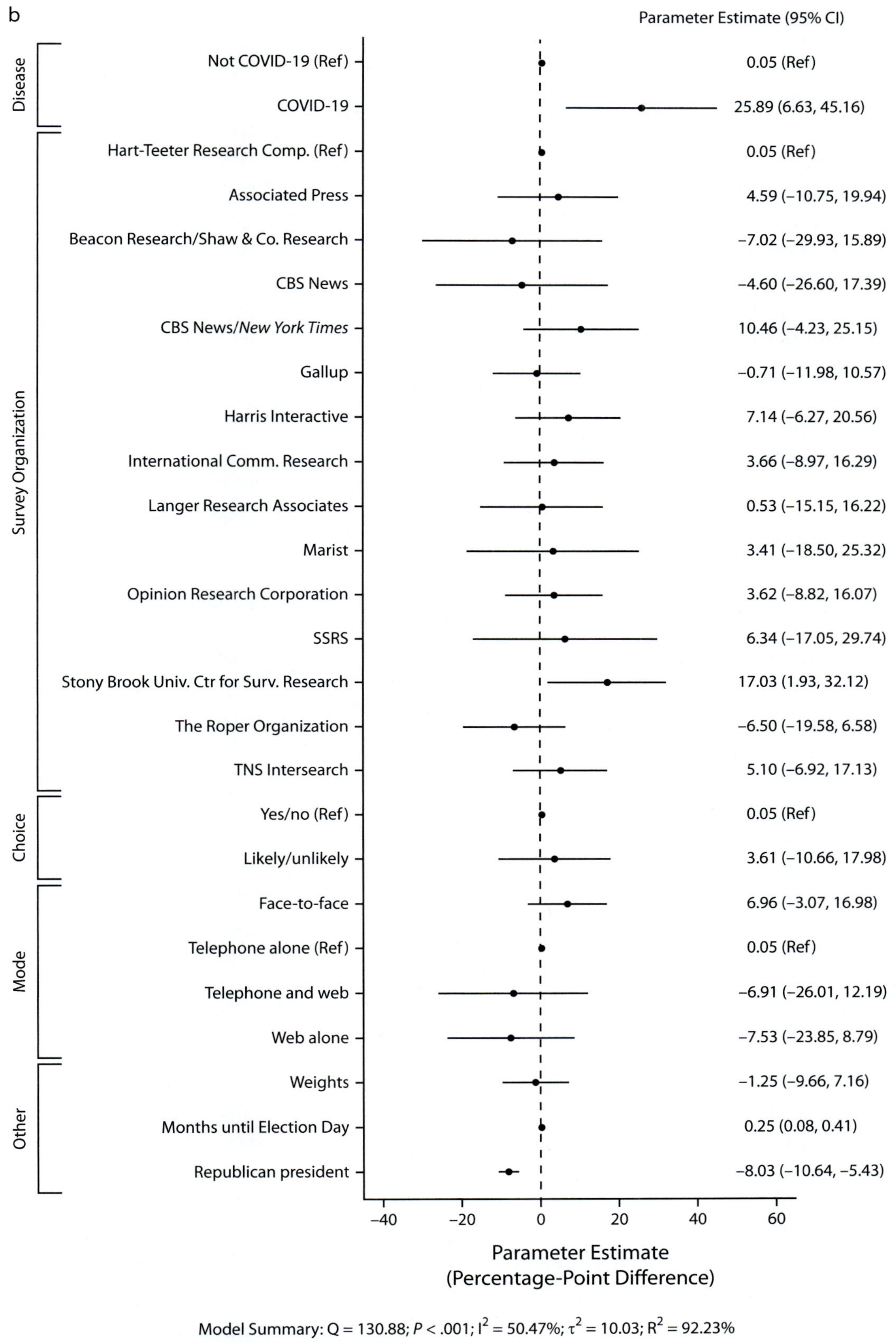

FIGURE 3— Continued

Note. CI = confidence interval; NORC = National Opinion Research Center; PRRRI = Public Religion Research Institute; SSRS = Social Science Research Solutions.

its scale and severity, these comparisons are not straw men. They include polls conducted just before midterm elections during the Ebola crisis, when President Obama's handling of the disease became a prominent campaign issue[32]; polls conducted a month after September 11, 2001, during a second round of terrorist attacks that used anthrax as a biological weapon; and during the HIV/AIDS epidemic, a disease shaped by homophobia, racism, and xenophobia. For vaccine hesitancy, the comparison also includes polls conducted a few months before the 1976 presidential election and polls before and after the release of faulty polio vaccines made at Cutter and Wyeth Laboratories, which accidentally used live virus and resulted in 204 cases of polio and 11 deaths among children.[33]

Even after adjustment for variation in question wording, response options, survey administration mode, sampling and weighting techniques, months until Election Day, and the party of the president in power, we find that COVID-19 was associated with 20 to 25 additional percentage points of polarization, compared with earlier disease outbreaks, and that this difference is statistically significant. Our results also indicate that outbreaks are not free from partisan differences regarding concern about infection. In fact, we should expect to see about 5 percentage points of separation during the average health crisis, with Democrats more concerned about infection. However, polarization during COVID-19 was considerably more extreme than in past outbreaks, representing a discrete jump in polarization that cannot be explained by gradual partisan separation over time. In fact, observed levels of polarization during COVID-19 were about 1.1 to 14.9 times higher than what prepandemic trends would predict, which indicates that past approaches to reducing societal divisions may not be effective. Additional research on strategies to reunify partisans is urgently needed.

Unprecedented levels of polarization may be influenced by the unique circumstances of the pandemic. The public's response to polarization among party elites is ordinarily limited by (1) party identification, (2) awareness of party differences on policy issues, and (3) issue salience, meaning that only those who think the issue is important pay attention.[34] However, COVID-19 was the most widespread pandemic in a century, raising the disease's salience, and it coincided with a contentious presidential election that encouraged people in the United States to understand party differences and cast their allegiance on the ballot. Together, these forces may have reduced protective factors normally present during disease outbreaks, leading to a surge in polarization.

Limitations

This study has several limitations. First, it examined 2 important prevention behaviors, for which the wording and response options in the polls remained stable over time. Other outcomes with shorter trends and less stable measures may have been less divisive during COVID-19 (e.g., contact tracing or quarantine). Second, the study only analyzed data available for download from the Roper Center. Although publication bias is not a concern, not all media outlets archive their data there, and news organizations only ask about outbreaks that capture the public's attention. Those that make national headlines may be more prone to polarization than others that do not garner polls, such as pertussis and mumps. However, this implies that our results may represent a conservative estimate of polarization between COVID-19 and non–COVID-19 disease outbreaks. Third, included polls demonstrated substantial heterogeneity. Although this can make it challenging to interpret results, it reflects the nature of public opinion during times of crisis. Lastly, it was not possible to account for variations in outbreak magnitude. This is important, given that COVID-19 was far more widespread in the United States than any other included outbreak. However, it was not possible to control for case counts leading up to each poll because of regional tracking of influenza.

Public Health Implications

From legislative gridlock and lagging risk protection to declining trust in government that can hamper public health efforts, political polarization can inhibit effective responses to outbreaks.[3,4,7] Fortunately, high levels of polarization, although they continue to linger, do not appear endemic to disease outbreaks and may be preventable. This indicates that research on new approaches to reducing societal divisions are urgently needed. However, progress on reducing polarization as it pertains to disease outbreaks may be jeopardized by funding freezes for health research and the revocation of grants to study vaccine hesitancy. More broadly, the effectiveness of public health efforts to prevent or mitigate future disease outbreaks may be diminished if they are perceived to be connected to politics or motivated by political gain.[35] AJPH

ABOUT THE AUTHORS

At the time of the study, Caitlin L. McMurtry and Rachana Cheu were with the Brown School, Washington University, St. Louis, MO.

CORRESPONDENCE

Correspondence should be sent to Caitlin McMurtry, Brown School, Washington University, MSC 1196-251-46, One Brookings Drive, St. Louis, MO, 63130 (e-mail: mcmurtry@wustl.edu). Reprints can be ordered at https://www.ajph.org by clicking the "Reprints" link.

PUBLICATION INFORMATION

Full Citation: McMurtry CL, Cheu R. Political polarization during disease outbreaks: a meta-analysis of archival survey data from polio to COVID-19. *Am J Public Health*. 2026;116(1):124–136.

Acceptance Date: June 18, 2025.

DOI: https://doi.org/10.2105/AJPH.2025.308226

ORCID iD:

Caitlin L. McMurtry https://orcid.org/0000-0003-2617-7085

CONTRIBUTORS

Both authors made substantial contributions to this article. C. L. McMurtry led the conceptualization, development, and drafting of this article. R. Cheu was instrumental in revising it and providing analytic, writing, and data acquisition assistance.

ACKNOWLEDGMENTS

C. L. McMurtry's work on this article was supported by the Dissertation Completion Fellowship at Harvard University.

We thank the staff—past and present—of the Roper Center for Public Opinion Research at Cornell University for the hard work they continue to invest in cataloguing, cleaning, and archiving public opinion data. Thanks also to the news and polling organizations that collect these data and share them with the Roper Center and with us, including, Mollyann Brodie and Ashley Kirzinger at KFF. Additionally, we thank Steven Worthington of the Institute for Quantitative Social Sciences (IQSS) at Harvard University, Rui Duan of Harvard T. H. Chan School of Public Health, and Laura Hatfield of the National Opinion Research Center (NORC) at the University of Chicago for their methodological mentorship. We are grateful for comments and feedback from seminar participants at Harvard University as well as conference participants at the National Research Service Award (NRSA) Trainees Research Conference, the American Public Health Association, and the American Political Science Association. Finally, we thank Robert Blendon, Jessica Cohen, and David Cutler for their help in developing and refining this dissertation paper. This study would not have been possible without their encouragement and support.

CONFLICTS OF INTEREST

The authors have no conflicts of interest to disclose.

HUMAN PARTICIPANT PROTECTION

Because this project analyzed existing anonymous data sets available through the Roper Center, the institutional review board at Washington University in St. Louis determined this study was not human subjects research (IRB ID #202506183).

REFERENCES

1. Barber M, McCarty NM. Causes and consequences of polarization. In: Mansbridge J, Martin CJ, eds. *Political Negotiation: A Handbook*. Washington, DC: Brookings Institution Press; 2016:37–90.
2. McCarty NM. The policy effects of political polarization. In: Pierson P, Skocpol T, eds. *The Transformation of American Politics: Activist Government and the Rise of Conservatism*. Princeton, NJ: Princeton University Press; 2007:223–255.
3. McCarty NM, Poole KT, Rosenthal H. *Polarization and Public Policy*. Cambridge, MA: MIT Press; 2006.
4. Rigby E, Wright GC. *The Policy Consequences of Party Polarization: Evidence From American States*. In: Thurber JA, Yoshinaka A, eds. *American Gridlock*. New York, NY: Cambridge University Press; 2015:236–255.
5. Iyengar S, Lelkes Y, Levendusky M, Malhotra N, Westwood SJ. The origins and consequences of affective polarization in the United States. *Annu Rev Polit Sci*. 2019;22(1):129–146. https://doi.org/10.1146/annurev-polisci-051117-073034
6. Hetherington MJ, Rudolph TJ. *Why Washington Won't Work*. Chicago, IL: University of Chicago Press; 2015.
7. Gadarian SK, Goodman SW, Pepinsky TB. Partisanship, health behavior, and policy attitudes in the early stages of the COVID-19 pandemic. *PLoS One*. 2021;16(4):e0249596. https://doi.org/10.1371/journal.pone.0249596
8. Allcott H, Boxell L, Conway J, Gentzkow M, Thaler M, Yang D. Polarization and public health: partisan differences in social distancing during the coronavirus pandemic. *J Public Econ*. 2020;191:104254. https://doi.org/10.1016/j.jpubeco.2020.104254
9. Bruine de Bruin W, Saw HW, Goldman DP. Political polarization in US residents' COVID-19 risk perceptions, policy preferences, and protective behaviors. *J Risk Uncertain*. 2020;61(2):177–194. https://doi.org/10.1007/s11166-020-09336-3
10. Fridman A, Gershon R, Gneezy A. COVID-19 and vaccine hesitancy: a longitudinal study. *PLoS One*. 2021;16(4):e0250123. https://doi.org/10.1371/journal.pone.0250123
11. Painter M, Qiu T. Political beliefs affect compliance with government mandates. *J Econ Behav Organ*. 2021;185:688–701. https://doi.org/10.1016/j.jebo.2021.03.019
12. Suhay E, Soni A, Persico C, Marcotte DE. Americans' trust in government and health behaviors during the COVID-19 pandemic. *RSF*. 2022;8(8):221–244. https://doi.org/10.7758/RSF.2022.8.8.10
13. Pagliaro S, Sacchi S, Pacilli MG, et al. Trust predicts COVID-19 prescribed and discretionary behavioral intentions in 23 countries. *PLoS One*. 2021;16(3):e0248334. https://doi.org/10.1371/journal.pone.0248334
14. COVID-19 National Preparedness Collaborators. Pandemic preparedness and COVID-19: an exploratory analysis of infection and fatality rates, and contextual factors associated with preparedness in 177 countries, from Jan 1, 2020, to Sept 30, 2021. *Lancet*. 2022;399(10334):1489–1512. https://doi.org/10.1016/S0140-6736(22)00172-6
15. Monfared IG. The connection between COVID-19 vaccine abundance, vaccination coverage, and public trust in government across the globe. *Vaccine*. 2022;40(43):6211–6217. https://doi.org/10.1016/j.vaccine.2022.09.011
16. Quinn SC, Parmer J, Freimuth VS, Hilyard KM, Musa D, Kim KH. Exploring communication, trust in government, and vaccination intention later in the 2009 H1N1 pandemic: results of a national survey. *Biosecur Bioterror*. 2013;11(2):96–106. https://doi.org/10.1089/bsp.2012.0048
17. Jamison AM, Quinn SC, Freimuth VS. "You don't trust a government vaccine": narratives of institutional trust and influenza vaccination among African American and white adults. *Soc Sci Med*. 2019;221:87–94. https://doi.org/10.1016/j.socscimed.2018.12.020
18. Tenforde MW, Self WH, Adams K, et al. Association between mRNA vaccination and COVID-19 hospitalization and disease severity. *JAMA*. 2021;326(20):2043–2054. https://doi.org/10.1001/jama.2021.19499
19. Janke AT, Mei H, Rothenberg C, Becher RD, Lin Z, Venkatesh AK. Analysis of hospital resource availability and COVID-19 mortality across the United States. *J Hosp Med*. 2021;16(4):211–214. https://doi.org/10.12788/jhm.3539
20. Poole KT, Rosenthal H. *Congress: A Political-Economic History of Roll Call Voting*. New York, NY: Oxford University Press; 1997.
21. Abramowitz A. *The Disappearing Center: Engaged Citizens, Polarization, and American Democracy*. New Haven, CT: Yale University Press; 2010.
22. Levendusky M. *The Partisan Sort: How Liberals Became Democrats and Conservatives Became Republicans*. Chicago, IL: University of Chicago Press; 2009.
23. Fiorina MP. *Unstable Majorities: Polarization, Party Sorting and Political Stalemate*. Stanford, CA: Hoover Institution Press; 2017.
24. Fiorina MP, Abrams SJ. Political polarization in the American public. *Annu Rev Polit Sci*. 2008;11(1):563–588. https://doi.org/10.1146/annurev.polisci.11.053106.153836
25. Jacobson GC. The electoral origins of polarized politics: evidence from the 2010 Cooperative Congressional Election Study. *Am Behav Sci*. 2012;56(12):1612–1630. https://doi.org/10.1177/0002764212463352
26. Ansolabehere S, Rodden J, Snyder Jr JM. Purple America. *J Econ Perspect*. 2006;20(2):97–118. https://doi.org/10.1257/jep.20.2.97
27. Baldassarri D, Gelman A. Partisans without constraint: political polarization and trends in American public opinion. *Am J Sociol*. 2008;114(2):408–446. https://doi.org/10.1086/590649
28. Levendusky MS, Malhotra N. (Mis)perceptions of partisan polarization in the American public. *Public Opin Q*. 2016;80(S1):378–391. https://doi.org/10.1093/poq/nfv045
29. Borenstein M, Hedges LV, Higgins JPT, Rothstein HR. *Introduction to Meta-Analysis*. 2nd ed. Hoboken, NJ: John Wiley & Sons; 2011.
30. Viechtbauer W. Conducting meta-analyses in R with the metafor package. *J Stat Soft*. 2010;36(3):1–48. https://doi.org/10.18637/jss.v036.i03
31. Flores AR. Examining variation in surveying attitudes on same-sex marriage: a meta-analysis. *Public Opin Q*. 2015;79(2):580–593. https://doi.org/10.1093/poq/nfv017

32. Campante FR, Depetris-Chauvin E, Durante R. The virus of fear: the political impact of Ebola in the US. *Am Econ J Appl Econ.* 2024;16(1):480–509.

33. Langmuir AD, Nathanson N, Hall WJ. The surveillance of poliomyelitis in the United States in 1955. CDC Report. November 9, 1955. Available at: https://stacks.cdc.gov/view/cdc/48111. Accessed August 1, 2025.

34. Layman GC, Carsey TM, Horowitz JM. Party polarization in American politics: characteristics, causes, and consequences. *Annu Rev Polit Sci.* 2006;9(1):83–110. https://doi.org/10.1146/annurev.polisci.9.070204.105138

35. SteelFisher GK, Findling MG, Caporello HL, et al. Trust in US federal, state, and local public health agencies during COVID-19: responses and policy implications. *Health Aff (Millwood).* 2023;42(3):328–337. https://doi.org/10.1377/hlthaff.2022.01204

Housing Status and Health in the United States: A National Study of Homeownership, Health Outcomes, and Access to Care

Shams Rahman, MD, PhD

See also Padgett, p. 29.

Objectives. To examine the impact of homeownership across multiple health and behavioral domains in the United States.

Methods. Using 2023 Behavioral Risk Factor Surveillance System data, I examined associations between homeownership and health across 5 domains, applying weighted logistic regression with sequential sociodemographic adjustments.

Results. Among 407 916 adults representing 235 million US residents, 72.3% reported living in owner-occupied housing. Renters were significantly younger, racially diverse, and twice as likely to report low income. Compared with homeowners, renters exhibited higher health risks, reduced health care access, and lower engagement in preventive services. Renters had higher odds of current smoking (adjusted odds ratio [AOR] = 1.17; 95% confidence interval [CI] = 1.13, 1.21), binge drinking (AOR = 1.08; 95% CI = 1.04, 1.13), poor or fair health (AOR = 1.21; 95% CI = 1.17, 1.26), and depression (AOR = 1.17; 95% CI = 1.13, 1.22) and lower odds of physical activity (AOR = 0.86; 95% CI = 0.84, 0.89). Health care access was more limited among renters, with lower odds of having health insurance (AOR = 0.75; 95% CI = 0.72, 0.78) or a personal doctor (AOR = 0.65; 95% CI = 0.63, 0.68). Preventive care gaps were pronounced between the 2 groups: renters had lower odds of receiving colonoscopy and sigmoidoscopy (AOR = 0.74; 95% CI = 0.71, 0.77) and routine checkups (AOR = 0.76; 95% CI = 0.74, 0.79).

Conclusions. Housing tenure stratifies health. Addressing housing in prevention frameworks is essential to improving US public health. (*Am J Public Health*. 2026;116(1):137–147. https://doi.org/10.2105/AJPH.2025.308278)

Stable housing and homeownership offer benefits, including financial stability, equity accumulation, and long-term well-being.[1] Despite past policy missteps, homeownership remains a pathway to health and economic security when supported by inclusive, sustainable policies.[1,2] Compared with renting one's home, owning one's home is linked to better overall health and lower prevalence of chronic conditions such as cardiovascular disease, diabetes, and stroke.[3,4] Homeownership also correlates with improved mental health, including reduced odds of depression, anxiety, cognitive decline, and functional limitations.[3] Homeownership may confer economic, psychological, and environmental advantages (e.g., residential stability and control) that support well-being.[3] It also buffers against rent increases or eviction, potentially reducing chronic stress.[5] These effects suggest that housing tenure (i.e., residential status defined as homeownership vs rental) can shape health behaviors and outcomes.[3,6]

Despite its potential health significance, homeownership is not equally attainable across society. Approximately two thirds of US households are owner occupied, but this figure masks large disparities by age, race/ethnicity, and socioeconomic status.[7] Homeownership climbs from about 39% among adults aged 35 years and younger to

AJPH January 2026, Vol. 116, No. 1

nearly 79% among those aged 65 years and older.[8] Racial and ethnic gaps are also stark: an estimated 74% of non-Hispanic White households own their homes, compared with 46% of Black and 50% of Hispanic households.[8] Socioeconomic factors are strongly linked to ownership too: households earning more than $130 000 per year have homeownership rates approaching 84%, nearly double the rate for those earning less than $25 000 per year (~46%).[9] Likewise, homeownership is more common among college graduates than less educated adults.[9]

These patterns reflect broader social and economic inequalities, underlining the importance of understanding how homeownership status might translate into differences in health-related factors. Given these disparities, homeownership functions not merely as an outcome of socioeconomic advantage but also as a structural determinant of health.[10] It reflects exposure to stability, neighborhood quality, and access to health-promoting resources, while potentially influencing psychosocial stress and health care access.[1]

The specific role of homeownership as an independent predictor of population health remains understudied. Previously, I showed that homeownership predicts better health, with lower rates of chronic conditions, even after adjusting for sociodemographic factors.[3] I also found that renters experienced disproportionately worse mental health outcomes, further underscoring the psychosocial benefits of stable housing.[6]

Building on my previous research, I broaden the scope to include preventive behaviors, functional limitations, and health care access. Using 2023 Behavioral Risk Factor Surveillance System (BRFSS) data, my objective was to examine whether owning a home, compared with renting, independently predicts health outcomes across multiple domains in a nationally representative sample of US adults.

METHODS

The 2023 BRFSS is a nationwide, state-based, cross-sectional telephone survey of noninstitutionalized US adults aged 18 years or older. It collects self-reported data on health behaviors, chronic conditions, health care access, and preventive service utilization. The BRFSS uses a dual-frame random-digit–dialing design with landline and cell phone samples. Most states apply disproportionate stratified sampling for landlines and simple random sampling for cell phones. Responses are weighted using iterative proportional fitting (raking) to reflect state-specific demographics, including age, sex, race/ethnicity, education, marital status, and homeownership. In 2023, the BRFSS surveyed more than 420 000 adults across all 50 states, the District of Columbia, and 3 US territories. Informed consent was obtained during interviews. Full methodology is detailed in the BRFSS technical reports (https://bit.ly/4ntGAC1). I included adults aged 18 years or older who completed the survey and had nonmissing data on housing status and relevant outcome variables in my analysis.

Study Measures

The primary exposure was homeownership, measured using the BRFSS variable RENTHOM1, which is based on whether the respondent's home was owned, rented, or occupied under another arrangement. I excluded participants reporting "other arrangement" (6.26%), "don't know" (0.48%), or "refused" (0.78%), totaling approximately 7.5% of the weighted sample. I also excluded 8 additional records (< 0.01%) with missing data.

To examine health-related effects of homeownership, I organized BRFSS variables into 5 theory-driven domains aligned with the social determinants of health framework:

1. Health care access and utilization and structural barriers,
2. Health risk and protective behaviors,
3. Prevalence of chronic health conditions,
4. Preventive health behaviors, and
5. Functional, physical, and mental health limitations.

These domains were conceptually informed by public health literature[11] and reflect pathways linking residential stability to health. I did not derive them from a single source but shaped them by theoretical relevance and the availability of variables in the data set. I grouped variables by construct (e.g., insurance, risk behaviors, disease burden), supporting both descriptive and adjusted analyses of housing-related health disparities.

Domain 1 captures structural vulnerabilities and access barriers affecting health care engagement. Domain 2 addresses modifiable risk and protective behaviors (e.g., tobacco use, alcohol use, activity, safety). Domain 3 focuses on chronic disease burden shaped by biological and social exposures. Domain 4 highlights preventive behaviors (e.g., immunizations, screenings) as markers of early detection. Domain 5 examines functional and mental health limitations reflecting lived health challenges. Together, these domains offer a policy-relevant framework linking housing tenure and social conditions to health.

Throughout this study, I used the term "health outcomes" to include both direct clinical conditions (e.g., diabetes) and health-related enabling indicators (e.g., insurance coverage and food stamp receipt) that reflect structural pathways linking housing to health.

Statistical Analysis

I conducted domain-based descriptive and regression-adjusted analyses to examine associations between homeownership status and multiple health outcomes using 2023 BRFSS data. All analyses accounted for the complex sampling design, applying weights, stratification, and primary sampling units to yield nationally representative estimates and variance estimation. I recoded selected BRFSS variables into binary outcomes to satisfy the requirements of the SAS software's statistical procedure PROC SURVEYLOGISTIC, which models binary dependent variables while accounting for complex survey design. I dichotomized "time since last routine checkup" (measured on a 1–4 scale) to distinguish recent from delayed or no checkups. I dichotomized "joint pain severity" (0–10 scale) at the sample median: less than 5 is low (2); 5 or more is high (1); I excluded invalid and missing values. I based recoding on conceptual relevance, distribution, and analytic simplicity. I modeled binary outcomes against homeownership status, adjusting for covariates.

I conducted weighted descriptive analyses to compare homeownership across demographic groups, including age, sex, race/ethnicity, education, income, employment, marital status, and urban versus rural residence. I calculated weighted prevalence estimates for each subgroup, stratified by homeownership. I tested group differences using the Satterthwaite-adjusted Rao–Scott χ^2 test, which adjusts for the BRFSS's complex sampling design and yields P values under multistage stratified sampling. I evaluated bivariate associations between homeownership and each binary health outcome using the Rao–Scott χ^2 test. I defined statistical significance as $P < .05$.

To account for confounding by age—which is strongly linked to both housing and health—I estimated age-adjusted prevalence using logistic regression with predictive margins. For each health outcome, I modeled homeownership as the exposure and age as a continuous covariate using SAS's PROC SURVEYLOGISTIC. I obtained adjusted prevalence estimates and 95% confidence intervals (CIs) via the LSMEANS statement with the ILINK option, which computes age-standardized predicted probabilities. For example, arthritis prevalence was modeled as a function of homeownership and age, with design-adjusted SEs.

I estimated adjusted odds ratios (AORs) and 95% CIs for associations between homeownership and each dichotomized health outcome using survey-weighted logistic regression. Two models were specified per health outcome: a partially adjusted model (age, sex, income) and a fully adjusted model (age, sex, income plus education, race/ethnicity, marital status, employment). I selected covariates a priori based on theoretical relevance and to reduce confounding by socioeconomic position. All analyses incorporated Centers for Disease Control and Prevention–recommended BRFSS methods, including raked weights, domain analysis, and design-consistent variance estimation.

Results were stratified by homeownership and organized by the 5 analytic domains. AORs and 95% CIs quantified the independent association between homeownership and health outcomes, adjusting for demographic and socioeconomic differences. As an additional step, I conducted sensitivity analyses treating having health insurance and receiving food stamps as covariates in the partial and full models. The results remained consistent, supporting my decision to treat them as outcomes reflecting structural pathways from housing to health. I performed analyses in SAS version 9.4 (SAS Institute, Cary, NC).

RESULTS

After exclusions, the final analytical sample comprised 407 916 adults, representing a weighted population of 235 008 118 persons. Weighted estimates showed that 72.3% lived in owner-occupied and 27.7% in rental housing, corresponding to approximately 235 million US adults (±0.14% SE). Table 1 presents weighted demographic and health characteristics by homeownership. Most differences were significant ($P \le .001$ unless noted). Renters skewed younger (51% aged 18–34 years vs 30.6% of homeowners aged ≥65 years), with no sex difference ($P = .81$). Homeowners were predominantly non-Hispanic White (65.8%), whereas renters had higher proportions of non-Hispanic Black (16.4%), Hispanic (6.7%), and non-Hispanic multiracial (33.4%) individuals. Education and income patterns diverged: 37.1% of homeowners were college graduates versus 19.9% of renters; 50.3% of renters earned less than $35 000 per year versus 20.5% of homeowners. Renters reported poorer general health, with more fair (18.7%) or poor (5.6%) health compared with homeowners (13.3% and 3.9%, respectively). Homeowners more often reported very good health (33.7%). Employment and retirement differed: 51.5% of renters were employed versus 46.5% of homeowners; 27.8% of homeowners were retired versus 7.0% of

TABLE 1— Demographic and Health Characteristics of Study Participants by Homeownership Status: Behavioral Risk Factor Surveillance System, United States, 2023

Characteristic	Homeowners, No.[a] (%)[b]	Renters, No.[a] (%)[b]	P[c]
Age, y			≤.001
18–24	8 139 106 (4.8)	13 886 718 (21.4)	
25–34	19 489 579 (11.5)	19 259 523 (29.6)	
35–44	27 766 141 (16.3)	12 384 151 (19.0)	
45–54	29 586 013 (17.4)	7 486 436 (11.5)	
55–64	33 037 684 (19.4)	6 048 730 (9.3)	
≥65	51 962 016 (30.6)	5 962 520 (9.2)	
Sex			
Male	82 316 471 (48.4)	31 431 727 (48.3)	.81
Female	87 664 069 (51.6)	33 596 531 (51.7)	
Race/ethnicity			≤.001
Non-Hispanic White	111 835 846 (65.8)	24 492 101 (37.7)	
Non-Hispanic Black	16 699 610 (9.8)	10 670 195 (16.4)	
Hispanic	9 442 974 (5.6)	4 360 261 (6.7)	
Non-Hispanic Asian	1 618 190 (1.0)	707 263 (1.1)	
Non-Hispanic other/multiracial	23 901 606 (14.1)	21 732 517 (33.4)	
Unknown	6 482 314 (3.8)	3 065 742 (4.7)	
Education			≤.001
< high school	12 869 886 (7.6)	13 761 093 (21.3)	
High school graduate	41 027 286 (24.2)	20 901 492 (31.2)	
Some college	52 720 861 (31.2)	17 843 509 (27.6)	
College graduate	62 818 611 (37.1)	12 857 949 (19.9)	
General health self-reported			≤.001
Excellent	27 557 826 (16.3)	9 632 156 (14.9)	
Very good	57 196 089 (33.7)	16 236 569 (25.1)	
Good	55 662 290 (32.8)	23 126 404 (35.7)	
Fair	22 508 388 (13.3)	12 128 480 (18.7)	
Poor	6 625 240 (3.9)	3 654 486 (5.6)	
Income, $			≤.001
≤15 000	4 100 605 (3.4)	6 902 766 (13.8)	
15 001–25 000	8 703 253 (7.1)	9 148 824 (18.3)	
25 001–35 000	12 149 812 (10.0)	9 109 588 (18.2)	
35 001–50 000	16 821 750 (13.8)	8 201 598 (16.4)	
50 001–75 000	42 315 805 (34.7)	11 669 666 (23.4)	
> 75 000	37 860 796 (31.0)	4 930 632 (9.9)	
Employment status			≤.001
Employed for wages	77 736 505 (46.5)	32 617 790 (51.5)	
Self-employed	17 266 700 (10.3)	5 753 650 (9.1)	
Out of work ≥1 y	2 613 456 (1.6)	2 475 924 (3.9)	
Out of work < 1 y	2 992 566 (1.8)	3 459 099 (5.5)	
Homemaker	8 668 145 (5.2)	3 895 897 (6.2)	
Student	3 394 243 (2.0)	4 561 705 (7.2)	
Retired	46 502 416 (27.8)	4 450 256 (7.0)	
Unable to work	7 923 744 (4.7)	6 095 688 (9.3)	

Continued

TABLE 1— Continued

Characteristic	Homeowners, No.[a] (%)[b]	Renters, No.[a] (%)[b]	P^c
Marital status			≤.001
Married	106 568 894 (63.2)	16 206 590 (25.2)	
Divorced	16 541 268 (9.8)	7 390 308 (11.5)	
Widowed	14 278 531 (8.5)	2 597 793 (4.0)	
Separated	2 509 067 (1.5)	3 230 516 (5.0)	
Never married	23 000 825 (13.6)	27 690 061 (43.0)	
Unmarried couple	5 845 322 (3.5)	7 245 062 (11.3)	
Urban/rural status			≤.001
Urban	155 797 539 (92.7)	62 040 672 (96.4)	
Rural	12 248 839 (7.3)	23 428 747 (3.6)	

[a]Weighted number of participants.
[b]Percentages are weighted and represent the distribution in each homeownership group. Percentages may not sum to 100% because of rounding.
[c]*P* values are from the Rao-Scott χ^2 test.

renters. Marital status also varied (63.2% of homeowners vs 25.3% of renters were married), as did urban residence (96.4% renters vs 92.7% homeowners).

Table 2 presents the unadjusted and age-adjusted prevalence of health outcomes and behaviors by homeownership status. Table 3 displays the corresponding AORs, derived from partially adjusted models (adjusting for age, sex, and income) and fully adjusted models (additionally adjusting for race/ethnicity, education, marital status, and employment). Results are organized by domain, revealing persistent differences between homeowners and renters across a broad range of health outcomes and behaviors.

Domain 1

Homeowners consistently showed more favorable health care access than renters (Table 2). Age-adjusted prevalence was higher among homeowners for having health insurance (95.9% vs 89.5%), having a personal doctor (91.6% vs 83.1%), and having had a routine checkup in the past year (85.0% vs 82.2%; all $P \leq .001$). Renters reported more care barriers, including cost-related avoidance (15.1% vs 6.9%) and lack of reliable transportation (14.0% vs 4.3%), as well as receipt of food stamps (25.2% vs 6.9%; all $P \leq .001$).

In adjusted analyses (Table 3), renters had significantly lower odds of health care access and higher odds of structural barriers. Compared with homeowners, renters had 25% lower odds of having health insurance (AOR = 0.75; 95% CI = 0.68, 0.83), 35% lower odds of having a personal doctor (AOR = 0.65; 95% CI = 0.61, 0.69), and 18% lower odds of having had a recent checkup (AOR = 0.82; 95% CI = 0.78, 0.87). They had higher odds of cost-related care delays (AOR = 1.39; 95% CI = 1.29, 1.49), lacking transportation (AOR = 1.51; 95% CI = 1.36, 1.68), and receiving food stamps (AOR = 1.55; 95% CI = 1.41, 1.71).

Domain 2

After age adjustment, renters had a higher prevalence of multiple health risk behaviors than homeowners (Table 2). Poor or fair self-rated health was nearly twice as common among renters (33.0% vs 17.2%; $P \leq .001$). Smoking rates were higher for renters than owners, both for current smoking (16.1% vs 10.0%) and having ever smoked (42.3% vs 37.3%; both $P \leq .001$). Alcohol use showed mixed patterns: overall use was lower among renters (41.6% vs 53.1%), but binge (10.5% vs 11.5%) and heavy (4.6% vs 5.5%) drinking were only slightly less common, although all differences were significant. Renters were less likely to report physical activity (62.0% vs 76.9%) and always wearing a seatbelt (93.7% vs 95.3%; both $P \leq .001$). In adjusted models (Table 3), renters had higher odds of poor or fair health (AOR = 1.21; 95% CI = 1.14, 1.28), current smoking (AOR = 1.17; 95% CI = 1.09, 1.24), ever smoking (AOR = 1.15; 95% CI = 1.10, 1.21), and binge drinking (AOR = 1.08; 95% CI = 1.02, 1.15). I observed no significant differences for alcohol use or heavy drinking. Renters had lower odds of physical activity (AOR = 0.86; 95% CI = 0.82, 0.91) and slightly higher odds of always wearing a seatbelt (AOR = 1.10; 95% CI = 1.00, 1.21).

Domain 3

Renters had higher age-adjusted prevalence of several chronic conditions than

TABLE 2— Unadjusted and Age-Adjusted Prevalence of Health Outcomes and Behaviors by Homeownership Status: BRFSS, United States, 2023

	Unadjusted Estimates			Age-Adjusted Estimates		
Outcome	**Homeowner, %**	**Renter, %**	**P[a]**	**Homeowner, %**	**Renter, %**	**P[a]**
Domain 1: health care access and utilization and structural barriers						
Had health insurance	95.1	82.1	≤ .001	95.9	89.5	≤ .001
Has personal doctor	89.1	68.7	≤ .001	91.6	83.1	≤ .001
Had routine checkup in past year	82.3	69.9	≤ .001	85.0	82.2	≤ .001
Could not see doctor because of cost	7.6	20.9	≤ .001	6.9	15.1	≤ .001
Lacked reliable transportation in past 12 mo	4.4	16.0	≤ .001	4.3	14.0	≤ .001
Received food stamps in past 12 mo	6.9	24.8	≤ .001	6.9	25.2	≤ .001
Domain 2: health risk and protective behaviors						
Has poor or fair health	17.2	24.4	≤ .001	17.2	33.0	< .001
Current smoker	9.9	15.3	≤ .001	10.0	16.1	≤ .001
Ever smoked	36.9	33.6	≤ .001	37.3	42.3	≤ .001
Alcohol use	54.0	48.7	≤ .001	53.1	41.6	≤ .001
Binge drinker	13.8	18.9	≤ .001	11.5	10.5	≤ .001
Heavy drinker	5.8	5.8	.1	5.5	4.6	≤ .001
Engages in physical activity	77.2	69.9	≤ .001	76.9	62.0	≤ .001
Always wears seatbelt	95.2	92.8	≤ .001	95.3	93.7	≤ .001
Domain 3: prevalence of chronic health conditions						
Arthritis	29.9	16.6	≤ .001	28.8	30.1	≤ .001
Depression	17.6	24.6	≤ .001	17.1	21.6	< .001
Asthma	14.1	16.9	≤ .001	13.8	15.4	≤ .001
Diabetes	14.3	10.9	≤ .001	13.3	17.9	≤ .001
Stroke	3.6	3.0	≤ .001	2.9	5.1	≤ .001
Obesity	69.8	65.3	≤ .001	70.4	68.9	≤ .001
Cancer	10.0	3.6	≤ .001	7.9	6.2	≤ .001
Domain 4: preventive health behaviors						
Tetanus/Tdap in past 10 y	64.7	53.9	≤ .001	64.3	51.6	≤ .001
Flu shot in the past year	64.3	56.8	≤ .001	64.5	57.6	≤ .001
Ever had pneumonia shot	71.0	62.1	≤ .001	71.7	63.8	≤ .001
Colonoscopy and sigmoidoscopy, aged 50–75 y	74.0	57.2	≤ .001	78.3	66.5	≤ .001
Ever been tested for HIV	36.3	47.3	≤ .001	35.0	39.4	≤ .001
Domain 5: functional, physical, and mental health limitations						
Serious difficulty walking or climbing	13.6	14.2	≤ .001	11.6	25.3	≤ .001
Activity limited because of arthritis	42.1	54.0	≤ .001	41.7	52.1	≤ .001
Severe joint pain	1.18	0.78	≤ .001	1.05	1.24	≤ .001
Has poor or fair physical health status ≥ 1 d	37.1	41.8	≤ .001	37.3	43.5	≤ .001
Has poor or fair mental health status ≥ 1 d	38.0	52.0	≤ .001	35.7	39.6	≤ .001

Note. BRFSS = Behavioral Risk Factor Surveillance System. Outcomes include clinical, behavioral, and structural access variables. Weighted unadjusted (crude) and age-adjusted prevalence estimates are presented for each health outcome by homeownership status (homeowners vs renters). I obtained age-adjusted estimates using logistic regression models with predictive margins, controlling for continuous age (_AGE80) and accounting for the BRFSS complex survey design and sampling weights. Percentages represent the estimated prevalence of each health outcome in each homeownership group.
[a]*P* values are from the Rao–Scott χ^2 test, which accounts for the BRFSS complex sampling design.

TABLE 3— AOR (95% CI) for Renters Compared With Homeowners for Health Outcomes: Behavioral Risk Factor Surveillance System, United States, 2023

Outcome[a]	Partially Adjusted Model,[b] AOR[c] (95% CI)	Fully Adjusted Model,[d] AOR[c] (95% CI)
Domain 1: health care access and utilization and structural barriers		
Had health insurance	0.65 (0.59, 0.71)	0.75 (0.68, 0.83)
Had personal doctor	0.61 (0.58, 0.65)	0.65 (0.61, 0.69)
Had routine checkup in past year	0.84 (0.80, 0.88)	0.82 (0.78, 0.87)
Could not see doctor because of cost	1.47 (1.37, 1.57)	1.39 (1.29, 1.49)
Lacked reliable transportation in past 12 mo	1.76 (1.59, 1.94)	1.51 (1.36, 1.68)
Received food stamps in past 12 mo	1.83 (1.68, 2.00)	1.55 (1.41, 1.71)
Domain 2: health risk and protective behaviors		
Had poor or fair health	1.36 (1.29, 1.43)	1.21 (1.14, 1.28)
Current smoker	1.18 (1.11, 1.25)	1.17 (1.09, 1.24)
Ever smoked	1.07 (1.02, 1.11)	1.15 (1.10, 1.21)
Alcohol use	0.97 (0.93, 1.01)	1.01 (0.96, 1.06)
Binge drinker	1.11 (1.04, 1.18)	1.08 (1.02, 1.15)
Heavy drinker	0.95 (0.87, 1.03)	0.97 (0.88, 1.06)
Engages in physical activity	0.79 (0.75, 0.83)	0.86 (0.82, 0.91)
Always wears seatbelt	1.04 (0.95, 1.14)	1.10 (1.00, 1.21)
Domain 3: prevalence of chronic health conditions		
Arthritis	0.89 (0.84, 0.93)	0.91 (0.86, 0.96)
Depression	1.11 (1.05, 1.16)	1.17 (1.10, 1.23)
Asthma	1.02 (0.97, 1.08)	0.99 (0.94, 1.05)
Diabetes	1.08 (1.01, 1.15)	1.00 (0.94, 1.07)
Stroke	1.26 (1.13, 1.39)	1.13 (1.01, 1.27)
Obesity	0.90 (0.86, 0.94)	0.91 (0.86, 0.96)
Cancer	0.90 (0.86, 0.94)	0.94 (0.86, 1.02)
Domain 4: preventive health behaviors		
Received tetanus/Tdap shots in past 10 y	0.84 (0.70, 1.01)	0.97 (0.79, 1.19)
Received flu shot in past year, aged ≥65 y	1.00 (0.91, 1.09)	1.06 (0.97, 1.17)
Ever received pneumonia shot, aged ≥65 y	0.91 (0.83, 0.99)	1.05 (0.97, 1.17)
Ever received colonoscopy and sigmoidoscopy, aged 50–75 y	0.76 (0.60, 0.95)	0.74 (0.58, 0.95)
Ever tested for HIV	1.27 (1.21, 1.32)	1.17 (1.11, 1.22)
Domain 5: functional, physical, and mental health limitations		
Has serious difficulty walking	1.42 (1.34, 1.52)	1.30 (1.21, 1.40)
Activity is limited because of arthritis	1.14 (0.98, 1.32)	1.04 (0.89, 1.23)
Has severe joint pain	0.97 (0.87, 1.08)	1.04 (1.03, 1.06)
Had poor or fair physical health ≥1 d	1.07 (1.03, 1.12)	1.12 (1.09, 1.20)
Had poor or fair mental health ≥1 d	1.12 (1.08, 1.20)	1.14 (1.09, 1.20)

Note. AOR = adjusted odds ratio; CI = confidence interval.
[a]Outcomes included clinical, behavioral, and structural access variables.
[b]The partially adjusted model controlled for age (continuous), sex, and income.
[c]Homeowners served as the reference group; AORs represent the odds of each outcome among renters compared with homeowners.
[d]The fully adjusted model additionally controlled for race/ethnicity, education, marital status, and employment status.

homeowners (Table 2), including depression (21.6% vs 17.1%), asthma (15.4% vs 13.8%), diabetes (17.9% vs 13.3%), and stroke (5.1% vs 2.9%; all $P \le .001$). Obesity was slightly more common among homeowners (70.4% vs 68.9%; $P \le .001$), whereas arthritis was more prevalent among renters (30.1% vs 28.8%; $P \le .001$). Cancer was more frequently reported by homeowners (7.9% vs 6.2%; $P \le .001$). In fully adjusted models (Table 3), renters had higher odds of depression (AOR = 1.17; 95% CI = 1.10, 1.23) and stroke (AOR = 1.13; 95% CI = 1.01, 1.27) and lower odds of arthritis (AOR = 0.91; 95% CI = 0.86, 0.96) and obesity (AOR = 0.91; 95% CI = 0.86, 0.96). I found no significant differences for asthma, diabetes, or cancer after adjustment.

Domain 4

Renters had lower uptake of several preventive services than homeowners (Table 2). After age adjustment, renters were less likely to report having received a tetanus or Tdap (tetanus, diphtheria, and acellular pertussis) vaccine in the past 10 years (51.6% vs 64.3%), a flu shot for adults aged 65 years or older (57.6% vs 64.5%), a pneumonia vaccine (63.8% vs 71.7%), and colonoscopy or sigmoidoscopy screening for adults aged 50 to 75 years (66.5% vs 78.3%). HIV testing was more common among renters (39.4% vs 35.0%). In fully adjusted models (Table 3), renters had lower odds of having had a colonoscopy or sigmoidoscopy (AOR = 0.74; 95% CI = 0.58, 0.95) and higher odds of HIV testing (AOR = 1.17; 95% CI = 1.11, 1.22); other vaccine outcomes were not statistically significant.

Domain 5

Renters reported higher age-adjusted prevalence of all limitations (Table 2). Serious difficulty walking was more common among renters (25.3% vs 11.6%), as were arthritis-related activity limitations (52.1% vs 41.7%) and severe joint pain (1.24 vs 1.05; all $P \le .001$). Renters also had higher prevalence of 1 or more day of poor or fair physical (43.5% vs 37.3%) or mental (39.6% vs 35.7%) health. Fully adjusted models (Table 3) showed renters had higher odds of serious difficulty walking (AOR = 1.30; 95% CI = 1.21, 1.40), severe joint pain (AOR = 1.04; 95% CI = 1.03, 1.06), poor or fair physical health (AOR = 1.12; 95% CI = 1.09, 1.20), and poor or fair mental health (AOR = 1.14; 95% CI = 1.09, 1.20). I found no statistically significant difference for arthritis-related activity limitation.

DISCUSSION

In this nationally representative analysis of 407 916 adults from the 2023 BRFSS—representing approximately 235 million US adults—homeownership emerged as a strong, independent correlate of good health and health care access. Across 5 domains, homeowners consistently exhibited better health profiles than renters, including lower behavioral risk, fewer chronic conditions, and greater preventive care utilization. These patterns persisted after adjusting for sociodemographic factors. This study offers one of the most comprehensive national assessments of the homeownership–health relationship.

Domain 1 findings underscored disparities in health care access linked to housing status. Homeownership reflects cumulative material advantage, facilitating health care engagement, lowering cost barriers, and providing logistical stability. By contrast, renters face housing precarity, income volatility, and competing demands that limit access to health care. These associations persisted after adjustment, suggesting that housing tenure may independently influence health care access beyond socioeconomic position. These findings support integrating housing security into public health frameworks and affirm homeownership as a stabilizing determinant for health care access and material well-being.[3,6] These disparities suggest that homeownership provides structural advantages—such as care continuity, financial flexibility, and transportation access—that facilitate health care engagement. Evidence links stable housing to better access and health outcomes, beyond income and education.[1,10] The persistent associations in my fully adjusted models support the interpretation that homeownership may offer benefits beyond socioeconomic status—likely reflecting reduced cumulative risk, enhanced residential stability, and pathways toward stronger spatial and community integration.[5]

Domain 2 showed that renters are more likely than homeowners to engage in adverse health risk behaviors, aligning with the literature identifying housing as a determinant of health behavior. Renters had significantly higher odds of reporting poor or fair self-rated health, smoking (current and ever), and binge drinking—all predictors of chronic disease and premature mortality. These results are consistent with research showing elevated risks among individuals facing housing instability or economic insecurity, which disproportionately affect renters.[10,12] Elevated smoking may reflect coping mechanisms tied to housing stress or neighborhood disorder.[13]

Interestingly, renters were more likely to report always wearing seatbelts—a finding warranting further investigation, possibly because of differences in transportation mode, risk perception, or community norms. The lack of significant differences in alcohol use and heavy drinking may reflect converging risk patterns across housing status.[14] Renters were also less likely to engage in regular physical activity, potentially owing to limited neighborhood walkability, safety concerns, or inadequate recreational infrastructure.[15,16] Differences in the built environment may also contribute to behavioral risk disparities, as homeowners often reside in areas with greater access to sidewalks, parks, and recreational infrastructure than do renters. These disparities suggest that homeownership may buffer health behaviors through material stability, environmental factors, and psychosocial resources. Interventions should consider housing tenure as a key axis of social vulnerability.

Domain 3 findings showed that elevated odds of depression and stroke among renters could be partially explained by the association of housing insecurity to chronic stress, social disconnection, and vascular dysregulation.[10,17,18] These conditions are sensitive to the psychosocial stressors that renters may disproportionately experience, such as financial volatility and residential instability. Conversely, the absence of disparities in asthma, diabetes, and cancer suggests that these conditions may be primarily driven by factors such as genetics and environmental exposures, which may not vary substantially by housing tenure. Lower odds of arthritis and obesity among renters could be driven by age structure, higher physical activity in labor-intensive jobs, or selective survival bias.[19]

These findings reinforce housing tenure as a socially patterned exposure with condition-specific effects, requiring social determinants of health frameworks beyond income or health care access alone.[1,15] Interestingly, homeowners reported higher prevalence of obesity and cancer. This may reflect greater access to health care and screening, leading to higher detection rates, rather than true higher incidence. It is also possible that lifestyle factors associated with aging or suburban living among homeowners contribute to these patterns.

Domain 4 findings revealed persistent disparities in preventive care access by housing tenure. Renters had lower odds of colonoscopy and sigmoidoscopy screening, aligning with the literature linking housing instability to underutilization of routine health care.[1,20,21] Structural barriers—such as discontinuous insurance, limited primary care access, and financial constraints—likely contribute to this gap.[22] By contrast, I found no significant differences for Tdap, influenza, or pneumonia vaccination after adjustment, suggesting that such services may be accessed via system-driven touchpoints (e.g., acute care, employer mandates) that are less dependent on housing stability. The elevated HIV testing rates among renters may reflect targeted outreach in high-density or vulnerable communities, where renters are overrepresented.[10,23,24] Together, these results underscore the service-specific influence of housing tenure on preventive care and the need to address housing as a structural determinant of health equity.

Domain 5 findings revealed substantial disparities in functional and mental health outcomes by housing tenure, with renters experiencing significantly worse outcomes than homeowners. Renters had higher odds of serious walking difficulty and frequent poor mental health—patterns consistent with studies linking housing instability to physical and psychological morbidity.[25–28] Multiple mechanisms may underlie these disparities; chronic stress exposure,[17] hazardous built environments,[29] and fragmented health care access[30] can erode functioning and increase distress. Financial strain and neighborhood disadvantage—more common among renters—may further amplify symptoms and disease burden.[2]

The absence of group differences in arthritis-related activity limitation likely reflects greater arthritis prevalence among older homeowners.[31] Although joint pain was more common among renters, its modest effect size suggests that broader contextual exposures—rather than disease-specific pathways—may be the dominant driver of functional limitations in this population. These findings underscore housing tenure as a critical structural context potentially shaping exposure to stressors, health care access, and physical environments with downstream consequences for both physical and mental health.

Taken together, my findings suggest that housing tenure is not merely a marker of social advantage but a pathway through which structural conditions shape health. Homeownership may offer stability, autonomy, and reduced stress, supporting healthier behaviors and care engagement. By contrast, renters often face cumulative stressors—precarity, financial strain, and neighborhood adversity—linked to poor health outcomes.

Importantly, the benefits of homeownership are not equally distributed. Research shows that housing markets, financial strain, and structural barriers—such as discriminatory lending and segregation—shape access and conditions of ownership.[4,32,33] These dynamics underscore the need for policies promoting affordable, stable, and equitable housing.

Strengths and Limitations

This study has several strengths, including use of recent, nationally representative data; extensive adjustment for sociodemographic confounders; and a domain-based analytic framework reflecting the multidimensional nature of health. The large sample supports statistical precision and generalizability. Nonetheless, limitations include the cross-sectional design, which precludes causal inference and limits temporal assessment. Unmeasured confounders—such as wealth, housing quality, and neighborhood context—may affect associations. Self-reported measures may introduce bias, and excluding "other" housing types may underestimate housing-related health disparities. Additionally, the BRFSS excludes individuals without access to a telephone, which may limit generalizability to certain low-income or disconnected populations.

Public Health Implications

These findings underscore key public health and equity implications. Integrating housing tenure into surveillance and health care could improve identification of at-risk populations.[30] Expanding affordable homeownership—through down payment assistance, subsidized loans, and antidisplacement protections—may offer health benefits beyond economic security.[34] Strengthening renter protections and health care–housing partnerships could help mitigate barriers related to access, cost, and transportation.[35] Housing policy must be central to equity efforts.[33]

Conclusions

This nationally representative analysis reinforces homeownership as a structural determinant of health in the United States. Renters experienced consistently worse health outcomes than homeowners across 5 domains: health care access and utilization and structural barriers, health risk and protective behaviors, chronic conditions, preventive health behaviors, and functional, physical, and mental health limitations. These disparities persisted after adjustment for sociodemographic factors, suggesting the independent health benefits of homeownership. Housing tenure is shaped by social and structural forces, including policy, market dynamics, and systemic inequities, and influences access to health-promoting resources and resilience against adversity. Integrating housing into surveillance, health care, and policy is essential. Addressing tenure-based disparities is a public health imperative. AJPH

ABOUT THE AUTHOR

Shams Rahman is with the College of Global Population Health, University of Health Sciences and Pharmacy in St. Louis, St. Louis, MO.

CORRESPONDENCE

Correspondence should be sent to Shams Rahman, 1 Pharmacy Pl, St. Louis, MO 63110 (e-mail: shams.rahman@uhsp.edu). Reprints can be ordered at https://www.ajph.org by clicking the "Reprints" link.

PUBLICATION INFORMATION

Full Citation: Rahman S. Housing status and health in the United States: a national study of homeownership, health outcomes, and access to care. *Am J Public Health*. 2026;116(1):137–147.

Acceptance Date: August 16, 2025.

DOI: https://doi.org/10.2105/AJPH.2025.308278

ACKNOWLEDGMENTS

The author thanks the Behavioral Risk Factor Surveillance System survey participants and the Centers for Disease Control and Prevention for providing the data.

CONFLICTS OF INTEREST

The author has no potential conflicts of interest with respect to the research, authorship, or publication of this article.

HUMAN PARTICIPANT PROTECTION

This study was exempt from institutional review board oversight because it used publicly available, de-identified Behavioral Risk Factor Surveillance System data (45 CFR 46.104[d][4]).

REFERENCES

1. Rolfe S, Garnham L, Godwin J, Anderson I, Seaman P, Donaldson C. Housing as a social determinant of health and wellbeing: developing an empirically-informed realist theoretical framework. *BMC Public Health*. 2020;20(1):1138. https://doi.org/10.1186/s12889-020-09224-0
2. Maqbool N, Viveiros J, Ault M. The impacts of affordable housing on health: a research summary. April 2015. Available at: https://nhc.org/wp-content/uploads/2017/03/The-Impacts-of-Affordable-Housing-on-Health-A-Research-Summary.pdf. Accessed September 30, 2025.
3. Rahman S, Steeb D. Homeownership matters: impact of homeownership on the prevalence of chronic health conditions in the United States. *Prev Chronic Dis*. 2024;21:230324. https://doi.org/10.5888/pcd21.230324
4. Munford LA, Fichera E, Sutton M. Is owning your home good for your health? Evidence from exogenous variations in subsidies in England. *Econ Hum Biol*. 2020;39:100903. https://doi.org/10.1016/j.ehb.2020.100903
5. Rohe WM, Stegman MA. The effects of homeownership on the self-esteem, perceived control and life satisfaction of low-income people. *J Am Plann Assoc*. 1994;60(2):173–184. https://doi.org/10.1080/01944369408975571
6. Rahman S, Steeb DR. Unlocking the door to mental wellness: exploring the impact of homeownership on mental health issues. *BMC Public Health*. 2024;24(1):3479. https://doi.org/10.1186/s12889-024-20842-w
7. USAFacts. What is the homeownership rate in the United States? 2024. Available at: https://usafacts.org/answers/what-is-the-home ownership-rate/country/united-states. Accessed April 6, 2025.
8. US Census Bureau. Housing vacancies and homeownership (CPS/HVS). July 28, 2025. Available at: https://www.census.gov/housing/hvs/data/reports.html. Accessed October 1, 2025.
9. Meli J, Rajadhyaksha A, Todorova Z. A growing divide: how income inequality affects US homeownership rates. October 13, 2020. Available at: https://www.ib.barclays/our-insights/a-growing-divide-how-income-inequality-affects-us-homeownership-rates.html. Accessed September 30, 2025.
10. Swope CB, Hernández D. Housing as a determinant of health equity: a conceptual model. *Soc Sci Med*. 2019;243:112571. https://doi.org/10.1016/j.socscimed.2019.112571
11. Flaubert JL, Le Menestrel S, Williams DR, Wakefield MK; National Academies of Sciences, Engineering, and Medicine. Social determinants of health and health equity. In: Wakefield MK, Williams DR, Le Menestrel S, Flaubert JL, eds. *The Future of Nursing 2020–2030: Charting a Path to Achieve Health Equity*. Washington, DC: National Academies Press; 2021:31–58.
12. Aidala AA, Wilson MG, Shubert V, et al. Housing status, medical care, and health outcomes

among people living with HIV/AIDS: a systematic review. *Am J Public Health*. 2016;106(1):e1–e23. https://doi.org/10.2105/AJPH.2015.302905

13. Ross CE, Mirowsky J. Neighborhood disadvantage, disorder, and health. *J Health Soc Behav*. 2001;42(3):258–276. https://doi.org/10.2307/3090214
14. Desmond M, Kimbro RT. Eviction's fallout: housing, hardship, and health. *Soc Forces*. 2015;94(1):295–324. https://doi.org/10.1093/sf/sov044
15. Krieger J, Higgins DL. Housing and health: time again for public health action. *Am J Public Health*. 2002;92(5):758–768. https://doi.org/10.2105/ajph.92.5.758
16. Yim B, Howland RE, Culp GM, Zhilkova A, Barbot O, Tsao T-Y. Disparities in preventable hospitalizations among public housing developments. *Am J Prev Med*. 2019;56(2):187–195. https://doi.org/10.1016/j.amepre.2018.08.019
17. Sweet E, Nandi A, Adam EK, McDade TW. The high price of debt: household financial debt and its impact on mental and physical health. *Soc Sci Med*. 2013;91:94–100. https://doi.org/10.1016/j.socscimed.2013.05.009
18. Hoke MK, Boen CE. The health impacts of eviction: evidence from the national longitudinal study of adolescent to adult health. *Soc Sci Med*. 2021;273:113742. https://doi.org/10.1016/j.socscimed.2021.113742
19. Bonauto DK, Lu D, Fan ZJ. Obesity prevalence by occupation in Washington State, Behavioral Risk Factor Surveillance System. *Prev Chronic Dis*. 2014;11:130219. https://doi.org/10.5888/pcd11.130219
20. Kushel MB, Gupta R, Gee L, Haas JS. Housing instability and food insecurity as barriers to health care among low-income Americans. *J Gen Intern Med*. 2006;21(1):71–77. https://doi.org/10.1111/j.1525-1497.2005.00278.x
21. Baggett TP, O'Connell JJ, Singer DE, Rigotti NA. The unmet health care needs of homeless adults: a national study. *Am J Public Health*. 2010;100(7):1326–1333. https://doi.org/10.2105/AJPH.2009.180109
22. Yabroff KR, Zhao J, Halpern MT, et al. Health insurance disruptions and care access and affordability in the US. *Am J Prev Med*. 2021;61(1):3–12. https://doi.org/10.1016/j.amepre.2021.02.014
23. Stergiopoulos V, O'Campo P, Gozdzik A, et al. Moving from rhetoric to reality: adapting Housing First for homeless individuals with mental illness from ethno-racial groups. *BMC Health Serv Res*. 2012;12(1):345. https://doi.org/10.1186/1472-6963-12-345
24. Hanna JJ, Saleh SN, Lehmann CU, Nijhawan AE, Medford RJ. Reaching populations at risk for HIV through targeted Facebook advertisements: cost-consequence analysis. *JMIR Form Res*. 2023;7:e38630. https://doi.org/10.2196/38630
25. Singh A, Daniel L, Baker E, Bentley R. Housing disadvantage and poor mental health: a systematic review. *Am J Prev Med*. 2019;57(2):262–272. https://doi.org/10.1016/j.amepre.2019.03.018
26. Pollack CE, Griffin BA, Lynch J. Housing affordability and health among homeowners and renters. *Am J Prev Med*. 2010;39(6):515–521. https://doi.org/10.1016/j.amepre.2010.08.002
27. Sandel M, Desmond M. Investing in housing for health improves both mission and margin. *JAMA*. 2017;318(23):2291–2292. https://doi.org/10.1001/jama.2017.15771
28. Cutts DB, Meyers AF, Black MM, et al. US housing insecurity and the health of very young children. *Am J Public Health*. 2011;101(8):1508–1514. https://doi.org/10.2105/AJPH.2011.300139
29. Saegert S, Evans GW. Poverty, housing niches, and health in the United States. *J Soc Issues*. 2003;59(3):569–589. https://doi.org/10.1111/1540-4560.00078
30. Taylor LA. Housing and health: an overview of the literature. *Health Aff Health Policy Brief*. June 7, 2018. https://doi.org/10.1377/hpb20180313.396577
31. Centers for Disease Control and Prevention. Vital signs: prevalence of doctor-diagnosed arthritis and arthritis-attributable activity limitation—United States. *MMWR Morb Mortal Wkly Rep*. 2017;66(9):246–253. https://doi.org/10.15585/mmwr.mm6609e1
32. Solomon D, Maxwell C, Castro A. Systemic inequality: displacement, exclusion, and segregation. August 7, 2019. Available at: https://www.americanprogress.org/article/systemic-inequality-displacement-exclusion-segregation. Accessed September 30, 2025.
33. Oliver M, Shapiro T. *Black Wealth/White Wealth: A New Perspective on Racial Inequality*. New York, NY: Routledge; 2013.
34. Saegert S, Fields D, Libman K. Mortgage foreclosure and health disparities: serial displacement as asset extraction in African American populations. *J Urban Health*. 2011;88(3):390–402. https://doi.org/10.1007/s11524-011-9584-3
35. Sandel M, Sheward R, Ettinger de Cuba S, et al. Unstable housing and caregiver and child health in renter families. *Pediatrics*. 2018;141(2). https://doi.org/10.1542/peds.2017-2199